ALZHEIMER'S DISEASE
A Handbook for Caregivers

ALZHEIMER'S DISEASE
A Handbook for Caregivers

RONALD C. HAMDY, MD, FRCP, FACP

Professor of Medicine,
Cecile Cox Quillen Professor of Geriatric Medicine and Gerontology,
Head, Division of Geriatric Medicine,
James H. Quillen College of Medicine,
East Tennessee State University;
Associate Chief of Staff, Extended Care and Geriatrics,
Veterans Affairs Medical Center,
Johnson City, Tennessee

JAMES M. TURNBULL, MD, FRCP(C)

Staff Psychiatrist, Central Appalachia Services, Inc.,
Kingsport, Tennessee;
Clinical Professor of Psychiatry and Family Practice,
James H. Quillen College of Medicine,
East Tennessee State University, Johnson City, Tennessee

WARREN CLARK, BSN, MS

Clinical Nurse Specialist,
Catawba Hospital,
Catawba, Virginia

MARY M. LANCASTER, RNC, MSN

Clinical Nurse Specialist—Gerontology,
Veterans Affairs Medical Center, Mountain Home, Tennessee;
Consultant, Center for Geriatrics and Gerontology;
Adjunct Clinical Instructor, School of Nursing,
East Tennessee State University, Johnson City, Tennessee

SECOND EDITION

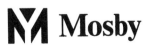 Mosby

St. Louis Baltimore Boston Chicago London Madrid Philadelphia Sydney Toronto

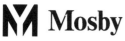

Dedicated to Publishing Excellence

Managing Editor: Jeff Burnham
Developmental Editor: Jolynn Gower
Project Manager: Patricia Tannian
Designer: Gail Morey Hudson
Manufacturing Supervisor: John Babrick

SECOND EDITION

Printed in the United States of America
Composition by Carlisle Communications, Ltd.
Printing/binding by R.R. Donnelley & Sons Company

Mosby–Year Book, Inc.
11830 Westline Industrial Drive
St. Louis, Missouri 63146

Library of Congress Cataloging in Publication Data

Alzheimer's disease: a handbook for caregivers / Ronald C. Hamdy . . . [et al.]. — 2nd ed.
    p.   cm.
    Includes bibliographical references and index.
    ISBN 0-8016-7282-1
    1. Alzheimer's disease. 2. Alzheimer's disease—Nursing.
3. Alzheimer's disease—Social aspects. I. Hamdy, R. C.
    [DNLM: 1. Alzheimer's Disease—nursing. 2. Alzheimer's Disease—psychology. 3. Caregivers. 4. Family. WM 220 A47765 1994]
RC523.A386 1994
618.97′6831—dc20
DNLM/DLC
for Lilbrary of Congress   93-11763
                                         CIP

93 94 95 96 97 / 9 8 7 6 5 4 3 2 1

Contributors

PATRICIA S. BROWN
Director, Area Agency on Aging,
First Tennessee Development District,
Johnson City, Tennessee

CURTIS B. CLARK, MD
Department of Family Medicine,
University of Tennessee, Health Service Center,
Jackson, Tennessee

WARREN CLARK, BSN, MS
Clinical Nurse Specialist,
Catawba Hospital,
Catawba, Virginia

MARK DOMAN, MD
Assistant Professor, Geriatric Medicine and Gerontology,
James H. Quillen College of Medicine,
East Tennessee State University;
Staff Physician, Geriatrics and Extended Care,
Veterans Affairs Medical Center,
Johnson City, Tennessee

NANCY ERICKSON, MBA
Director, Education Services,
Alzheimer's Association, Inc.,
Chicago, Illinois

GARY S. FIGIEL, MD
Associate Professor, Department of Psychiatry,
Emory University,
Atlanta, Georgia

J. HOWARD FREDERICK, MD
Clinical Professor of Family Practice and Geriatrics,
University of Texas, Health Sciences Center,
San Antonio, Texas

KEVIN F. GRAY, MD
Departments of Psychiatry and Neurology,
University of Texas Southwestern Medical Center
Dallas Veterans Affairs Medical Center,
Dallas, Texas

RONALD C. HAMDY, MD, FRCP, FACP
Professor of Medicine,
Cecile Cox Quillen Professor of Geriatric Medicine and Gerontology,
Head, Division of Geriatric Medicine,
James H. Quillen College of Medicine,
East Tennessee State University;
Associate Chief of Staff, Extended Care and Geriatrics,
Veterans Affairs Medical Center,
Johnson City, Tennessee

LARRY HUDGINS, MD
Associate Professor, Geriatric Medicine and Gerontology,
James H. Quillen College of Medicine, East Tennessee State University;
Staff Physician/Geriatrics and Extended Care,
Veterans Affairs Medical Center,
Johnson City, Tennessee

LISSY F. JARVIK, MD, PhD
Distinguished Physician, Professor of Psychiatry, Psychogeriatric Unit,
West Los Angeles Veterans Affairs Medical Center and Neuropsychiatric Institute
and Hospital, University of California,
Los Angeles, California

MARY M. LANCASTER, RNC, MSN
Consultant, Center for Geriatrics and Gerontology;
Adjunct Clinical Instructor, School of Nursing, East Tennessee State University,
Johnson City, Tennessee;
Clinical Nurse Specialist—Gerontology,
Veterans Affairs Medical Center,
Johnson City, Tennessee

ELEANOR P. LAVRETSKY, MD, PhD
Research Psychopharmacologist,
West Los Angeles Veterans Affairs Medical Center,
Neuropsychiatric Institute and Hospital, University of California,
Los Angeles, California

DANIEL MERRICK, MD
Associate Professor, Department of Internal Medicine,
East Tennessee State University,
Johnson City, Tennessee

MARGUERITE METTETAL, BS
District Public Guardian for the Elderly,
First Tennessee Area Agency on Aging,
Johnson City, Tennessee

CHARLES B. NEMEROFF, MD, PhD
Professor and Chairman, Department of Psychiatry,
Emory University,
Atlanta, Georgia

KIM SALYER, MA
Research Assistant, Division of Geriatric Medicine,
James H. Quillen College of Medicine, East Tennessee State University,
Johnson City, Tennessee

PATRICK SLOAN, PhD
Clinical Associate Professor, Department of Psychiatry and Behavioral Sciences,
Department of Internal Medicine, James H. Quillen College of Medicine,
East Tennessee State University;
Clinical Psychologist, Veterans Affairs Medical Center,
Johnson City, Tennessee

ZEBBIE C. TIPTON, BA
Research Technician, Division of Geriatric Medicine,
James H. Quillen College of Medicine, East Tennessee State University,
Johnson City, Tennessee

ELIZABETH A. TURNBULL, BA
Research Assistant, J&S Turnbull Consulting,
Johnson City, Tennessee

JAMES M. TURNBULL, MD, FRCP (C)
Staff Psychiatrist, Central Appalachia Services, Inc.,
Kingsport, Tennessee;
Clinical Professor of Psychiatry and Family Practice,
James H. Quillen College of Medicine, East Tennessee State University,
Johnson City, Tennessee

SHARON TURNBULL, BS (N), MPH, PhD
Consultant, J&S Turnbull Consulting,
Johnson City, Tennessee;
Clinical Associate Professor of Family Practice and Psychiatry,
East Tennessee State University,
Johnson City, Tennessee

LYNDA WEATHERLY, RN, MSN, C–ANP
Assistant Professor of Nursing,
Jackson State Community College;
Facilitator, Alzheimer's Family Support Group,
Jackson–Madison County General Hospital,
Jackson, Tennessee

MICHAEL L. WOODRUFF, PhD
Professor of Anatomy, James H. Quillen College of Medicine,
East Tennessee State University;
Associate Dean for Research and Graduate Studies,
East Tennessee State University,
Johnson City, Tennessee

To
our patients with Alzheimer's disease
and to
their relatives and caregivers
from whom we have learned and continue to learn so much.

Foreword from first edition

The full tragedy of Alzheimer's disease, which affects one out of every ten Americans over the age of 65, was impressed upon me during a series of Congressional hearings I chaired in 1984. At a hearing in Tennessee, a woman whose husband suffers from Alzheimer's offered testimony I will never forget. "A few months ago," she began, "my husband asked me to go into the bedroom—we needed to talk privately, he said. I went to the room and closed the door. Turning to me with tears in his eyes he asked, 'Am I losing my mind, honey? Am I going crazy?'" She went on: "My life can be described as a funeral that never ends . . . I want my husband back."

That women is not alone. Two to three million "never-ending funerals" are sapping the strength of both victims and their families across America. A concerted effort is long overdue to defeat this disease which erodes the mental and physical health of the patient before his or her time. Part of the solution lies in research to uncover the causes of the disease and develop treatments for it. Just as crucial, however, is assuring that those who take care of patients with Alzheimer's know as much about the problem as possible.

That is one reason I am so pleased with *Alzheimer's Disease: A Handbook for Caregivers*, which contains a wealth of practical information about the effects of Alzheimer's on the patient's day-to-day life. The book offers detailed descriptions of the stages of the disease, the options for treatment, and the effects of other mental and physical characteristics upon the expression of Alzheimer's. It also offers valuable suggestions for approaching issues such as nutrition, sleep habits, and therapy. The book is a perfect bridge between those who know most about the disease—and those who know most about the patient.

Congress, by establishing regional centers devoted to the research and treatment of Alzheimer's, has taken one step in the right direction. The medical faculty at East Tennessee State University, by creating this fine book, has taken another. Perhaps, through more efforts like these, we can begin to lift some of the fear and uncertainty that surround this national tragedy.

Albert Gore, Jr.
Vice President of the United States

Preface

This is the second edition of a book that was written in response to requests from caregivers in our community. Based on comments and suggestions from our readers, we have considerably expanded the text and have included new chapters on such subjects as brain imaging, dementia, psychopharmacology, specific drug therapy, programming for activities, and promising areas of research.

Although the revised edition is intended primarily for nurses, most of the content will be valuable to caregivers who do not have a nursing degree. A comprehensive glossary explains almost all the technical terms used. Although the authors have attempted to be as accurate as possible with regard to drug dosages, readers are advised to consult the *Physician's Desk Reference* before prescribing.

Alzheimer's disease has been called "the disease of the century." It occurs in up to 3 million Americans, mostly people over the age of 65. It may be the harshest of all the incurable diseases because it hits its victims twice. First the mind dies, and the simplest tasks, such as eating with a knife and fork, telling time, or putting on a dress, become insurmountable. Then the body dies. Victims become unable to walk or control their body functions. In the end the victim lies curled in a fetal position, gradually sinking into coma and death.

Alzheimer's disease is even more devastating for the families and caregivers of its victims. The caregivers drive themselves to physical and emotional exhaustion while rendering continuous care and experiencing the anguish of seeing a loved one turned into a person who no longer remembers who he or she is.

While researchers struggle to understand the disease and look for drugs that will slow its progress, it is becoming increasingly clear that patients with Alzheimer's disease are not beyond help. In the early stages of the disease, aids to memory, behavior therapy, day care centers, respite care, and some simple understanding of how the disease works can postpone the day when the victim must be placed in a nursing home.

We recognized the need for a comprehensive book that would address many of the issues faced by caregivers who help the victims of this devastating illness. Although the disease affects more women than men, we have chosen to use the male pronoun throughout the text. We hope that this book will prove of real value to those who are expected to care for this growing population.

Ronald Hamdy
James M. Turnbull
Warren Clark
Mary M. Lancaster

Acknowledgments

We thank all our colleagues who have referred to us patients with dementing illnesses and Alzheimer's disease, thus allowing us to gain a wider experience in this field. We also thank the patients' relatives and caregivers, who have given us so much information and insight on the illness and its impact on their lives. We thank the staff of the Mosby Company, in particular Jeff Burnham, Jolynn Gower, and Patricia Tannian, for their work on this book. Finally, we thank Kathy Whalen, Jewel Greene, and Janice Lyons for their painstaking secretarial work and efficient help in producing this manuscript.

Contents

THE NORMAL BRAIN

1

Structure and function of the normal brain

Michael L. Woodruff

First and foremost, Alzheimer's disease is an illness of the brain. For this reason the health care professional who treats patients with Alzheimer's disease needs to be familiar with the structure of the brain in order to understand how it is affected by the disease. In addition, because research concerning the causes of Alzheimer's disease increasingly involves the cellular and molecular level of brain function, it is important for the health care professional to develop a clear understanding of the cell biology of the neuron. This chapter presents information about the normal brain that will allow professionals who have not received specific advanced training in neurobiology to appreciate more clearly the changes, both gross and cellular, that occur in the brain affected by Alzheimer's disease.

FUNCTIONAL ELEMENTS OF NERVOUS SYSTEM
Neurons and Neuroglia

Like all organ systems of the body, the central nervous system (brain and spinal cord) is built from individual cells. The two general categories of cells within the central nervous system (CNS) are neurons and neuroglia (Fig. 1-1, *A* and *B*). The neuroglia provide physical and metabolic support to the neurons. One type of neuroglial cell, the oligodendrocyte, forms the myelin sheath of the nerve fibers. Among its other functions myelin electrically insulates the nerve fiber and is necessary for proper conduction of the nerve action potential. The other type of neuroglial cell, the astrocyte, serves many functions, including formation of scar tissue within the brain and spinal cord in response to injury.

3

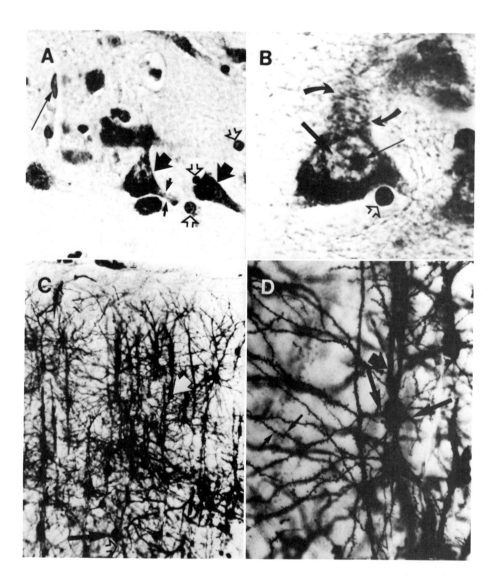

Neuroglia are obviously important for normal brain functioning (e.g., multiple sclerosis is caused by loss of CNS myelin); however, the neuron is the functional unit of the CNS. The death of neurons leads to neurological disorders such as Alzheimer's disease, Huntington's disease, and Parkinson's disease.

Fig. 1-1. A, Photomicrograph of thionine-stained cells from human neocortex shows large pyramidal neurons (*solid arrowheads*), neuroglial nuclei (*open arrowheads*), and nuclei of endothelial cells (*long arrow*) that form capillaries of brain. **B,** Nuclei of neurons (*large straight arrow*) are lightly stained relative to cytoplasm of cell body but contain darkly stained nucleolus (*thin straight arrow*). Only nuclei of neuroglial cells stain (*open arrowheads* in **A** and **B**), but these cells have long processes that surround neurons and their axons and dendrites. Two smaller black arrowheads in **A** and curved arrows in **B** point to pyramidal cell dendrites. High-power magnification shows that Nissl substance of cell body extends into dendrite. Axons are not seen with Nissl stain. **C** and **D,** Photomicrographs of neocortical neurons highlighted with Golgi stain, which penetrates entire neuron. Solid arrow in **C** indicates cell body of large pyramidal neuron located in fifth layer of neocortex. Only one axon emerges from a neuron (*open arrowhead* in **C**). Apical dendrite emerges from top of soma (*dark arrowhead* in **D**) and extends toward surface of brain. Several basilar dendrites emerge from bottom of soma and extend laterally and downward. Dendritic spines (*small arrows* in **D**) also can be seen in **C** and **D**.

Neuron cell body

The approximately 100 billion neurons found in the brain of a young adult can be placed into hundreds of categories based on shape, pattern of connectivity to other neurons, and transmitter content. However, all neurons have basic structural features in common.

The cell body, or soma, essential for sustaining the neuron is composed of the nucleus and the perikaryon. The components of the nucleus, with the exception of the nucleolus, appear diffuse when viewed through a light microscope (see Fig. 1-1, *A* and *B*). These components are the chromosomes that embody the genes containing the deoxyribonucleic acid (DNA) that specifies patterns of protein synthesis. The particular DNA that codes for production of the sites where protein synthesis occurs (i.e., the ribosomes) is contained within the nucleolus. When viewed through a light microscope, the nucleolus of a neuron stained with a dye such as thionine, which deeply colors nucleic acids, appears as a dark sphere within a lightly stained nucleus.

The perikaryon consists of the cytosol, which contains a variety of subcellular elements. These elements, which can be seen only under an electron microscope, include both smooth and rough endoplasmic reticulum (ER), the Golgi apparatus, lysosomes, mitochondria, and secretory granules. Microtubules and neurofilaments are also abundant in the perikaryon and comprise the neurofibrils of the cytoskeleton. The rough ER condenses when brain tissue is prepared for staining. The condensed rough ER appears as Nissl substance when Nissl-stained neurons are viewed through the light microscope (Fig. 1-1, *A* and *B*).

The various subcellular components of the perikaryon have distinct purposes. The lysosomes are bound by a membrane that protects the cell from the more than 50 digestive enzymes contained in lysosomes. These enzymes digest worn-out cellular components, including organelles such as mitochondria. The number and size of lysosomes increase with age, and lipofuscin may be found within lysosomes. This yellowish pigment is probably the accumulation of insoluble cellular debris. The amount of lipofuscin contained within a neuron increases with age but does not appear to impair the neuron.

The mitochondria are membrane-bound organelles responsible for energy production in all cells, including neurons. Mitochondria form adenosine triphosphate (ATP), which produces energy from sugars and fats. Impaired mitochondrial function is deleterious to the neuron, and there is some evidence that mutation by free radicals of DNA responsible for production of mitchondria might lead to cell death within the substantia nigra and thereby cause Parkinson's disease.

The ribosomes are granules in which cell proteins are formed. Information for correct synthesis of proteins appropriate for the neuron is contained within the DNA of the nucleus. This information is coded into RNA within the nucleus by a process called transcription. The transcribed information is then carried from the nucleus by messenger RNA (mRNA), which crosses the nuclear membrane through pores and enters the cytoplasm of the perikaryon. The mRNA interacts with ribosomes to form cell proteins by a process known as translation. Many ribosomes attach to endoplasmic reticulum within the perikaryon to form the rough ER, but others are free. Proteins for the neurofibrils that make up the neuronal cytoskeleton are formed on the free ribosomes. In addition, all the enzymes used to catalyze various neuronal functions are formed on free ribosomes. The combination of free ribosomes and the mRNA that encodes for these proteins is called a polyribosome, or polysome. After their formation the proteins that develop on polysomes undergo little modification. Proteins that will be used as secretory products of the cell (e.g., neurotransmitters) or that will become part of the major membrane systems of the cell are formed on the rough ER. These proteins undergo extensive modification after they have been formed. These posttranslational modifications occur within both the rough and the smooth ER and in the Golgi apparatus.

The Golgi apparatus functions to finalize assembly of the specific proteins to be used in the various major membrane systems of the neuron. Once completed, these membrane constituents are released from the Golgi apparatus and are transported to their specific destinations within the cell.

Dendrites and axons

As a cell, the neuron includes not only the cell body but processes known as dendrites and axons (see Fig. 1-1, *C* and *D*). The dendrites and the axon of the cell are bound by the same plasma membrane that surrounds the cytoplasm of the soma. However, dendrites and axons have specialized functions, and they differ from each other in appearance.

The internal structure of dendrites, especially the part of large dendrites that lies close to the cell body, resembles that of the perikaryon (see Fig. 1-1, *B*). The cytoplasm of dendrites contains the same type of neurofibrils found in the cell body as well as both rough and smooth ER and a Golgi apparatus. Therefore dendrites have the capacity for a certain amount of protein synthesis. CNS neurons typically have several dendrites (see Fig. 1-1, *C* and *D*). The extensive dendritic tree provides a large area where incoming axons may synapse. The presence of structures known as dendritic spines (see Fig. 1-1, *D*) contributes to this surface area and provides specialized points where axon terminals from other neurons may synapse.

Dendrites and the cell body receive input from other neurons via axons. Each neuron gives rise to only one axon. However, axons branch extensively and end in multiple terminals called boutons. Because the axon lacks both types of ER and ribosomes, it is incapable of synthesizing proteins. The axon contains neurofibrils in the form of neurotubules, neurofilaments, and microfilaments. As part of the cytoskeleton, these neurofibrils give form and structure to the axon as well as the cell body and dendritic tree. However, they also provide the physical substrate for movement of substances through the cell and its axon. The process whereby substances are transported through the length of the axon is known as axoplasmic transport or flow.

Axoplasmic Transport

The cell body is the trophic center of the neuron. For example, all the macromolecules necessary for sustaining the axon are produced in the cell body. Therefore these substances must be transported, often over "long" distances, from the soma to their destination. Axoplasmic transport accomplishes this job.

Three basic types of axoplasmic transport have been identified according to speed and direction of the flow. The first is fast anterograde (cell body to axon terminal) transport. Newly made membrane-bound cell organelles, such as mitochondria and synaptic vesicles, are transported along the axon by fast anterograde axoplasmic flow. These organelles move in a stepwise or saltatory manner by cross-linking to microtubules with the adenosine triphosphatase (ATPase) kinesin. The microtubules that run the length of the axon serve as a track on which the membrane-bound neuronal organelles appear to "walk" with "feet" made of kinesin molecules. The microtubules travel comparatively quickly since the rate of fast axoplasmic flow is greater than 400 mm/day.

Slow axoplasmic transport is the second category, and its approximate rate ranges from 0.2 to 5 mm/day. Components of the axonal cytoskeleton, enzymes, and other cytosol proteins are transported in the anterograde direction by slow axoplasmic flow. Slow axoplasmic flow can be divided into two subcategories based on rate and type of protein transported.

The final category of axoplasmic transport is called fast retrograde transport. As the name suggests, this type of transport goes from axon terminal to cell body. Dynein provides the cross-link to neurotubules that enables retrograde transport to occur at a rate of approximately 200 to 300 mm/day. The primary function of retrograde axonal transport is to return scavenged materials from the axon terminals to the cell body for digestion in lysosomes. However, trophic substances produced by target cells and needed by the cell body that is parent to the axon are also transported by retrograde axonal transport. Nerve growth factor is an example of such a substance. Lack of this substance may be partly responsible for the degeneration of the cholinergic neurons of the basal forebrain that occurs in Alzheimer's disease (see Chapter 7). Finally, retrograde transport provides a mechanism that gives certain viruses (e.g., herpes simplex, rabies, and polio) access to the CNS.

TRANSMISSION OF INFORMATION WITHIN BRAIN

The purpose of nervous tissue is the transmission of information between neurons. The transmission, accomplished chemically at specialized sites known as synapses, is the result of two types of electrical events. The small, relatively localized, nonpropagating postsynaptic potentials (PSPs) occur across the membrane of dendrites and cell body, and the propagated action potential (AP) occurs across the membrane of the axon. The frequency and temporal pattern of the AP represent the basic information code for the axon. The generation of an AP is the result of changing the voltage potential that exists across the neuron cell membrane.

Resting Membrane Potential

Every axon, cell body, and dendrite maintains a separation of electrical charges across its membrane known as the resting membrane potential. The magnitude of this potential is determined by the relative distribution of positively or negatively charged ions near the extracellular and intracellular surfaces of the cell membrane. The important ions for maintenance of the resting membrane potential and for generation of the AP are positive sodium (Na^+) and potassium (K^+) ions and negative chloride (Cl^-) and organic (A^-) ions. The positive ions are called cations, and the negatively charged ions are called anions. During the resting state K^+ is more highly concentrated within the cell than in the extracellular space, whereas Na^+ and Cl^- have higher extracellular concentrations. The organic anions are mostly proteins and organic acids. They never leave the intracellular space and are largely responsible for the fact that in the resting state the inside of the neuron is about -60 to -70 mV relative to the outside.

However, the inside of the cell would not remain negative relative to the outside if Na^+ were able to move freely across the membrane. Two factors should drive Na^+ into the cell. First, if the membrane were freely permeable to Na^+, the lower concentration of Na^+ inside the cell would compel this cation to enter the cell to equalize its concentration on both sides of the membrane. Second, electromotive force would compel Na^+ to enter the negatively charged inside of the cell to reduce the voltage gradient if free movement of this cation were not prevented.

Two factors prevent Na^+ from entering the cell and K^+ from leaving it. First, although some Na^+ ions leak into the cell and some K^+ ions escape from the intracellular space, in the resting state the cell membrane is not freely permeable to either of these cations. Also, an active "pump" works to drive Na^+ out of the cell and return K^+ to its proper intracellular location.

At rest the cell membrane is not freely permeable to Na$^+$ and K$^+$ because selective channels for these ions through the membrane are not open during the resting state. These channels comprise proteins that span the membrane and open when voltage is applied to them. Hence they are called voltage-gated channels. Nonselective, nongated channels also exist, and some Na$^+$ and K$^+$ ions move across the membrane through these channels. However, the second mechanism that maintains resting cation concentrations operates to extrude the Na$^+$ ions from the cell and return K$^+$ ions to the inside of the axon. This mechanism is the Na$^+$/K$^+$ pump. This pump requires energy to maintain the resting membrane potential and to return the cell membrane to the resting state in response to the generation of the AP.

Effect of Neurotransmitters on Membrane Potential

The sequence of events that leads to opening of the voltage-gated Na$^+$ channels in the axon begins at the synapses of the dendrites and cell body. Neurotransmitter molecules are released from the axon terminals that end at these synapses. These molecules bind to receptor sites on the postsynaptic membrane of the dendrites and cell body. Postsynaptic neurotransmitter receptors are highly localized on the cell membrane. Receptors for inhibitory neurotransmitters are more highly concentrated on the cell body than on dendrites, whereas receptors for excitatory neurotransmitters are more highly concentrated on dendrites.

When the neuron is at rest, no current flows along the cell membrane. Neurotransmitters change that condition by binding to their specific receptors on the cell membrane and causing ion channels to open. Since these channels are chemically gated, the presence or absence of a transmitter determines the conformation of the proteins that comprise the channels and the flow of ions across the membrane. The ions carry charges across the cell membrane, and this ionic current changes the resting membrane potential.

If the transmitter is inhibitory, channels open and allow chlorine anions (Cl$^-$) to enter the cell and K$^+$ ions to leave the cell. The movement of Cl$^-$ and K$^+$ makes the inside of the cell more negative relative to the outside, and an inhibitory postsynaptic potential (IPSP) is generated. The cell membrane is hyperpolarized relative to its resting condition and less likely to produce an action potential. Gamma-aminobutyric acid (GABA) and glycine are the most prevalent inhibitory transmitters in the brain. Both of these transmitters open Cl$^-$ channels and induce membrane hyperpolarization.

Excitatory neurotransmitters act on their receptors to open calcium cation (Ca^{++}) channels, and Ca^{++} enters the cell. This action decreases the relative negativity of the cell membrane and causes a membrane depolarization known as the excitatory postsynaptic potential (EPSP). Glutamate is the most ubiquitous excitatory transmitter in the CNS, and most neurons, from the alpha motor neurons of the spinal cord to the pyramidal neurons of the hippocampus, have glutamate receptors. Input (afferent) pathways to these neurons release glutamate, and EPSPs are generated in the dendrites of the target neurons.

Although glutamate is a naturally occurring neurotransmitter, excessive amounts of this substance can contribute to brain damage caused by hypoxia, neurodegenerative diseases such as Huntington's chorea, and epileptic seizures. For example, seizures that involve the temporal neocortex can excite the neurons in this region that send axons to the hippocampus. The terminal boutons of these axons employ glutamate as their neurotransmitter. The excessive excitation of the seizure can cause these terminals to release abnormally high amounts of glutamate, which can kill the target cells. The result could be some amount of impairment in the ability to form new memories.

Inhibitory and Excitatory Postsynaptic Potentials

Each neuron receives a combination of excitatory and inhibitory inputs onto its dendrites (mostly EPSPs) and its cell body (mostly IPSPs). The electrical currents generated by the transmitter-induced movement of ions across the cell membrane spread along the dendritic and somatic membranes and open voltage-gated channels. PSPs do not propagate as do APs; instead, the electrical potentials lessen in strength the farther they spread from the synaptic site where they were initiated.

At any given moment a neuron is bombarded by numerous excitatory and inhibitory inputs. The individual EPSPs and IPSPs that result from this bombardment decay over time, and across the space of the membrane their combined activity may be sufficient to change the polarity of the cell membrane in the region where the axon arises. The summation of the EPSPs and IPSPs in this area—the axon hillock—determines whether or not an AP will be generated.

An AP is generated if EPSPs sufficiently outweigh IPSPs in summation and the voltage across the membrane at the axon hillock becomes approximately 8 to 10 mV more positive than the -60 to -70 mV maintained in the resting state. This positive voltage shift opens voltage-gated sodium channels, and Na^+ ions flow into the cell at a rate far greater than the Na^+/K^+ pump can negate. The sudden influx of Na^+ increases the membrane potential almost to the value it would have if it were entirely determined by Na^+ distribution across the membrane. The rapid change in positive voltage of the first 0.5 ms of the AP opens the voltage-gated K^+ channels, and K^+ rapidly exits the cell. The reduction of intracellular concentration of this cation counteracts the effects of Na^+ influx and reverses the increasing positivity of the AP. Sodium channels close as the K^+ efflux moves the membrane potential back toward the resting level. K^+ channels remain open long enough not only to allow the membrane potential to return to normal but also to create a brief hyperpolarization during which the axon cannot produce an AP. The K^+ channels then close, and the Na^+/K^+ pump rapidly restores the cations to their resting concentrations. The entire sequence of events that underlies the electrical change lasts only about 0.002 sec.

The sequence of events just described is restricted to a small portion of the axon. Axons may be as long as a meter, and the AP must, and does, propagate the entire length of the axon in order to cause the release of neurotransmitters from the presynaptic axon terminals. This action occurs because the voltage changes produced at a restricted part of the axon membrane cause current to flow from the adjacent segment of the axon. This current flow changes the voltage across the membrane at the adjacent segment, Na^+ channels open, and the process described here begins in the axon closer to the terminal.

When the AP invades the terminal bouton, the change in membrane potential causes neurotransmitter molecules to be released into the synaptic cleft between the presynaptic and postsynaptic membranesbranes. These molecules find their receptors on the postsynaptic cell, and the process of PSP generation begins.

ORGANIZATION OF CENTRAL NERVOUS SYSTEM

Comprehension of the neuron as a cell is important in understanding the pathological nature of Alzheimer's disease because it acts at the level of the subcellular elements of the neuron. However, neuron loss in Alzheimer's disease does not occur diffusely in all brain structures. The clinical signs and symptoms of the disease are caused by a pattern of neuron loss in different regions of the brain. Therefore a basic knowledge of the anatomy of the CNS is important in understanding Alzheimer's disease.

Basic Divisions

The two principal divisions of the CNS are the brain and the spinal cord. The brain can be divided into the brainstem and the forebrain. The brainstem comprises the medulla, the pons, and the midbrain. The forebrain includes the cortex, the thalamus, the hypothalamus (Fig. 1-2), and a collection of subcortical nuclei related, anatomically and functionally, either to the limbic system or to the basal ganglia. The cerebellum has major anatomical connections with the spinal cord, the brainstem, and the forebrain (especially the neocortex). Therefore it is not readily categorized, either anatomically or functionally, with the other gross divisions of the brain.

Basic Neural Circuits and Long Axonal Pathways

The structure of the spinal cord provides the basis of all movement. It is also responsible for transmission of sensory information from the body to the brain. Bundles of axons that either transmit sensory information concerning the body surface, viscera, joints, or muscles to the brain or carry motor commands from the brain to the spinal cord form the outer part of the cord. Because the axons are myelinated, they appear white in fresh spinal cord. The neuron cell bodies of the spinal cord are internal to the long axon tracts of the cord. The cell bodies, which lack myelin, are gray in color in fresh spinal cord.

As noted earlier, neurons can be categorized in many ways. However, two categories are especially useful and are represented by neurons of the spinal cord. Some neurons extend their axon away from the region of the brain or spinal cord in which they are found and therefore conduct information away from the locale of their parent cell body. These neurons are known as principal neurons. Two examples of principal neurons are the motor neurons of the ventral (anterior) horn of the spinal cord, which give rise to peripheral motor nerves, and the sensory neurons of the dorsal horn, which create the pathways that conduct pain input from the spinal cord to the brain. The second type of neuron is an interneuron, or local circuit neuron. The axon of this

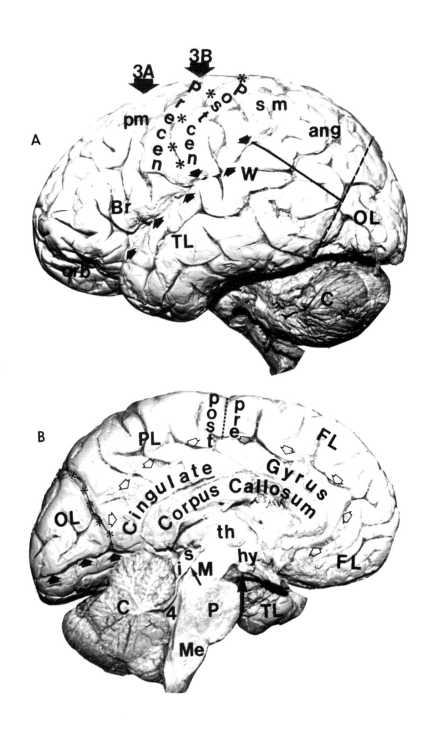

Fig. 1-2. A, Lateral aspect of human brain shows some important areas of brain. Asterisks demarcate central fissure, and arrowheads indicate course of lateral (sylvian) fissure. Solid black line represents approximate division between parietal lobe and temporal lobe. Broken line indicates approximate separation between occipital lobe and other lobes. Large dark arrows at superior surface of brain indicate level from which cross sections shown in Fig. 1-3 were taken. **B,** Medial aspect of hemisphere shown in **A.** Open arrowheads indicate course of cingulate sulcus. Arrow that appears in midbrain indicates cerebral aqueduct; large arrow at base of hypothalamus shows mammillary body. Broken line indicates approximate division of medial extension of precentral (*pre*) and postcentral (*post*) gyri. Dark arrowheads delineate calcarine fissure surrounded by primary visual cortex. Asterisks indicate parietooccipital fissure. Abbreviations: *ang,* angular gyrus; *Br,* Broca's area; *C,* cerebellum; *FL,* frontal lobe; *hy,* hypothalamus; *i,* inferior colliculus of midbrain; *M,* midbrain; *Me,* medulla; *OL,* occipital lobe; *orb,* orbital frontal cortex; *P,* pons; *PL,* parietal lobe; *pm,* premotor area; *Postcen,* postcentral gyrus; *Precen,* precentral gyrus; *s,* superior colliculus of midbrain; *sm,* supramarginal gyrus; *th,* thalamus; *TL,* temporal lobe; *4,* fourth ventricle.

neuron remains within the region of the cell body. The complexity of the connections of interneurons determines the complexity of information processing by the CNS.

Some of the circuits formed by interneurons of the spinal cord are the basis for posture and locomotion; other local circuit spinal cord neurons inhibit pain input or enhance the ability to localize touch on the surface of the skin. However, the ability of the spinal cord to integrate sensory information and motor activity is limited. Bundles of axons running from the spinal cord to the brain or coming from the brain to the spinal cord are necessary for normal function.

Divisions of Brain

The medulla, pons, midbrain, and cerebellum (see Fig. 1-2) represent the next stage in the hierarchy of complexity of the brain. The cerebellum receives input from the spinal cord about limb position, extent of muscle contraction, and amount of tension on the tendons. It also receives input from the neocortex about decisions made in the motor and premotor cortex and in the visual and auditory sensory modalities. The primary function of the cerebellum is to coordinate movement. Damage to the cerebellum, or to its input, may result in decomposition of movement so that normally smooth movements become jerky and irregular. Hands may tremble during movement (intentional tremors), and the ability to accurately place a limb without overshooting or undershooting the target may be lost (dysmetria). There also may be a decrease in resistance to passive movement of the limbs (hypotonia). However, cerebellar damage does not cause weakness (paresis) or paralysis of voluntary movement.

The medulla, pons, and midbrain contain most of the cranial nerve nuclei. Collections of cell bodies within the CNS that have a common function, receive common input, give rise to common output, and share other physical features are called nuclei. Most of the subcortical brain structures are organized into nuclei. Some cranial nerve nuclei give rise to motor axons that control somatic musculature of the head and neck, whereas others are the source of the cranial part of the parasympathetic nervous system. Still other cranial nerve nuclei receive sensory input from the viscera or the head and neck. Thus some parts of the brainstem are functionally equivalent to the gray matter of the spinal cord but serve the head and neck rather than the body.

Reticular formation

The cranial nerve nuclei are embedded within the reticular formation of the brainstem. The reticular formation comprises distinct nuclear subdivisions. Some of the reticular formation nuclei, particularly those located in the medulla and the caudal pons, send axons to the spinal cord to influence autonomic function and to bias somatomotor reflexes. Nuclei of the reticular formation also send axons to the forebrain, and these axons are involved in modulation of the levels of consciousness and attention. For example, parts of the reticular formation interact to produce the different stages of sleep and the cortical electrical rhythms that accompany varying mental states.

Electrical rhythms of neocortex

The electrical rhythms of the neocortex are recorded from the surface of the scalp, and this recording is called an electroencephalogram (EEG). The EEG is a recording of the summed PSPs of the neocortical neurons within range of the recording electrode; that is, the neurons of the neocortex actually produce the EEG. However, the frequency and the waveforms of the EEG are determined by interaction among the neocortex, the thalamus, and the reticular formation. The main waveforms of the EEG are delta, theta, alpha, and beta. Although the amplitude of these waveforms varies, with delta typically being the largest and beta the smallest, the frequency is the defining characteristic of the EEG rhythms. Delta has a frequency of 0.5 to 4 Hz (cycles/sec) and is associated with slow-wave sleep. Theta has a frequency of 4 to 7 Hz and is related to profound relaxation; when recorded from the temporal lobe, it also may reflect memory processing. Alpha (8 to 13 Hz) is associated with a wakeful but relaxed state, and beta (13 to 30 Hz) is related to both alert attending and rapid eye movement (REM) sleep.

Reticular formation input to the thalamus is more involved in appearance of beta than of the slower EEG rhythms. For example, increased activity in the reticular formation disrupts the cyclical excitatory-inhibitory interaction between the cortex and the thalamus that produces the alpha rhythm. This disruption causes the EEG to enter beta from alpha. Thus reticular formation bombardment of the thalamus causes the synchronous alpha rhythm to become desynchronized.

The EEG becomes desynchronized during an awake vigilant state and also during REM sleep. Although the EEG is very similar in these two situations, the reticular formation nuclei and the neurotransmitter systems involved appear to be different. Increased activity in the locus ceruleus, the neurons of which use norepinephrine as a neurotransmitter, and the median raphe nucleus, the neurons of which use serotonin as a transmitter, appears to stimulate waking activities and to inhibit REM sleep, whereas increased activity of cholinergic neurons in the region of the rostral pons and the caudal midbrain seems to trigger REM sleep. In addition to playing a role in maintenance of vigilance, the locus ceruleus and the raphe nuclei may interact with the cholinergic neurons of the reticular formation to produce the alternation between non-REM (NREM) and REM sleep that constitutes a normal sleep pattern.

Normal sleep begins with an episode of NREM, or slow-wave, sleep. During NREM the EEG shows delta frequency activity broken by bursts of synchronous high-voltage alphalike sleep spindles. These EEG events are paced by the thalamus, but experimental evidence suggests that activity of the neurotransmitter serotonin in the preoptic area of the hypothalamus may trigger slow-wave sleep, presumably under the influence of the suprachiasmatic nucleus of the hypothalamus. Neurons of the suprachiasmatic nucleus are sensitive to the light/dark cycle and control circadian rhythmicity of many of the responses of the body and brain.

Therefore nuclei of the reticular formation that use norepinephrine, serotonin, or acetylcholine as their transmitters participate in the regulation of the sleep/waking cycle and in modulation of arousal during waking. The ability of the brain to synthesize these three transmitters decreases in older age, and it is possible that this decline contributes to the disruption of sleep that is a prevalent complaint of older people.

The number of neurons that produce these transmitters and the markers for the presence of these transmitters in the axons and terminals show a much larger decrease in patients with Alzheimer's disease than in the normal aging population. Some data indicate that decreases in these transmitters, especially loss of cholinergic neurons and other cholinergic markers, are related to the cognitive deficits associated with Alzheimer's disease (see Chapter 7). In addition, because of these transmitters' regulation of EEG changes associated with different states of consciousness, changes in their activity also may be responsible for the significant shift toward slower than normal dominant EEG frequencies during both waking and REM sleep states found in patients diagnosed as having Alzheimer's disease.

Thalamus

One function of the thalamus is to pace the continuous electrical activity of the entire neocortex while it is under the influence of the brainstem reticular formation. However, the thalamus performs other roles in its relationship with the neocortex and with other subcortical structures. A principal function of the thalamus is to transmit sensory information to the neocortex. Several individual nuclei relay specific sensory information to definite sections of the neocortex. The lateral geniculate nucleus (see Fig. 1-3, *B*) receives input from the retina through the second cranial nerve, integrates this input, and transmits it to the visual cortex of the occipital lobe (see Fig. 1-2, *A*). The medial geniculate nucleus transmits auditory information to the transverse gyri of the superior temporal lobe, and the ventral posterior lateral and medial nuclei receive somatosensory input from the medial lemniscus and ascending trigeminal pathways, integrate this information, and transmit it to the postcentral gyrus of the parietal lobe. Other nuclei of the thalamus, such as the pulvinar and dorsomedial nuclei, receive input from several sensory modalities, associate this input, and relay it to the association areas of the parietal (pulvinar nucleus) and prefrontal (dorsomedial nucleus) lobes (see Fig. 1-2, *A*).

The ventrolateral and ventroanterior nuclei of the thalamus represent the primary link between the output of the basal ganglia (Fig. 1-3) and the primary motor cortex of the precentral gyrus and premotor area of the frontal lobe (see Fig. 1-2, *A*). The anterior nuclear complex serves a similar function for the limbic system and the cortex. Therefore the thalamus acts as an integrative relay from subcortical structures to the neocortex for sensory, motor, arousal, motivational, and emotional systems.

Hypothalamus

The hypothalamus is a relatively small part of the brain (less than 1% of its volume). It is located just below, or ventral to, the thalamus (see Fig. 1-2, *B*). The hypothalamus modulates the autonomic nervous system, the hormonal systems controlled by the pituitary gland, and the diffuse neural structures involved, as indicated earlier in the sleep/waking cycle.

Different regions and nuclei of the hypothalamus have different functions. These functions can be deduced from the effects of stimulation of various hypothalamic areas or the effects of their destruction. For example, destruction of the ventromedial hypothalamus will produce overeating (hyperphagia), which leads to obesity, whereas destruction of the lateral hypothalamus will lead to cessation of eating and drinking.

The anatomical connections and the neurotransmitter content of the various hypothalamic nuclei also may predict their function. In addition to the neurotransmitters, the nuclei of the hypothalamus produce many peptides that may participate in the endocrine function of the hypothalamus or may be released at a neural synapse to serve as neurotransmitters or neuromodulators. For example, neurons in the supraoptic and paraventricular hypothalamic nuclei produce oxytocin and vasopressin. Some of these neurons extend their axons to the posterior lobe of the pituitary gland, where these substances are released directly into the systemic circulation. Oxytocin and vasopressin act as circulatory hormones to produce uterine contractions during labor. Oxytocin induces milk injection during lactation, and vasopressin causes the kidney to conserve water and increase blood pressure. Other neurons in these two nuclei also produce oxytocin and vasopressin but they extend their axons to nuclei of the medulla, thus influencing the autonomic nervous system. These axons synapse in these sites, and oxytocin and vasopressin act as neuromodulators or neurotransmitters on the target neurons.

Other peptides produced by hypothalamic neurons are transported down the axons of these neurons; they are released into the local portal circulation of the median eminence. This circulation extends only to the anterior pituitary gland, where these peptides serve to cause or prevent the release of pituitary hormones into the general circulation. For example, neurons in the hypothalamus produce growth hormone–releasing hormone (GHRH). GHRH moves in vesicles down the axons of these neurons to the median eminence, where it is released into the portal circulation. When GHRH reaches the anterior pituitary, it causes release of growth hormone. Other neurons in the hypothalamus produce a peptide known as somatostatin. Somatostatin follows the same route as GHGH, but it inhibits the release of growth hormone.

Corticotropin-releasing hormone (CRH), another hormone produced in the hypothalamus, causes release of a hormone from the anterior pituitary. This hormone is adrenocorticotropic hormone (ACTH), which stimulates release of corticosteroids by the adrenal gland. Some of the neurons that produce CRH also make vasopressin. If vasopressin reaches the anterior pituitary with CRH, ACTH release is facilitated. Prolonged stress, either physical or mental, and aging increase the release of vasopressin and ACTH. The resulting high levels of glucocorticoids released by the adrenal cortex into the blood can be toxic to certain areas of the brain, especially the hippocampus. It is possible that hyperactivity within this system is involved in hippocampal cell death associated with aging and Alzheimer's disease.

Limbic system structures

In 1949 Paul MacLean introduced the modern concept of the limbic system. Several subcortical and cortical structures are included in the limbic system. These include the amygdala and the hippocampus, which are found beneath the cortex of the medial surface of the temporal lobe; the cingulate gyrus, which extends around and close to the corpus callosum (see Figs. 1-2, *B*, and 1-3); the orbital frontal cortex; the mammillary nuclei of the hypothalamus (see Fig. 1-2, *B*); the anterior nuclear group of the thalamus (see Figs. 1-2, *B*, and 1-3, *B*); and their interconnections among all of these structures.

Many of the functions of the limbic system are related to hypothalamic functions. For example, the amygdala is involved in modulation of emotional behavior. Stimulation of the amygdala can cause aggression and rage responses, whereas its destruction is associated with placidity, increased oral activity, and hypersexuality, a constellation of behaviors known as the Klüver-Bucy syndrome. Destruction of the orbital frontal cortex (Fig. 1-2, *A*) also may lead to flattening of affect, and destruction of the anterior cingulate cortex has been used as a treatment for chronic pain. Following this type of neurosurgery, some patients with terminal cancer report that they still feel pain as a sensation but that it has lost its affective component. However, the loss of general affective response and motivation associated with orbital frontal damage does not occur with restricted removal of the anterior cingulate.

Although the hippocampus (see Fig. 1-3, *B*) originally was included as part of the emotional circuitry of the limbic system, it has been well documented that this structure is involved in the formation of new memories. Although damage to the hippocampus, whether as part of a degenerative disease such as Alzheimer's disease or by surgical means or vascular insult, produces impairment in the formation of new memories, the hippocampus is not the site of memory storage. Rather, this structure is involved in the processing of information that will be stored in the neocortex as a memory.

Basal ganglia

The basal ganglia of the forebrain properly include the caudate nucleus, the putamen, and the globus pallidus. However, because of their close anatomical and functional relationship with these structures, the substantia nigra and the subthalamic nucleus (see Fig. 1-3, *B*) are included in this discussion of the basal ganglia.

The basic function of the basal ganglia is to modulate movement. However, the basal ganglia do not accomplish their function through direct pathways to the spinal cord motor neurons. Instead, the output of the basal ganglia, which arises almost entirely from the globus pallidus, is relayed through the ventrolateral and ventroanterior nuclei of the thalamus to motor areas of the cortex that give rise to the descending motor pathway. Therefore paralysis may occur when the motor cortex is damaged, but not when basal ganglia structures are damaged or degenerate. The consequences of damage to basal ganglia include involuntary movement and tremors, slowness of movement (bradykinesia), and changes in muscle tone (including rigidity).

Loss of the individual structures of the basal ganglia produces distinct combinations of these fundamental disturbances in movement. For example, death of the dopamine-containing neurons of the substantia nigra results in Parkinson's disease. Although the cause of Parkinson's disease has not been established, its signs include varying degrees of bradykinesia, rigidity of the body and facial muscles, and tremors that are worse at rest than during movement. Normally the dopaminergic neurons of the substantia nigra extend their axons to the putamen and the caudate nucleus. Together the putamen and the caudate nucleus are known as the neostriatum. It is thought that since the dopaminergic nigrostriatal pathway degenerates in Parkinson's disease, the loss of the inhibition normally provided to the neostriatum by this pathway is the cause of the increased muscle tone (rigidity) and observed tremors.

Spasmodic but coordinated involuntary movements of the distal

Fig. 1-3. Coronal (frontal) cross sections made approximately at plane indicted by dark arrows in Fig. 1-2, *A*, reveal internal structures of brain discussed in text. Asterisks in **A** indicate position of anterior limb of internal capsule. Asterisks in **B** show lateral fissure. Body of lateral ventricles is located inferior to corpus callosum. Two lateral ventricles are separated by septal area in **A** and body of fornix in **B**. Inferior horns of lateral ventricles are superior and lateral to hippocampus. Third ventricle is space separating two halves of thalamus. *an*, Anterior nuclear group of thalamus; *cau*, caudate nucleus; *cc*, corpus callosum; *cg*, cingulate gyrus; *dm*, dorsomedial nucleus of thalamus; *Hpc*, hippocampus; *ic*, posterior limb of internal capsule; *LGN*, lateral geniculate nucleus of thalamus; *p*, pons; *sn*, substantia nigra; *snu*, subthalamic nucleus; *TL*, temporal lobe.

---

parts of the upper limbs and abrupt movements of the face characterize the early stages of Huntington's disease chorea. Huntington's disease is caused by an inherited abnormality on chromosome 4. The chorea is the result of loss of acetylcholine- and GABA-containing neurons that normally produce IPSPs in the neostriatum. As the disease progresses, much of the forebrain becomes involved in the neuropathological process and profound dementia results.

The final and most extreme example of this type of movement disorder is produced by hemorrhagic damage to the subthalamic nucleus. Typically such damage occurs on only one side, and the contralateral limbs flail violently about in uncontrollable, ballistic movements.

The subthalamic nucleus normally exerts its influence via its connections with the globus pallidus, and the excitatory neurotransmitter glutamate is the neurotransmitter. The globus pallidus provides the principal output from the basal ganglia. The transmitter between the globus pallidus and the thalamus appears to be the inhibitory neurotransmitter GABA, but the transmitter from the thalamus to the cortex is excitatory. Thus the net influence of the basal ganglia, as represented by its output, is inhibition of an excitatory drive to the neocortex.

Neocortex

The external surface of the neocortex is composed of neuron cell bodies and appears gray in fresh tissue. The cortical white matter, which is found beneath the gray matter, is composed of bundles of axons that enter or exit the gray matter. Some of these axons continue to form part of the internal capsule. The internal capsule is the large white matter structure comprising virtually all the axons that carry information to or from the cortex. This capsule is entirely subcortical. Its anterior limb (see Fig. 1-3, *A*) divides the caudate nucleus from the

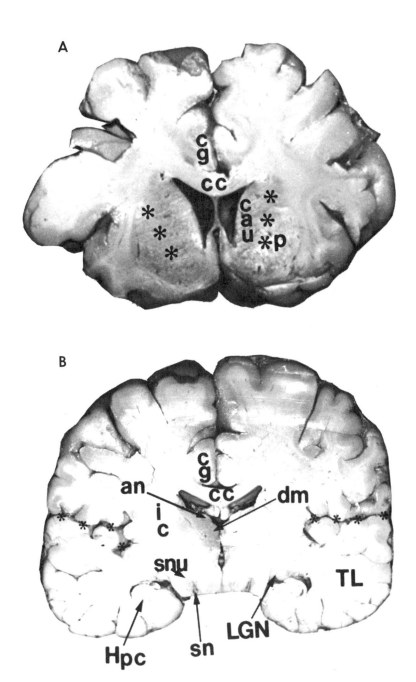

putamen, and its posterior limb (see Fig. 1-3, *B*) separates the thalamus from the globus pallidus and the putamen. Because all input and output of the cortex travel through the internal capsule, damage to this structure produces severe clinical deficits. For example, both the output of the motor cortex and the input to the sensory cortex from the somatosensory nuclei of the thalamus travel through the posterior limb of the internal capsule; therefore a stroke that destroys this limb will produce paralysis or paresis and sensory loss.

Other axons in the deep cortical white matter carry information from one area of the cortex to other areas in the same lobe. These routes are called association pathways. An example is the arcuate fasciculus, which connects parts of the superior temporal cortex to the frontal lobe. The arcuate fasciculus is particularly important in the left hemisphere because it connects the receptive speech area of the posterior superior temporal and the posterior inferior parietal cortices to the expressive speech area of the posteroinferior frontal convolution and the premotor area. Because of this anatomical relationship, destruction of the left arcuate fasciculus produces conduction aphasia and bilateral apraxia. These deficits in higher cortical function are discussed in detail in Chapters 2 and 3.

The final type of axon found in the deep white matter of the cortex crosses the midline of the brain to synapse on neurons in the cortical gray matter located directly opposite. Collectively these axons comprise the corpus callosum (see Figs. 1-2, *B*, and 1-3). Destruction of the corpus callosum prevents communication of the two hemispheres. It may produce apraxia in the hand opposite the language-dominant hemisphere and some types of agnosia. The effects of callosal destruction are discussed further in Chapter 2.

The neocortex is divided into four visible lobes—frontal, parietal, temporal, and occipital. The frontal lobe contains the motor and premotor cortex and the prefrontal and orbital areas (see Fig. 1-2, *A*). The orbital frontal cortex is associated with the limbic system, and damage to this area may result in affective changes. Damage to the prefrontal regions disrupts the ability to formulate plans and perform other higher cognitive functions. The parietal cortex is made up of primary somatosensory cortex and association cortex, which are involved in various visuospatial functions, including recognition of body scheme as it relates to space. In addition to visual association cortex, the occipital cortex contains primary visual cortex in and around the calcarine fissure (see Fig. 1-2, *B*). The inferior portion of the temporal lobe is involved in complex visual association, whereas the remainder of this lobe handles associations from several modalities. The primary auditory cortex is located in the superior temporal lobe; in left hemisphere language-dominant people, the posterosuperior temporal lobe is involved in recognition of language. More information concerning the neocortex can be found in Chapter 2.

When the microscopic structure of the neocortex is studied, six cell layers can be observed. These cell layers are distinguished by the predominant cell type. The most superficial layer of the neocortex, the plexiform layer, is relatively cell free (see Fig. 1-1, *C*), but it contains dendrites and axons. The second layer, the external granule layer, contains predominantly small neurons referred to as granule cells. The third layer, the external pyramidal layer, is made up of the pyramidal neurons. The fourth layer is called the internal granule layer because it consists of granule neurons. The fifth layer, which comprises pyramidal neurons, is known as the internal pyramidal layer. The sixth layer, the multiform layer, includes relatively large neurons of varying shapes.

The human neocortex appears convoluted. The surface of a convolution is called a gyrus (plural: gyri), and the grooves between the gyri are referred to as sulci (singular: sulcus). A large, prominent sulcus may be called a fissure. Many of the gyri are associated with specific functions. For example, the gyrus located immediately anterior to the central fissure, the precentral gyrus (see Fig. 1-2, *A*), contains the primary motor cortex; the gyrus immediately posterior to the central fissure, the postcentral gyrus, is primary somatosensory cortex. Although these gyri are close to each other, their histological structure differs. In the precentral gyrus, the large pyramidal neurons of the fifth layer give rise to the motor pathway that reaches the spinal cord, and the fifth layer is very thick in the precentral gyrus. In the postcentral gyrus, the granule cells of the fourth layer receive the axon terminals from the somatosensory nuclei of the thalamus. In contrast with the precentral gyrus, the fourth layer is thicker, whereas the fifth layer is thinner.

These examples demonstrate that differences in function may accompany at least some variations in cortical structure. Further, as discussed in Chapter 7, in patients with Alzheimer's disease neuron death is more likely to occur in some layers of the affected lobes of the cortex than in others.

BIBLIOGRAPHY

Cave CB, Squire LR: Equivalent impairment in spatial and nonspatial memory following damage to the human hippocampus, *Hippocampus* 1:329-340, 1991.

Coben LA, Danziger WL, Berg L: Frequency analysis of the resting awake EEG in mild senile dementia of the Alzheimer type, *Electroencephalogr Clin Neurophysiol* 55:372-380, 1983.

Coben LA, Danziger WL, Storandt M: A longitudinal EEG study of mild senile dementia of the Alzheimer type: changes at 1 year and at 2.5 years, *Electroencephalogr Clin Neurophysiol* 61:101-112, 1985.

Corkin S: A prospective study of cingulotomy. In Valenstein E, editor: *The psychosurgery debate*, San Francisco, 1980, WH Freeman.

Côté LJ, Kremzner LT: Biochemical changes in normal aging in human brain. In Mayeux R, Rosen WG, editors: *The dementias: advances in neurology*, vol 38, New York, 1983, Raven Press.

DiMonte DA: Mitochondrial DNA and Parkinson's disease, *Neurology* 41(suppl 2):38-42, 1991.

Hefti F: Is Alzheimer's disease caused by a lack of nerve growth factor? *Ann Neurol* 13:109-110, 1983.

Hobson JA: Sleep and dreaming, *J Neurosci* 10:371-382, 1990.

Jones EG, Cowan WM: Nervous tissue. In Weiss L, editor: *Histology: cell and tissue biology*, ed 5, New York, 1983, Elsevier Biomedical.

Kelly DD: Sleep and dreaming. In Kandel ER, Schwartz JH, Jessel TM, editors: *Principles of neural science*, ed 3, New York, 1991, Elsevier.

MacLean PD: Psychosomatic disease and the "visceral brain": recent developments bearing on the Papez theory of emotion, *Psychosom Med* 11:338-353, 1949.

Milner B: Amnesia following operation on the temporal lobes. In Whitty CW, Zangwill OL, editors: *Amnesia*, London, 1966, Butterworth.

Mountcastle VB: An organizing principle for cerebral function: the unit module and the distributed system. In Schmitt FO, Worden FG, editors: *The neurosciences: fourth study program*, Cambridge, Mass, 1979, The MIT Press.

Nakagawa-Hattori Y and others: Is Parkinson's disease a mitochondrial disorder? *J Neurol Sci* 107:29-33, 1992.

Peters A, Palay SL, Webster H DeF: *The fine structure of the nervous system*, New York, 1991, Oxford University Press.

Prinz PN and others: EEG markers of early Alzheimer's disease in computer-selected tonic REM sleep, *Electroencephalogr Clin Neurophysiol* 83:36-43, 1992.

Sapolsky RM, McEwen BS: Adrenal steroids and the Hippocampus: involvements in stress and aging. In Isaacson RL, Pribram KH, editors: *Hippocampus*, vol 3, New York, 1986, Plenum.

Schwartz JH: The cytology of neurons. In Kandel ER, Schwartz JH, Jessel TM, editors: *Principles of neural science*, ed 3, New York, 1991, Elsevier.

Schwartz JH: Synthesis and trafficking of neuronal proteins. In Kandel ER, Schwartz JH, Jessel TM, editors: *Principles of neural science,* ed 3, New York, 1991, Elsevier.

Schwartz WH, Gainer H: Suprachiasmatic nucleus: use of ^{14}C-labeled deoxyglucose uptake as a functional marker, *Science* 197:1089-1091, 1977.

Steriade M: Alertness, quiet sleep, dreaming. In Peters A, editor: *Cerebral cortex,* vol 9, New York, 1991, Plenum Press.

Vallee RB: Mechanisms of fast and slow axonal transport, *Annu Rev Neurosci* 14:59-92, 1991.

2

Higher brain functions

Patrick Sloan

This chapter presents an overview of normal brain functions with emphasis on higher brain (cortical) functions in humans. How these functional brain systems operate and how dementia, particularly Alzheimer's disease, interferes with or impairs these functions is explained to prepare the reader for subsequent chapters.

For centuries it has been known that the human brain is the primary organ of thought and emotion. Scientists now understand that the brain grows to weigh approximately 3 pounds by the time an individual reaches age 30, and then it slowly begins to shrink. By using the human brain's capacity for planning, problem-solving, and communication, we have been able to travel to the moon, but there is still much to be learned about how the brain actually works. Much of what we already know about the brain is based on brain pathology. In order to understand better how a brain disease such as Alzheimer's disease affects brain functioning, it is important to begin with a basic understanding of the normal brain and its functions.

NERVE CELLS

The brain comprises approximately 140 billion cells, 20 billion of which are directly involved in information processing. Each of these information-processing cells has up to 15,000 direct physical connections with other brain cells. In fact, the brain is an organ that is far more complex and more sophisticated than a mainframe computer.

Nerve cells are made up of different types of cells. Regardless of the type, each nerve cell (neuron) has a body, a stem (axon), and connecting branches (dendrites). Neurons within the brain are interconnected and operate primarily on the basis of electrical and chemical activity (see

Chapter 1). Through the combination of these two types of activity, a great amount of information is communicated among cells, both within specific areas and throughout all parts of the brain.

The cells' bodies give the brain a gray appearance on gross inspection; hence the term "gray matter." The outer layer of the brain, which is called the cortex or neocortex, is mainly composed of cell bodies. The connective nerve tissue cells are called neuroglias or glia cells. Because the axons of nerve cells bind easily to lipids (fat), they have a white appearance; hence the term "white matter." The white sheaths help to speed conduction of nerve impulses. White tracks or fibers run from the outer layer of the cortex throughout the brain. Gray matter and white matter are discussed frequently in the study of brain functioning.

BRAIN STRUCTURE

Structurally, the brain is divided into hemispheres—a left half and a right half—that are connected by a large bundle of white matter called the corpus callosum. The two halves are essentially symmetrical in appearance but are not alike in function.

Scientists use various methods of conducting studies of brain structure and function, including the comparative, the cytoarchitectonic, and the physiological approach. The comparative approach studies the brains of lower animals to learn about the structure and function of the human brain through comparison. Mammals are often studied because, like man, they have a larger neocortex than lower animals. The cytoarchitectonic approach deals with the structure of cells, their differences, and how they are distributed throughout the brain. Some areas of the brain have six layers of cells, whereas other areas have only three layers. These cells can be mapped to show differentiation in brain structure, which roughly corresponds to brain function. The physiological approach studies nerve structure and the electrical and biochemical activity of neurons. The study of electrical activities of nerve cells and how they are conducted has led to the development of instruments that produce recordings of brain function, such as the electroencephalogram and evoked potentials.

When a nerve cell is stimulated, an electrical impulse is generated and moves along the nerve cell. When the impulse reaches the end of the nerve cell, it stimulates the production and release of chemical compounds called neurotransmitters. Acetylcholine is one neurotransmitter that has been studied extensively in regard to Alzheimer's disease. In fact, a deficiency in this neurotransmitter has been noted in some patients with Alzheimer's disease. Acetylcholine is normally present in various parts of the brain and seems to be involved in the establishment of memories in the cortex. Acetylcholine's precursor, choline, is contained in certain food substances, such as lecithin, which have been given to patients with Alzheimer's disease in an attempt to improve memory. Unfortunately, these studies have not been generally successful in terms of clinical treatment, although they have been most helpful in improving our understanding of the neurochemical processes that occur in the brain.

Other neurotransmitters that have received much attention in the past few decades are dopamine, noradrenaline, serotonin, and enkephalins, a type of endorphins. Neurons that contain certain neurotransmitters appear to be organized in systems, and researchers try to relate these systems to particular brain functions. Chemicals in drugs that are used for medicinal or recreational purposes can either increase or decrease the natural activity of these neurotransmitters, and much has been learned about how certain drugs affect behavior. Drugs that affect cognitive activity, or psychoactive drugs, act on neurotransmitters in different ways, depending on the neurotransmitter system affected. Researchers continue to report on the effectiveness of certain drugs in improving cognition, such as tacrine and selegiline hydrochloride, which are used in the treatment of Parkinson's disease and have been reported to improve attention and episodic memory in Parkinson's disease and early Alzheimer's disease.

Stimulant drugs, such as amphetamines, release noradrenaline and block its reabsorption (reuptake) in the nerve cells. Stimulants cause a general increase in arousal. Antidepressants, such as desipramine and fluoxetine, block the reuptake of noradrenaline and serotonin, respectively, causing an antidepressant effect. Antipsychotic drugs, such as chlorpromazine, block the transmission of dopamine, creating a tranquilizing effect. Sedative-hypnotic drugs, such as alcohol, benzodiazepines, and barbiturates, reduce anxiety when administered at low doses but produce sedation or coma at higher doses. These drugs decrease the activity of neurotransmitter systems that produce arousal, such as noradrenaline, and also affect gamma-aminobutyric acid (GABA) receptors.

It should be noted that the neurotransmitter systems in normal elderly persons may be more vulnerable to the effect of psychoactive drugs. This vulnerability may be even greater if brain disease (e.g., dementia) has altered the normal numbers or the activity of brain cells. Drug and neurotransmitter interactions also can cause a variety of complex reactions, which is why physicians should exercise great care in prescribing psychoactive drugs for persons with suspected dementia.

Some neurotransmitters are made naturally within the brain. Endorphins, which may act as either tranquilizers or stimulants, are examples. The release of some endorphins is thought to be generated by physical exercise; for example, the "runner's high" that joggers describe is probably a result of the stimulation of these opiatelike substances. Acupuncturists believe that needles can be used to stimulate the flow of endorphins, which then act as natural anesthetics in some patients.

CENTRAL NERVOUS SYSTEM

The central nervous system is composed of the spinal cord and the brain. The neocortex, the outer covering of the brain, is the main focus of this discussion of higher brain (cortical) functions because it makes up about 80% of the human brain and separates humans from the lower animals. Only about 1.5 to 3 cm thick, the neocortex covers an area of up to 2500 cm. The brain is folded and wrinkled so that all of its surface area fits neatly in the human skull. The many ridges (gyri), grooves (fissures), and shallow grooves (sulci) that make up the cerebral cortex give the brain its wrinkled appearance.

The brain and the spinal cord are nourished by cerebrospinal fluid, which flows around the spinal cord and into the brain in a system of cavities called ventricles. In the normal brain the cerebrospinal fluid is produced, circulates, and is reabsorbed freely. The ventricles can be viewed on a computed tomographic (CT) scan, a computer-generated x-ray "picture" of the brain. If a decrease in brain tissue (i.e., neurons) occurs, the ventricles may become enlarged to fill the unoccupied space that results. This shrinking of cortical matter is called cortical atrophy. Cortical atrophy and the resulting enlarged ventricles sometimes occur in persons with dementia and therefore can offer clues in diagnosis. However, they are not an unequivocal indication of the presence of dementia because many normal elderly persons show signs of cortical atrophy as a function of normal aging.

HEMISPHERES AND LOBES

Structurally, the neocortex can be divided several ways. The simplest way, and the one most often publicized in the popular media, is to divide it into two halves, the left and the right cerebral hemispheres. Each hemisphere specializes in different functions, but both typically work in conjunction with each other. Whether the brain is considered as a whole or as two halves, it can be divided further into four basic divisions or lobes. Basically, these lobes are structural divisions at the deepest fissures. The frontal lobe constitutes the front (anterior) half of the brain. In the back (posterior) portion of the brain is the parietal lobe. The parietal lobe is evident on the outside (lateral) surface and overlaps into the middle (medial) surface of the cortex. The temporal lobe rests behind the temple, and the occipital lobe is located at the posterior pole above the cerebellum.

The task becomes more complicated when we try to divide the brain in terms of its functions because the brain operates in an integrated fashion. Although certain neocortical regions or zones specialize in particular brain functions, the brain works as an integrated functional unit. It can be compared with a symphony orchestra. Each individual instrument has its own sound and function, but when the orchestra plays together, these instruments become part of the unified activity of playing a musical piece.

BRAIN FUNCTIONS

One way of mapping brain functions is to stimulate the brain with tiny electrodes and record what happens when certain parts of the brain are touched. This method has shown that, in terms of primary motor and sensory function, the brain works largely in a contralateral fashion. The side of the body that moves (motor function) or brings in information (sensory information) is on the opposite side from the half of the brain in which this information is handled. In essence, the left half of the brain "controls" the right side of the body, and vice-versa. Although the relationship is not quite that simple, for general purposes it can be thought of in that way. This concept is not to be confused with the popular notion of "right brain" or "left brain" individuals, based on a predominance of specialized abilities. The latter refers to complex higher cortical functions related to thinking or personality style. For example, some people are thought to have better verbal skills (i.e., "left brain" functions) than visuospatial or artistic ones (i.e., "right brain"), or vice-versa; hence the terms "left brain" and "right brain" people. The specialized abilities of each hemisphere are described later in this chapter. Basic sensory and motor functions will not be addressed in detail; instead, the focus will be on complex higher brain (cortical) functions.

Various models have evolved in the attempt to map and describe different brain functions. More than two centuries ago it was thought that certain brain functions could be localized to certain parts of the head. The "science" of phrenology tried to relate brain functions to the conformation of the head. Cautiousness, combativeness, benevolence, and language skills were thought to be located in certain areas. However, phrenology became outdated as neuroanatomical research developed. Yet it is interesting to note that the phrenologists labeled the language area as being alongside the eye because the subject of study was a soldier who had received a wound through the left eye and was unable to speak. They thought that speech was related to the eyes and that the two were causally connected. In retrospect, we know that the soldier's injury probably resulted in a lesion in the posterior part of his left frontal lobe. Paul Broca, a French physician, subsequently discovered that this area controls verbal output. In fact, this type of expressive language disorder later came to be called Broca's aphasia (i.e., without language). Its counterpart, receptive or comprehension aphasia, the inability to understand language, was described a few years later by Karl Wernicke, the physician who localized the lesion that caused this disorder to the superior temporal gyrus of the dominant (usually left) hemisphere.

With the advent of sophisticated radiologic techniques, it has become possible to study brain functions in new ways. One important method is positron emission tomography (PET) scanning, in which a person is injected with glucose that contains radioisotopes. A computer-enhanced view of the brain highlights areas of high and low glucose usage through different colors. Although the CT scan affords a look at the structure of the brain, the PET scan offers a view of the actual brain functions in terms of what parts of the brain are active and inactive during certain types of mental activities, such as thinking, speaking, looking, and listening.

Another way of analyzing brain functions that is relatively inexpensive and does not require the use of highly sophisticated equipment (e.g., a cyclotron) is through a systematic study of cognitive and emotional behavior, the neuropsychological evaluation. This type of evaluation allows us to study what the brain actually does indirectly, by examining what a person can and cannot do on various behavioral tasks (i.e., tests) of sensory, motor, and higher cortical functions, such as those of attention, concentration, memory, thinking, problem-solving, and expression of emotions.

HIGHER BRAIN (CORTICAL) FUNCTIONS

In general, the front part of the brain, which is composed of the frontal lobes, is associated with the programming and execution of motor functions. At more complex levels of functioning, the frontal lobes orchestrate attention, thinking processes, planning, organizing, and abstract reasoning. The posterior part of the brain, made up of the parietal lobes, is related to sensory perception, which involves taking in information from the environment. At more complex levels, the parietal lobes are specifically associated with the monitoring and organizing of all sensory input—visual, auditory, tactile, and kinesthetic. This association makes sense geographically because the parietal lobe lies between the temporal and the occipital lobes. The temporal lobe is responsible for audition, and the occipital lobe is primarily involved with vision. Therefore the parietal lobe is a conveniently located "switching station" for information. In short, one can think of the four basic lobes and their respective functions in the following way: frontal/motor, parietal/sensory, temporal/auditory, and occipital/visual.

To describe the various levels of brain functions further, the model developed by A. R. Luria can be used. Luria studied thousands of brain-damaged individuals and compared their brain functions to those of normal persons. He divided levels of brain activity into functional units. These units are related to areas, or zones, within the brain and to theoretical levels of functioning. Luria called these primary, secondary, and tertiary levels of brain function. The primary level refers to immediate sensory and motor input and output. The secondary level relates to the association among or between the primary zones. The tertiary level involves both the zones that overlap and the higher levels of integration and organization of brain functions. Luria's model helps to explain brain functions from the simplest to the most complex.

Fig. 2-1 illustrates the integration of various levels of brain function in the speaking of a heard word from the perspective of a lateral, or side, view of the left cerebral hemisphere. First, one must be awake at the primary level of arousal, a precursor to the activation of the primary projection areas of the brain. Projection refers to the actual recording or reception of sensory information. Once the person is aroused, the temporal lobe is the primary projection area for audition. In order to repeat a word that has been heard, the person first must have normal functioning of the auditory cortex in the left temporal lobe. After the sound has been sensed, the signal is carried to Wernicke's area in the temporoparietal area, where it is translated or decoded from a sound into a recognizable word. The passage of this

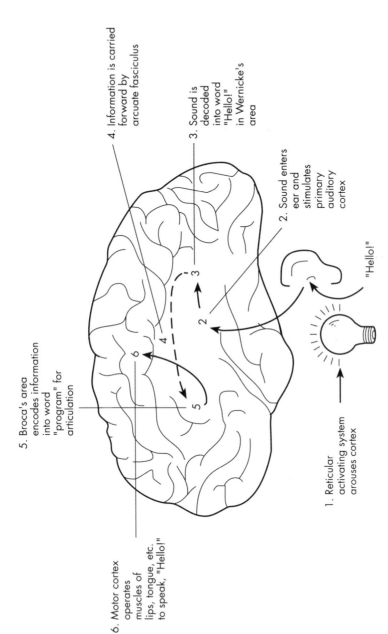

5. Broca's area encodes information into word "program" for articulation

4. Information is carried forward by arcuate fasciculus

3. Sound is decoded into word "Hello!" in Wernicke's area

2. Sound enters ear and stimulates primary auditory cortex

6. Motor cortex operates muscles of lips, tongue, etc. to speak, "Hello!"

1. Reticular activating system arouses cortex

"Hello!"

Fig. 2-1. Speaking a heard word. Process is depicted in order of sequence (counter-clockwise). (Modified from Geschwind N: *Sci Am* 241:180-199, 1979.)

signal and its translation involve the secondary level of association. In turn, the message is carried forward by the white matter tracks (arcuate fasciculus) to Broca's area in the frontal lobe. In Broca's area the signal is translated or encoded into its spoken form. This area is directly adjacent to the motor strip, which controls the lips, tongue, vocal cords, and palate so that the word can be verbalized.

This communication between primary and secondary levels of the brain involves the tertiary level of complex brain functioning, represented by actual thinking and recognizing what we are doing as we do it. The tertiary level also includes forethought and conscious appreciation of this process. These processes require intact "working memory," which allows acquisition, retention, and retrieval of memories and information necessary to orchestrate such complex cortical functions. Because Alzheimer's disease often affects the temporoparietal areas of the brain selectively and prominently, the working memory, language, and visuoconstructive functions are usually disrupted in various combinations and degrees, as described further in Chapter 3.

In order for a person to say a written word or name an object, the image must be projected onto the visual cortex of the occipital lobe (Fig. 2-1). The image is then carried forward into the association area of the parietal lobe and passed to the motor speech area, resulting in a verbal response. Any disruption in the structures or processes that govern these functions is likely to create problems such as visual agnosia (i.e., inability to recognize familiar objects or symbols) or difficulty in naming objects, both common symptoms in Alzheimer's disease. This connection seems to be a fairly simple, straightforward process, and it is not difficult to assign a functional-anatomical correlation to these particular higher cortical functions if the anatomical structures and their basic functions are understood. The examples presented show that we have a relatively well-understood neurologic basis for both vision and audition. However, we do not yet have a clear understanding of the neurologic basis for cognition, or complex thinking. These examples highlight the complexity of the processes within and among the various functional units and levels of the brain in the execution of complex behavior.

In order to discuss higher cognitive processes, certain brain structures and their basic functions need to be described and related to the complex brain activities called higher brain, or cortical, functions. For instance, what processes are involved when a person not only hears and sees what is going on around him but also organizes the various events simultaneously? This processing includes understanding various perceptions and ideas congruently and planning one's next action or some future action. For all of the motor, sensory, and associative processes to respond and act smoothly, the various brain functions must be working both independently and in concert. This process is sometimes referred to as the "executive" function of the cortex. Some researchers have described the breakdown in multiple brain areas associated with Alzheimer's disease as "dysexecutive syndrome," in which these higher integrative powers are impaired as a result of multiple brain lesions throughout the cortex.

Cerebellum

The cerebellum lies under the cerebral hemispheres and facilitates the coordination and regulation of motor movements and, to some extent, cognitive activity. The cerebellum is an organ of synergy. Its functions can be best described by demonstrating how they are negatively affected by alcohol. Excessive alcohol intake interferes with the synergy of the cerebellum. The result is difficulty with gait and the coordination of smooth movements, such as touching one's finger and nose in a rapidly alternating fashion or walking a straight line. The cerebellum, which has far-reaching connections into the brain and spinal cord, predominantly coordinates the movement of independent parts of the body into a smoothly operating whole.

Reticular Formation

The reticular formation, which lies between the brainstem and the cortex, is responsible for activation, arousal, awakening, and attention. At a basic level, the reticular activating system must be working in order to awaken and arouse the cortical structures so that they will be ready to respond and operate; that is, the cortex must be aroused by the reticular system in preparation for receiving and sending messages. This system both awakens and keeps the brain "in tone" to receive sensory information and execute motor and cognitive activity.

Cranial Nerves

Situated around the brainstem, the cranial nerves are special sensory and motor nerves that communicate sensations and movements of the face, eyes, tongue, and vocal cords. These nerves will not be described in detail here, but the reader can review their specific locations and functions in any good neurology text.

Basal Ganglia

The basal ganglia, which are composed of cell bodies, are important structures related to the motor functions. Symmetrically arranged, the basal ganglia lie under the frontal cortex and have many connections to the cortex above and midbrain structures below. Loss of brain cells or neurochemicals in the basal ganglia and their connections can cause severe motor problems and, to a lesser extent, cognitive problems. Parkinson's disease, for example, affects nerve cells and neurochemicals in the basal ganglia, specifically the substantia nigra, and results in difficulties with posture, gait, and initiation and speed of motor activity.

The basal ganglia also are involved in the learning and programing of behavior. Activities that are well learned and rehearsed over the course of life become somewhat "automatic." For example, the complex motor skills involved in walking, eating, or driving become so ingrained that a person does not need to think consciously in order to perform them. Some of these complex but well-programed activities apparently are relegated to the basal ganglia. This function may help to explain why some complex behaviors may be retained in persons with dementia long after severe loss of memory or language has occurred.

Thalamus

The thalamus is an important structure located among the bundles of the basal ganglia situated at the top of the brainstem. It is the central relay center for input and output of sensory and motor messages. The thalamus must be working normally for all the information that enters the relay station to reach the cortex and then to be relayed to the spinal cord, which mediates the movement of the extremities. The thalamus also is involved in higher cortical functions, including memory and the coordination of complex acts associated with various sensory inputs.

Limbic System

Needs, instincts, drives, and emotions are considered part of the functions of the deeper structures of the brain, which comprise the limbic system (limbic lobe). These structures are referred to as a system because its functions are thought to be related and working together. Part of the limbic system, the amygdala, is instrumental in emotional functioning. This structure is sometimes removed surgically in persons with epilepsy when the seizures are refractory to anticonvulsant medication. The hypothalamus, another part of the limbic system that rests deep within the brain, generates drives such as hunger and sex. The hypothalamus also helps to regulate sleep, body temperature, emotions, and endocrine function. The pituitary gland, for example, which is very important to endocrine function, is located in very close proximity to the hypothalamus. In addition to emotional and instinctual activities, the limbic system is involved in cognitive activities. Finally, this system is important in both the recording and the generation of memories.

INTEGRATION AND SPECIALIZATION OF HIGHER BRAIN (CORTICAL) FUNCTIONS

In moving from the deeper brain structures and their functions to the cortex, we encounter complex cognitive functions referred to as higher cortical functions. Examples of these functions are the processes involved in logical thinking, association, memory, and problem-solving. Many interconnections exist between the limbic system and the cortex, as well as within the cortex itself, and all these connections contribute to the network of higher cortical functions. As with the instruments in an orchestra, all the deeper and higher brain structures need to be both functional and working in concert in order for the music (i.e., thought, behavior) to evolve as effective and synthesized.

By using electrodes to probe the brains of patients who are undergoing surgery (one can be awake during brain surgery since the brain does not have pain receptors), researchers have shown that different parts of the brain control different types of cognitive functions as well as simple motor movements. Activities such as speech and the production of different types of verbal activity (e.g., nouns and verbs) are located in different brain areas. It has even been found, for example, that bilingual people control words differently and in different parts of their brains than do people who use only one language.

We know that in most people language is predominantly controlled by the left cerebral hemisphere. Therefore after a massive stroke on the left side of the brain, patients not only are paralyzed on the right side of the body but also tend to lose speech function. The left hemisphere is thought of as specialized for language and abilities related to language, such as reading, listening to and remembering verbal material, and logical thinking. Because language is predominantly controlled by the left side of the brain, it is not surprising that

Broca's area is situated between the left temporal lobe, where verbal memories are generated and stored, and the motor strip, which controls the output of speech. Even in most left-handed people, who make up approximately 10% of the population, language is still "located" in the left cerebral hemisphere. Cases have been reported in which language was found to be distributed in both cerebral hemispheres or managed predominantly by the right hemisphere. These instances usually resulted from familial (i.e., genetic) left-handedness or early developmental brain injury. More typically, however, the right hemisphere is thought to contribute to language functions less in direct or "linguistic" ways than through its involvement in attentional, organizational, or synthesizing activities.

The right cerebral hemisphere is typically more specialized for visuospatial functions that involve a significant configural component, such as recognizing the parts of a puzzle as a whole picture, the ability to follow directions on a map, or the ability to look at a design and then build the object from constructional materials. The right hemisphere is thought to be more specialized for holistic, musical, and other nonverbal activities, such as recognizing and appreciating emotionality and solving problems or puzzles by using nonverbal concepts. However, the right hemisphere also contributes to the synthesis, pacing, or organization of language functions, with emphasis noted on the integrative capacities and functions of the two hemispheres taken as a whole. In general, functions of the right hemisphere have been described as "creative" or "artistic"; those of the left hemisphere are identified as "logical" or "analytical." The right hemisphere also is involved in the recognition and expression of emotionally toned responses or behavior, such as facial expressions.

Although the two hemispheres of the brain and other brain areas are specialized for certain functions, the entire cerebral cortex governs cognition (i.e., thinking, mental activity). The cerebral cortex, sometimes called the association cortex, includes the frontal, parietal, temporal, and occipital lobes and other brain areas, such as the cingulate gyrus and the hippocampus of the limbic system, which are not directly involved in primary, sensory, and motor abilities. Although different brain regions are specialized for certain activities, some functions are distributed throughout the brain. Memory is a prime example. For instance, we know that the basal nucleus of Meynert, located deep within the brain, is greatly involved in generating mental activity and is specifically instrumental in the establishment of memories throughout the cerebral cortex.

Fig. 2-2 illustrates the projected lines of communication from the basal nucleus to the distant areas of the cortex. This communication

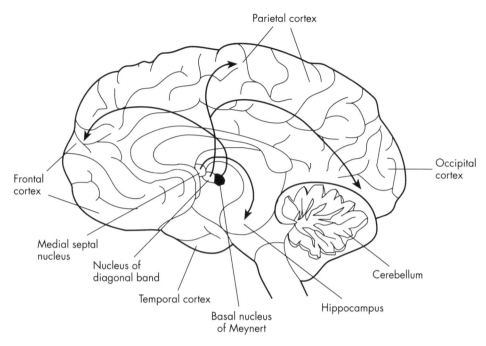

Fig. 2-2. Projections of pathways from basal nucleus of Meynert to distant areas of cortex.

is mentioned because patients with Alzheimer's disease often have an unusually large number of neurofibrillar tangles and senile plaques in the basal nucleus of Meynert, and these pathological cells and their related alterations in neurochemical activity interfere with the transmission of information into the higher levels of the brain. These examples demonstrate that the disruption of normal brain functions can be related to disease processes that affect specific brain areas and their connections. This relationship is an extremely important concept in the study of diseases that cause abnormal behavior.

The parietal and frontal lobes seem to be especially important in complex higher cortical functions. We know that the parietal lobes are the hub of sensory information and association. In fact, the inferior, or lower, portion of the left parietal lobe is believed to be the "association area of association areas." As noted earlier, this brain area must be working normally for a person to be able to speak and understand language and to read and write. The corresponding parietal lobe in the right cerebral hemisphere must be functioning normally for a person to be able to follow directions on a map accurately, read a clock, and construct objects (e.g., sewing a dress, building a birdhouse, or dressing oneself). In patients with Alzheimer's disease who have right parietal lobe dysfunction, it is not unusual to note dressing apraxia (i.e., inability to dress oneself because of disturbance of body schema, hemispatial attentional problems, or visuoconstructive difficulties). The parietal lobes are also involved in organizing information and communicating it to the frontal lobes.

The frontal lobes constitute much of the area in the neocortex. The functions of the frontal neocortex are complex, and they are the least well understood and least measured functions of the brain. We know that the frontal lobes are involved in the initiation and execution of motor behavior. They also are instrumental in the normal functioning of higher thought processes, such as planning, abstract reasoning, trial-and-error learning, decision-making, complex thinking, and problem-solving. In addition, the frontal lobes modulate intellectual insight, judgment, and expression of emotions. Luria compared a farmer with frontal lobe damage to a person in danger of starvation, not because the farmer would fail to eat from the cupboard as long as there was food, but because he had lost his ability to plan ahead. Since the farmer would not initiate the planting of next year's crops, eventually he would not be able to replenish the cupboard and therefore he would starve.

SUMMARY

With this chapter's description of normal brain functions, it is easier to understand why patients with Alzheimer's disease have difficulty with cognitive functions. Early in the disease a larger distribution of neurofibrillar tangles and senile plaques occurs in the hippocampus and the temporal and parietal lobes than in other brain areas. This early-stage disruption in normal brain functions results in predominant impairment in memory, language, and constructional abilities. As the disease progresses, the frontal lobes and their connections may be affected. This degeneration can result in behavioral changes, such as loss of initiative, spontaneity, and the ability to plan and organize behavior, as well as other personality changes.

Based on the information presented in this chapter, normal brain functioning can be defined as a situation in which all the different brain structures and their functions are working properly, both independently and in concert. This state is, of course, relative to the individual and his or her cultural surroundings. This definition is analogous to how we attempt to define normal intelligent behavior through the use of such methods as intelligence tests and other neuropsychological instruments. David Wechsler, who developed the intelligence tests often used in assessing patients with suspected dementia, stated that the tests do not measure intelligence per se. Instead, he noted, the tests simply correlate with other more widely accepted criteria of intelligent behavior. Thus the normal brain and its functions are defined in the context of the individual, his or her peer group, and the culture within which the individual lives. The neuropsychological assessment of brain functions used in the evaluation of dementia is discussed in Chapter 3.

BIBLIOGRAPHY

Bannister R: *Brain's clinical neurology,* New York, 1985, Oxford University Press.

Becker JT, Bajulaiye O, Smith C: Longitudinal analysis of a two-component model of the memory deficit in Alzheimer's disease, *Psychol Med* 22:437-445, 1992.

Begley S, Carey J, Sawhill R: How the brain works, *Newsweek,* Feb 7, 1983, pp 40-47.

Chusid JG: *Correlative neuroanatomy and functional neurology,* Los Altos, Calif, 1976, Lange Medical Publications.

Gazzaniga MS: *The bisected brain,* New York, 1970, Appleton-Century-Crofts.

Geschwind N: Disconnection syndromes in animals and man, *Brain* 88:237-294, 1965.

Geschwind N: Specializations of the human brain, *Sci Am* 241:180-199, 1979.

Heilman KM, Bowers D, Valenstein E: Emotional disorders associated with neurological diseases. In Heilman KM, Valenstein E, editors: *Clinical neuropsychology,* New York, 1985, Oxford University Press.

Katzman RD: Alzheimer's disease, *N Engl J Med* 314:964-973, 1986.

Kolb B, Whishaw IQ: *Fundamentals of human neuropsychology,* San Francisco, 1980, WH Freeman.

Lees AJ: Selegiline hydrochloride and cognition, *Acta Neurol Scan* 84:91-94, 1991.

Lezak MD: *Neuropsychological assessment,* New York, 1985, Oxford University Press.

Luria AR: *Higher cortical functions in man,* New York, 1966, Basic Books.

Luria AR: *The working brain,* New York, 1973, Basic Books.

McKhann G and others: Clinical diagnosis of Alzheimer's disease, *Neurology* 34:939-944, 1984.

Snyder SH: Basic science of psychopharmacology. In Kaplan HI, Sadock BJ, editors: *Comprehensive textbook of psychiatry,* vol 4, Baltimore, 1985, Williams & Wilkins.

Wechsler D: *The measurement and appraisal of adult intelligence,* Baltimore, 1958, Williams & Wilkins.

Zandi T: Changes in memory processes of dementia patients. In Zandi T, Ham RJ, editors: *New directions in understanding dementia and Alzheimer's disease,* New York, 1990, Plenum Press.

3

Neuropsychological assessment of dementia

Patrick Sloan

This chapter focuses on the neuropsychological evaluation of brain dysfunction, particularly in dementia. The clinical neuropsychological evaluation attempts to describe, by quantitative measurement and qualitative observation, the behavioral expression of brain dysfunction. This approach to assessment is historically rooted in clinical, physiological, and experimental psychology; behavioral neurology; and testing and measurement. Clinical neuropsychology has become a well-recognized subspecialty in recent years. Most practitioners are clinical psychologists with training in neuropsychology or geropsychology. The term "neuropsychologist" is reserved for board-eligible or board-certified (American Board of Professional Psychology of the American Psychological Association) practitioners with additional predoctoral and/or postdoctoral training in the neurosciences. Most clinical psychologists can perform cognitive screening tests, but the practitioner's experience with the elderly, dementia, and neuropsychology determines the degree to which specific assessments of higher cortical functions can be rendered.

The goal of the evaluation is to measure and describe what the patient can and cannot do on various tasks of motor, sensory, cognitive, and emotional functioning, which are, in turn, correlated with activities of daily living.

The typical evaluation attempts to address the following questions
1. Is there evidence of brain dysfunction?
2. If so, is the degree of impairment mild, moderate, or severe?
3. Is there a particular pattern of impairment?

4. Are the degree and the pattern consistent with a specific diagnosis (e.g., Alzheimer's disease or another type of dementia)?

The answers to these questions address issues regarding the course, prognosis, and management/treatment of the patient and his or her caretakers.

Neuropsychologists use a variety of tests or a battery of tests and tasks to address these questions. The advantage of standardized tests is that they typically meet scientific standards of reliability and validity, and therefore they can be replicated and interpreted among various practitioners. The greatest statistical strength of most of the tests is their ability to distinguish between groups of patients with and without brain impairment, including various types and degrees of brain dysfunction. Patients are also tested thoroughly in motor, sensory, cognitive, and emotional functioning; this battery of tests assesses a variety of brain functions in depth. This approach provides systematized observations of subtle cognitive and behavioral changes that may not be readily identifiable or quantifiable through a typical bedside neurological or psychiatric examination, for example, those of the more complex higher cortical functions. Finally, because the tests record subtle or specific changes in mentation, they are well suited for measuring such changes over time, an ideal approach in the study and management of progressive illnesses such as dementia.

CLINICAL EVALUATION PROCEDURES

In evaluation, an attempt is made with neuropsychological measures to "map" the brain in terms of its various integrated functional systems. A typical test battery comprises a number of tests that may require a minimum of 3 hours total. Testing time can be longer in persons who are less severely impaired. An evaluation costs approximately the equivalent of a computed tomographic (CT) scan or a magnetic resonance imaging (MRI) head scan. Except for patients who are in the very early stages of disease, most patients suspected of having dementia are not able to undergo several consecutive hours of testing because of cognitive impairment and fatigue. In my experience it is typical that patients, because of health, demographic, and cost factors, may be available for only one testing session limited to 3 hours or less. Thus the neuropsychologist must make good use of a selected number of measures that have been shown empirically to reveal dementia and to distinguish it from other causes of brain dysfunction.

The typical evaluation incorporates information available from the medical, neurological, and social history combined with the standard clinical psychological procedures. These procedures include interviews with the patient, family, and friends or associates; behavioral observations; and mental status examination. Specific psychometric procedures are added to these routine procedures. The specific procedures may include an individually administered intelligence test and other standardized tests. The latter include tests of attention, concentration, verbal and nonverbal memory, language, motor and somatosensory functions, and specific higher order cognitive functions, such as complex reasoning, learning, and problem-solving skills.

Studies have shown that there are a number of brief cognitive screening instruments available, such as the Modified Blessed Dementia Scale and the Mini Mental State Examination (MMSE), which are reliable in differentiating persons with and without dementia. The Modified Blessed Dementia Scale, for example, has been correlated with neuropathological findings indicative of Alzheimer's disease. Another brief checklist, the Hachinski Ischemic Score, has been shown to help differentiate Alzheimer's disease from multiinfarct dementia in patients with known histological diagnoses. The use of these brief scales is an example of the basic neuropsychological approach of quantitatively measuring cognitive impairment and empirically correlating such impairment with different types of dementia.

The MMSE assesses orientation, attention, concentration, memory, and basic dominant and nondominant hemisphere functions but not nearly to the extent or depth of formal neuropsychological assessment. In 1987 Tierney and associates found that four different brief cognitive tests differentiated between patients with Alzheimer's disease and normal elderly subjects but not among the different types of dementias. They recommended that additional cognitive testing be done for such discriminations. Cognitive screening tests can provide helpful measures of rate of deterioration in patients with Alzheimer's disease. Some experts have argued for inclusion of clinical ratings measures and tests of specific cognitive capacities, particularly when drugs are being evaluated for their efficacy in the treatment of Alzheimer's disease because of possible fluctuation in performance on any given test at a particular time. The MMSE has been used successfully in differentiating dementia from depression, and the Mattis Dementia Rating Scale has been validated in staging of dementia and has been correlated with clinical ratings of dementia on the Instrumental Activities of Daily Living Scale for use in making level-of-care decisions and research investigations of the natural course of dementia illnesses.

Neuropsychologists go beyond these basic screening measures in order to evaluate cognitive and emotional functioning more systematically and in depth. Most neuropsychologists use a group of tests designed to measure brain impairment. The particular tests, or battery of tests, usually reflect the individual neuropsychologist's training and experience, but typically they include tests that have demonstrated empirical utility. Some of the best-known tests constitute or are selected from neuropsychological test batteries constructed by and named for reputable neuropsychologists and their colleagues, such as Ward Halstead, Ralph Reitan, Arthur Benton, A.R. Luria, and Luria-Nebraska. Most practitioners have their own favorite tests and batteries, but they should be able to defend on empirical and ethical grounds the use of their instruments. The most well known standardized neuropsychological test batteries are the Halstead-Reitan, Luria's tests, and Benton's battery. Each of these tests has its strengths and weaknesses; however, their authors prefer that they be given in entirety, which often requires multiple hours and testing sessions. Yet these tests and their derivatives, such as the Luria-Nebraska battery, are usually too lengthy for the typical dementia patient unless the disease is in its very early stages. Thus practitioners use parts of these batteries or other selected instruments.

The case studies presented later in this chapter, which are taken from my experience, illustrate specific issues in neuropsychological assessment of dementia. In addition, the unique utility of neuropsychological testing was illustrated in a recent important study of the genetic markers for Alzheimer's disease. This study suggested that a certain protein in the spinal fluid of patients with familial Alzheimer's disease is associated with the disease process that causes neuritic plaques in the central nervous system. One of the symptom-free, gene-carrying family members in the study was detected as having impairment in visual and verbal recent memory, information processing, and conceptual reasoning that was revealed only by neuropsychological testing.

DIFFERENCES BETWEEN DEMENTIA AND NORMAL AGING

In normal aging a certain amount of deterioration in cognitive abilities and psychomotor speed is expected. Changes in functions such as perceptual abilities, attention, information-processing speed, and memory have been described in detail. Of particular note are diminution of, or lapses in, memory, sometimes called benign forgetfulness of senescence, and progressive slowing of reaction times. In dementia, however, these changes are not merely a function of accelerated normal aging; they represent pathological processes in the brain and their consequences. Metaanalyses of reaction times of patients with Alzheimer's disease and normal elderly controls have shown that Alzheimer's disease produces a generalized slowing of cognitive processing that increases with task complexity uniformly for cognitive operations, regardless of the task. The degree of background slowing in the electroencephalograms (EEGs) of patients with Alzheimer's disease also correlates with the degree of cognitive impairment.

Studies have attempted to document the changes in neuropsychological functioning associated with the disease processes in various brain areas and correlate them in meaningful ways with Alzheimer's disease or other types of dementia. Neuropsychological test results are correlated with neurofibrillar counts in the nucleus basalis of Meynert, and counts in that area are closely related to disease severity and duration and neurofibrillar counts in other regions. These test results are also useful in distinguishing Alzheimer-type dementia from vascular forms of dementia. Patients with Alzheimer's disease score lower on various aspects of verbal memory and visuospatial functions.

Great attention has been paid to memory and language impairment in dementia because these changes are commonly the earliest and most prominent clinical symptoms of the disease, particularly in Alzheimer's disease. Most current theorists and researchers describe memory processes along a continuum that includes three parts—acquisition, retention, and retrieval. Neuropsychologists attempt to measure functions related to these processes. Memory loss in patients with Alzheimer's disease is multifactorial, and changing performance in memory patterns over time indicates that multiple independent systems are deteriorating rather than one specific cortical lesion being responsible for the memory loss. Deficits in all three areas (acquisition, retention, and retrieval) have been described in patients with Alzheimer's disease. Language impairment, particularly anomia, has been suggested as a predictor of fast decline in Alzheimer's disease.

Testing with a clock-drawing task has shown that patients with Alzheimer's disease make more conceptual errors whereas patients with Huntington's disease make more motor errors. The motor errors correspond to the destruction of the subcortical caudate nucleus in Huntington's disease, as opposed to the cortical impairment in Alzheimer's disease. Impaired insight in patients with Alzheimer's disease is best predicted by neuropsychological measures of continuous performance and visual reproduction, reflecting prefrontal dysfunction and anosognosia of right hemisphere dysfunction, respectively. The use of neuropsychological measures suggests a functional-anatomical correlate for insight.

In 1983 Fuld stated that the most common diagnostic differentiation posed to neuropsychologists is evaluating for Alzheimer's disease versus multiinfarct dementia. Fuld's work has been seminal for three reasons. First, Fuld and her colleagues have successfully used neuropsychological tests to discriminate between groups of patients with dementia and normal elderly persons. Second, they have found different patterns of performance on these tests among different subtypes of dementia. Third, they have correlated these patterns with neuropathological findings and current theoretical understanding of dementia processes.

The third edition of the *Diagnostic and Statistical Manual of the American Psychiatric Association–Revised* (DSM-III-R) lists the diagnostic criteria for dementia as demonstrable evidence of impairment in short- and long-term memory and impairment in at least one other area of higher cortical functioning. The latter includes impairment in abstract thinking or judgment and other disturbances such as aphasia (disorder of language), apraxia (inability to carry out motor activities despite intact comprehension and motor function), agnosia (failure to recognize or identify objects despite intact sensory function), constructional difficulty (e.g., inability to copy designs), and personality change. To constitute a diagnosis of dementia, these impairments must interfere significantly with work, social, or interpersonal relationships.

CLINICAL DIFFERENTIATION OF ALZHEIMER'S DISEASE

Neuropsychological tests have been useful in showing that patients with Alzheimer's disease perform more poorly on standardized tests than do patients with multiinfarct dementia, who, in turn, perform more poorly than do normals. In addition to having a greater degree of general cognitive impairment, patients with Alzheimer's disease differ from patients with multiinfarct dementia on these tests in other characteristic ways. For example, although individual patients with Alzheimer's disease may perform somewhat differently from one another on the tests, their relative strengths and weaknesses typically remain consistent from initial diagnosis through the end stages of the disease. Therefore a patient with Alzheimer's disease who has predominant impairment in nonverbal memory and visuoconstructive ability but relatively good verbal skills will show these relative strengths and weaknesses over the course of the illness, regardless of how severe the impairment becomes. Patients with multiinfarct dementia, on the other hand, will show more variation in test patterns from patient to patient and within the same patient over a period of time than do patients with Alzheimer's disease. This difference is presumably a result of the multifocal nature and "stuttering" course of multiinfarct dementia.

In a series of studies published in 1983, Fuld used some subtests of the Wechsler Adult Intelligence Scale (WAIS) to identify characteristic patterns of performance among various groups of persons with and without dementia. Based on previous studies showing a cholinergic deficiency in patients with Alzheimer's disease, Fuld found that a particular pattern of performance revealed in a previous study could be used to identify two consecutive groups of Alzheimer's disease patients in another study. She derived this characteristic test pattern from the one found in a group of normal young adults with a temporary cholinergic deficiency induced by the drug scopolamine. The "Fuld profile" of the WAIS was highly specific for Alzheimer's disease among 138 consecutive referrals for dementia, producing only two false positives (two patients selected to have Alzheimer's disease who did not). Furthermore, although the profile resembles that expected in normal aging, the actual profile was found in less than 1% of 390 normal elderly people without dementia who were 75 to 85 years of age. Thus the profile is reasonably sensitive because it allows identification of about 50% of all testable patients with Alzheimer's disease but is highly specific for the disease. The utility of the psychometric approach is further enhanced by the fact that the WAIS is such a commonly used and well-known IQ test, it is both content- and age-appropriate for elderly persons, and it is a thorough yet nonthreatening test for most patients. The first case study presented (see box, p. 51) illustrates the Fuld profile. The other case studies describe some of the most common diagnostic issues and clinical considerations encountered in the neuropsychological assessment of dementia.

Text continued on p. 59

SENILE DEMENTIA OF ALZHEIMER TYPE

A 69-year-old, right-handed, retired professional man with an 18-month history of cognitive decline was referred as an outpatient for neuropsychological evaluation of dementia after an extensive medical evaluation proved unremarkable. There was no history or symptoms of cerebrovascular disease. Although the man's attention and concentration were adequate, he showed prominent memory loss for both recent and well-learned (i.e., remote) information. His WAIS scores revealed global intellectual decline (verbal IQ, 94; performance IQ, 82; full scale IQ, 88), given his estimated premorbid level of above-average to superior intellect (average IQ, 90 to 110). Age-corrected scores on each of the selected WAIS subtests were consistent with the Fuld profile:

A = Vocabulary + Information ÷ 2
B = Digit Span + Similarities ÷ 2
C = Digit Symbol + Block Design ÷ 2
D = Object Assembly
A = Vocabulary + Information ÷ 2
D = Object Assembly
Fuld profile = A > B > C ≤ D; A > D

Interpretively, these scores tell us that this man's vocabulary and general fund of information were relatively well preserved, although the scores were still lower than expected for his educational and vocational experience. This situation is understandable because these well-learned areas of knowledge are retained well and are the last to deteriorate in either normal aging or dementia illness. The man's ability to recite strings of digits forward and backward (Digit Span) and his analysis of verbal similarities (e.g., How are an orange and a banana alike?) showed more impairment than did his scores on the Vocabulary and Information subtests. The Digit Span and Similarities subtests reflect auditory processing/immediate memory and abstract reasoning, respectively. These more complex cognitive functions are more likely to deteriorate earlier in Alzheimer's disease. Similarly, the man's performance on timed tasks requiring visuospatial organization and visuomotor coordination and speed, the Digit Symbol substitution task and the visuoconstructive Block Design subtest, showed even more impairment. Finally, his ability to construct puzzles of familiar objects (i.e., Object Assembly) demonstrated less impairment than the last two pairs of subtests but more impairment than the first pair, a finding that is consistent with empirical data from Fuld's studies of Alzheimer's patients. With the respective pairs of tests represented by a letter, this man's age-corrected scores for the seven WAIS subtests corresponded to Fuld's profile (i.e., A > B> C< D; A > D), which is suggestive of Alzheimer's disease.

This man also made one or more "intrusive" persevering errors, which have been found frequently among patients with dementia and are suspected to be characteristic of Alzheimer's disease. These are errors in which the patient gives an inappropriate response to a question by carrying forward (i.e., intruding) a response to a previous question despite the occurrence of other responses in between. For example, having correctly named the current president earlier in the test, the man was asked,

Continued.

Senile Dementia of Alzheimer Type—cont'd

after several intervening questions, the name of a character in a brief story that had been read to him. He answered again with the name of the president, which was grossly incorrect for the question asked.

The remainder of the neuropsychological tests revealed no particular pattern of sensorimotor or cognitive asymmetries suggestive of localized or lateralized brain dysfunction; that is, there were no findings suggestive of focal brain disease such as those found in patients with a brain tumor or stroke. Memory and other global intellectual impairments were prominent, and there were no significant motor findings suggestive of "subcortical" disease. The man's wife described personality changes of decreased spontaneity and initiative. The history and neuropsychological findings in this case were consistent with those of patients with Alzheimer's disease, which is the most definitive statement that can be made on the basis of the clinical neuropsychological evaluation since Alzheimer's disease can be confirmed neuropathologically only at autopsy.

MULTIINFARCT DEMENTIA

A 53-year-old, right-handed, disabled laborer with an eighth grade education was referred for neuropsychological evaluation of dementia on admission to an inpatient psychiatry service. The patient was brought to the hospital by police, who reported that he was confused and had been rummaging through a large trash dumpster. His history included treatment for chronic hypertension and several episodes of suspected transient ischemic attacks. On testing several days after admission, the patient's orientation, attention, concentration, and verbal memory (immediate, recent, and remote) were all commensurate with his education, despite his recent disorientation and confusion. Nonverbal recall for figures and visuoconstructive drawings was extremely impaired. The WAIS profile did not correspond to Fuld's profile for Alzheimer's disease. Instead it suggested mild global decline and specific impairment in functions served by the right cerebral hemisphere. Asymmetries were found on the sensorimotor examination, such as decreased tapping speed of the index finger on the left hand and impaired ability to recognize numbers written on the left fingertips (i.e., agraphesthesia). The Hachinski Ischemic Score was elevated and was positive for several markers suggestive of cerebrovascular disease (e.g., abrupt onset, history of hypertension, stuttering course, and focal neurological symptoms). The clinical neuropsychological evaluation was strongly suggestive of right cerebral hemisphere dysfunction and multiinfarct dementia, and a thorough neurological evaluation for suspected stroke was recommended. Concurrent neurological examination, EEG, CT scan, and noninvasive blood flow studies suggested an infarct in the distribution of the right middle cerebral artery and bilateral carotid artery disease. Treatment was handled accordingly, and the patient continued to improve to reach a plateau in cognitive functions.

Multiinfarct Dementia—cont'd

A pattern of multiple infarcts, either clearly identifiable or subtle, is typical of multiinfarct dementia. These appear in a patchy distribution of deficits on the neuropsychological examination and tend to plateau after each event, with each episode causing more dysfunction than the previous one. Typically, however, the course is one of a less severely progressive and rapid decline than in the typical patient with Alzheimer's disease, unless a large stroke occurs in the process. Yet, even when a large stroke occurs, unaffected areas of the brain often remain relatively functional. This picture is somewhat contrary to the global diminution in cortical function seen in Alzheimer's disease, particularly in its middle to late stages. In mixed cases, having evidence of both Alzheimer's disease and multiinfarct dementia, this distinction is more difficult to determine.

SUBCORTICAL DEMENTIA

After 48 hours of confusion and hallucinations possibly related to her medication (levodopa for Parkinson's disease), a 73-year-old, right-handed woman was referred for evaluation of dementia as a medical inpatient. She was alert, oriented, and accurately described her previous confusion, which was clearing. The woman's mental status examination revealed good attention, concentration, and recent recall for her age and situation. Mood and personality were bright and well preserved despite marked difficulty with initiating motor and cognitive activity. Her face was masked, she was motorically rigid, and she could write only with great difficulty because of the rigidity. Because the patient was bedfast, extensive testing was impossible. Bedside examination, however, revealed no significant impairments of language, motor praxis (the learned aspects of movement), calculation, or visuospatial perception, although the patient showed some mild impairment in complex cognitive functions and in drawing, writing, and movement. The latter included rigidity and micrography (small handwriting), typical of Parkinson's disease.

Although dementia could not be ruled out by this evaluation, the subcortical motor impairment was far more prominent than any cortical cognitive manifestations, and the patient did not appear to have Alzheimer's disease. These findings increased the likelihood that her recent delirium was related to the suspected medication problem, which could be explored further by her neurologist without undue concern about an interfering cortical dementia. The patient was referred for subsequent reevaluation as an outpatient but could not avail herself of such testing because of her progressive Parkinson's disease.

• • •

A 67-year-old, right-handed man with a professional degree was referred as a medical inpatient for evaluation of dementia because he answered most of the resident physician's questions with "I can't remember." Formal testing immediately

Continued.

Subcortical Dementia—cont'd

revealed good attention, concentration, and apparent cognitive awareness. When asked to recite a brief story that had been read to him, however, he said, "I can't remember." When given a clue that the story was about a scrubwoman (the Anna Thompson story from the Wechsler Memory Scale), he immediately recited most of the details of the story in chronological sequence. Because the patient was clearly cooperative and did not appear significantly depressed, his difficulty in memory was revealed as *initiating* recall, or retrieval, not one of acquisition or retention of information. This phenomenon has been called "forgetting to remember" and is thought to be related to neurochemical dysfunction and structural impairments in subcortical areas. The remainder of the tests, including the WAIS, revealed relatively mild diminution of complex higher cortical functions. However, as with the woman in the preceding case study, severe impairments in motor function were found. These included significant slowing, stooped posture, rigidity, and oculomotor changes. The difficulties with eye movements were revealed by the neurologist to be typical of a subcortical disease that affects gray matter structures, progressive supranuclear palsy. As a result of the neuropsychological evaluation, it was recommended that the patient be given verbal cues, or "boosts," to help him initiate action, both motor and cognitive, which helped significantly in his communication and self-esteem. As an equally important measure, it was encouraged that the patient be socially stimulated and that he not be assumed to be more cortically impaired than he actually was, an all too common response to patients who have dementia and sometimes to elderly persons without dementia.

Difficulty with initiating and sustaining language, memory and other cognitive activity, and motor activity is typical of subcortical diseases. Although diseases such as progressive supranuclear palsy, Parkinson's disease, and Huntington's disease usually include dementia as a complication, the cortical involvement commonly occurs later in the disease process and is overshadowed by various motor symptoms earlier. Since the clinical neuropsychological evaluation includes both motor and cognitive tasks, relative quantification is useful in plotting the course of such diseases, response to medication, and the degree of motor versus cognitive impairment at various stages. Although there has been some controversy about the clinical distinction between cortical and "subcortical" dementias, neuropsychological test batteries carefully designed to quantify clinical differences have produced results that do differentiate these dementia syndromes.

AIDS DEMENTIA COMPLEX

A 58-year-old, right-handed clerk was referred as a medical inpatient for neuropsychological evaluation with a diagnosis of acquired immunodeficiency syndrome (AIDS). The intern, who had treated many AIDS patients, requested formal evaluation of cortical functions for what was described as "hazy" mentation. A common disorder that is unique to patients with AIDS and is characterized by progressive dementia with accompanying motor and behavioral problems is called the AIDS dementia complex. Consistent with this condition, the patient's testing revealed mild to moderate global cognitive impairment. As with many patients who have AIDS, this man was mildly ataxic (difficulty walking and with fine motor execution), dysarthric (slurred speech), and "foggy" in attention, concentration, and mentation, but he had no outstanding or focal cognitive dysfunctions.

Although the AIDS dementia complex usually develops after other complications of AIDS, in some patients progressive dementia with motor and behavioral disturbances has been described as one of the first manifestations of the disease. As in many patients with AIDS who show only mild physical symptoms early in the illness, the dementia in this man was already apparent. Although this patient was somewhat reactively depressed, as expected, depression could not account for the degree of cognitive impairment found. The patient had characteristic difficulty with concentration and recent memory, mental slowing, and an inability to perform complex activities of daily living such as finding his way around the hospital. Although the AIDS virus is known to attack the cerebral cortex directly, the effects of the disease are typically most apparent in the white matter and the subcortical gray matter. Therefore motor problems—particularly ataxia, leg weakness, and tremor—are often presumed to be an early sign in the complex, as seen in this patient. Clinically, the early cognitive and behavioral manifestations are more typical of the subtler subcortical dementias than of the cortical dementias. However, in its later stages the AIDS dementia complex can be nonsubtle in its destruction of the brain. This complex, with its cognitive, motor, and behavioral problems, can complicate severe cases of AIDS and appear either in isolation or as part of the AIDS-related complex with a variety of central nervous system complications. The course can be a rapidly deteriorating one characterized by severe dementia with mutism that occurs within a few weeks or months, or it can be a milder, less precipitous one that lasts many months or longer than a year.

This case illustrates the importance of the evaluation of emotional functioning in the clinical neuropsychological examination. Although this man was initially very stoical and denied his illness, as rapport was established during interviewing and personality testing, his emotional lability became more apparent and his concerns about his illness, his family, and himself were expressed. Although the testing established a good cognitive baseline against which future data could be compared, the evaluation also led to psychotherapeutic consultation with the patient, family, and staff. As the patient's mentation deteriorated, assessment of emotional issues took prominence over cognitive measurement in assisting both patient and family.

ALCOHOL AMNESTIC DISORDER AND ASSOCIATED DEMENTIA

A 63-year-old, right-handed machinist was referred for neuropsychological evaluation as an inpatient on the intermediate medicine service. He was still unable to walk, presumably because of peripheral neuropathy and ataxia following a brief stay on an acute care medical ward for treatment of delirium. The medical evaluation was unremarkable, and alcoholism and inadequate nutritional intake were denied by the patient. Careful review of the patient's past medical record and interviews with relatives, however, revealed a strong likelihood of chronic and recent alcohol abuse and inadequate nutrition. Testing on consecutive days showed intermittent disorientation for time and place and deficits in concentration despite overall cognitive lucidity, facile conversational speech, and gregarious, shallow affect. No significant asymmetries were noted on sensorimotor examination, and complex higher cognitive functions showed only mild impairment, most apparent in visuoperceptual and visuomotor skills. Memory was grossly impaired, with recent memory more affected than remote, and the patient frequently confabulated (filled in) missing details in memory. Except for poor memory, the test data suggested only mild global impairment. However, this patient frequently misidentified the examiner as being one of several familiar acquaintances and confabulated totally erroneous explanations of such matters as previous meetings or locations. For example, he misconstrued one meeting that took place on the acute care medical ward as having occurred at a hospital in a distant state several weeks before the meeting actually occurred. He was inappropriately euphoric and nonchalant regarding his inaccuracies of memory, offering weak rationalizations for them. These behaviors were in striking contrast to his generally appropriate behavior on the ward and his overall mildly impaired test performance.

All these characteristics are fairly typical of the patient with alcohol amnestic disorder, or Korsakoff's syndrome. As a unique entity, this disorder is relatively rare among chronic alcoholics. However, the clinical distinctions among chronic substance abusers with varying degrees of dementia are not usually clear-cut because difficulties in memory are frequently the most prominent dysfunction relative to other higher cortical functions. Korsakoff's syndrome is thought to be related to the deleterious effects of thiamine deficiency (and probably the alcohol itself) on deep-brain structures, whereas the milder forms of global dementia are associated with overall cortical deterioration. Yet, on neuropsychological testing, it is most common to find at least mild impairment in cognitive functions among chronic substance abusers, particularly in memory, visuoconstructive skills, and visuomotor speed. It is not uncommon to see the clinical picture predominated by amnestic disorder features, whether or not full-blown Korsakoff's syndrome is present. Similarly, in those patients who meet the diagnostic criteria for alcohol amnestic disorder, some degree of mild dementia is almost always present, as in the case described here. Research has shown that deficits in recent and remote memory, in the absence of other higher cortical dysfunction, are the hallmarks of alcohol-related dementias. These memory deficits have specific characteristics that can be differentiated from those seen in Alzheimer's disease through neuropsychological testing. Dementia associated with alcoholism is diagnosed when impairment involves other cognitive functions besides memory and is sufficient to interfere with social or occupational functioning.

DEPRESSION AND OTHER PSEUDODEMENTIAS

A 66-year-old, right-handed, retired administrative assistant was referred as a psychiatric inpatient for treatment of depression. He had a family history of affective disorder and had become clinically depressed after his recent retirement and the death of his wife. On interview, he was psychomotorically slowed, was generally oriented (with effortful questioning), and appeared sad and despondent. His response to formal testing was generally cooperative but slowed. He frequently stated "I don't know" to questions, and he could not be motivated to respond. No sensorimotor asymmetries were noted, and constructional drawings were adequate though sparse. Attention and concentration were severely impaired. Verbal recall was adequate for recent news events, although the patient did poorly on formal memory tests. Abstract reasoning and topographical direction-finding were intact. The history, clinical behavior, and cognitive test data strongly suggested depression rather than dementia, although the latter could not be ruled out. Personality testing suggested depression, not confusion. Vigorous treatment of depression was recommended.

On reevaluation a few weeks later, the patient's cognitive performance, psychomotor speed, and mood had improved measurably. A key diagnostic determinant in this man's history was that his cognitive impairment occurred abruptly after his losses (i.e., work and spouse). If his cognitive impairment had occurred first and in an insidious manner, since depression occurs frequently after a person recognizes progressive cognitive impairment, dementia and secondary, or reactive, depression would have been suspected more strongly.

Since virtually any medical illness can masquerade as dementia, a thorough history and a complete medical evaluation are precursors to good diagnosis and treatment; the latter can be a means of identifying many treatable causes of dementia (i.e., pseudodementia). Neuropsychological testing is useful because it can help distinguish between cognitive impairment and emotional paralysis, as in depression, and can document quantitatively recovering or diminishing cognitive functioning over time. Memory complaints, for example, are very common among depressed elderly adults, and neuropsychological testing has been demonstrated to differentiate among patients with Alzheimer's disease, depression, and normal control subjects on such factors as the rate of forgetting. Contrary to anecdotal lore suggesting that patients with dementia do not appear depressed, patients in the early stages of the condition are frequently depressed to at least a mild degree, as shown by neuropsychological testing. In addition, many patients in chronic medical or psychiatric populations have varying degrees of dementia, particularly milder forms, that accompany their chronic medical or psychiatric problems. The medical group includes, but is not limited to, patients with cancer and those with vascular, lung, systemic, or neurological disease. The psychiatric group may include patients with accompanying mild dementia, but it is particularly composed of patients with chronic schizophrenia, an affective disorder, or a substance abuse disorder.

FOCAL LESIONS POSING AS DEMENTIA:
ANGULAR GYRUS SYNDROME

A 52-year-old, right-handed, disabled auto mechanic with a high school education was referred as a medical outpatient because of memory problems and unpredictable behavior over the past 2 years. No definitive focal event was identified for this man, who had a history of hypertension and occasional dizzy spells. However, on close questioning, his wife recalled that he had one spell of dizziness after which his behavior seemed different. A long premorbid history of intermittent alcohol abuse and antisocial behavior, such as overspending and debauchery, complicated the history of behavioral change. There was no clear history of affective disorder. The man had been examined by physicians but had not had a thorough evaluation for dementia.

The patient was gregarious yet evasive on interview, but his conversational speech suggested problems with language functions, with comprehension being more affected than expression (fluency). For example, he engaged in overlearned, repetitive phrases such as, "You know what I mean," "That's the way it goes," and otherwise had rather "empty," disjointed speech that approximated accuracy of phrasing (i.e., paraphasia). The patient had difficulty comprehending simple and complex commands and sometimes responded inappropriately. Reading, writing, calculation, and finger recognition were all impaired. Screening with the WAIS quickly revealed fairly good, though impaired, visuospatial and visuoconstructive skills on the Block Design subtest but severely impaired language skills on the Vocabulary subtest. Further testing of language and other cognitive functions supported the hypothesis of a posterior left cerebral hemisphere focal lesion, and a full medical workup with a CT head scan was recommended to the referring resident physician. As suspected, the CT scan revealed a lesion in the superior temporal gyrus of the left hemisphere, which was subsequently determined to be an old infarction (stroke) in Wernicke's area, probably involving connecting pathways to the angular gyrus area, that resulted in the syndrome of receptive/comprehension aphasia. Since this man's condition had apparently not progressed significantly over the past 24 months, his condition was strongly suspected to be a case of a focal lesion appearing as Alzheimer's disease.

Approximately one half of patients with multiinfarct dementia are believed to have angular gyrus syndrome, which is a symptom complex resulting from lesions to the posterior left hemisphere. These symptoms, as in the case described here, include fluent aphasia and difficulty in reading, writing, calculating, recognizing fingers, and constructing. Although memory for verbal information is impaired, these patients typically can engage in complex social activities and continue to know their way around. This situation was true in the case of this patient, who continued to frustrate his wife by demonstrating goal-directed yet sociopathic behavior.

MALINGERING AND PSYCHOLOGICAL DYSFUNCTION

Occasionally, patients feign or exaggerate cognitive problems, particularly when there is the possibility of secondary gains, such as decrease in personal responsibilities, escape from family conflict, or compensation for illness or incapacity. The neuropsychological evaluation is valuable because the standardized tests involved are good tools for detecting atypical patterns of performance, and malingering usually produces distinctly atypical patterns. For example, most patients are naive about what variables constitute either a normal performance or an abnormal one, particularly in terms of what behavior and responses are typical of patients with Alzheimer's disease or those with multiinfarct dementia, the most common types of dementia. The Fuld profile on the WAIS is one example of empirical data of which the typical patient would be unaware and unable to replicate. This principle of interpretation is also true of both the qualitative and the quantitative aspects of the evaluation; that is, malingering behavior is often quite unusual in one or more ways.

My experience has shown that one is more likely to encounter patients who are exaggerating or distorting real problems or deficits rather than faking illness altogether. The exaggeration is usually fairly obvious: the patient tends to endorse any and all symptoms inquired about, and the symptom patterns and presentations do not follow known neuroanatomical pathways or functions. Deficits that are not consistent with neuroanatomical pathways and that are not reproducible on repeated trials are the hallmarks of malingering. In addition, overly dramatic behavior is often evident, and test performance is disparately impaired compared with clinical behavior. For example, the patient may discuss his medical history in detail; however, on subsequent testing he may be unable to cite personal identity, perform the simplest tasks, or recall any details from a brief story, or he may feign an impairment that would be seen in only the most severe dementia. Other nonverbal indications of manipulation, evasion, or deception, such as inconsistencies in information or behavior, are usually apparent.

Distinguishing malingering or obvious psychological dysfunction (e.g., conversion hysteria) from true brain dysfunction is usually less difficult than distinguishing subtle psychological factors affecting behavior (e.g., very mild depression, anxiety, or somatization disorders) that may complicate and "overlie" real neurological dysfunction. Because these and other psychological symptoms, such as irritability, fatigue, and emotional lability, are characteristic of both dementia and psychological disorders and may occur in combination, the subtle distinctions are difficult. Therefore a standardized group of tests in the hands of an experienced neuropsychologist is of unique utility. As the growing body of literature in clinical neuropsychology expands and the number of practicing neuropsychologists increases, availability of these evaluations and use of these services will likely be more prevalent.

EMOTIONAL FACTORS

As shown by the case studies presented here, in the typical neuropsychological evaluation of dementia, much of the focus is on assessment of cognitive factors. Yet the importance of evaluating emotional variables should not be underestimated. Not only is such evaluation important when emotional variables are involved in the primary differential diagnosis, but the patient's and the family's or caretaker's reaction to the condition in question is always of critical importance, particularly in regard to treating and coping with the condition. It is typical that the neuropsychologist and other members of the interdisciplinary team will eventually devote as much time, or more time, to working with the family or caregiver of the affected patient as with the patient.

Assessment of emotional factors can take two forms of evaluation. One is of the patient; the other is of the family system. In the former, the patient's objective mental status includes evaluation of emotionality. This evaluation may include formal testing of emotional variables and observations of emotionality during interviewing and cognitive testing. In the early stages of dementia, the patient may be able to complete self-report inventories of feeling/personality, such as the Minnesota Multiphasic Personality Inventory (MMPI). More typically, the patient is too impaired to complete long questionnaires. Thus projective tests, such as the Rorschach test, may be useful. Although the Rorschach is not a good test of brain dysfunction per se, it can be helpful in eliciting and documenting empirically how a person with dementia is perceiving his environment. For example, the Rorschach test helps to determine whether or not the person is experiencing good contact with reality, how strongly he is affected by emotionality, and how effectively he is coping with it. Other projective tests may be used in a similar way, particularly when the variables in question are not sufficiently revealed by the other aspects of the evaluation. Such instruments may also help clarify the patient's subjective experience of emotionality in relation to his own personality or coping style, which can help to individualize the treatment plan, particularly regarding personal and family psychotherapeutic interventions.

For example, the evaluation of a 57-year-old man with mild multiinfarct dementia and a right cerebral hemisphere stroke revealed that he was having significant difficulty in maintaining sustained attention and emotional control. The man quickly changed topics of conversation, was impatient, and laughed or cried disinhibitedly at the slightest stimulation. His emotionality during the cognitive testing provided ample data for later education of him and his wife in helping them to cope with his problems. Personality testing with the patient and joint interviews with him and his wife helped to elucidate emotional strengths and weaknesses and communication patterns. For instance, personality testing revealed this patient's paternalistic relationship with his wife, his compulsive need to organize his environment, and the painful emotion he felt by being emotionally out of control. This information was most helpful in constructing his individual treatment plan and the psychotherapeutic strategies for the couple.

SUMMARY

The neuropsychological evaluation of dementia is typically a comprehensive endeavor involving various methods, instrumentation, and focuses. The diagnostic aspects of the evaluation center on cognitive factors, because of their historical and natural role, whereas the treatment aspects involve greater emphasis on emotional, interpersonal, and family factors. The evaluation requires a combination of clinical skill, precise measurement, and psychotherapeutic acumen. Any given referral question may require one or more aspects of the evaluation to be emphasized. The foregoing description and case studies have highlighted both the traditional and the developing issues to be addressed in the typical neuropsychological evaluation of dementia.

REFERENCES

American Psychiatric Association: *Diagnostic and statistical manual of mental disorders (Third edition, revised)*, Washington, DC: 1987, The Association.

Bayles KA, Kaszniak AW: *Communication and cognition in normal aging and dementia*, Boston, 1987, Little, Brown.

Bayles KA, Trosset MW: Confrontation naming in Alzheimer's patients: relation to disease severity, *Psychol Aging* 7:197-203, 1992.

Becker JT, Bajulaiye O, Smith C: Longitudinal analysis of a two-component model of the memory deficit in Alzheimer's disease, *Psychol Med* 22:437-445, 1992.

Benson DF, Cummings JL, Tsai SY: Angular gyrus syndrome simulating Alzheimer's disease, *Arch Neurol* 39:616-620, 1982.

Benton AL and others: *Contributions to neuropsychological assessment*, New York, 1983, Oxford University Press.

Blennow K, Wallin A: Clinical heterogeneity of probable Alzheimer's disease, *J Geriatr Psychiatry Neurol* 5:106-113, 1992.

Blessed G, Tomlinson BE, Roth M: The association between quantitative measures of dementia and of change in the cerebral grey matter of elderly subjects, *Br J Psychiatry* 114:787-781, 1968.

Boller F and others: Predictors of decline in Alzheimer's disease, *Cortex* 27:9-17, 1991.

Brid M, Luszcz M: Encoding of specificity, depth of processing, and cued recall in Alzheimer's disease, *J Clin Exper Neuropsychol* 13:508-520.

Claman DL, Radebaugh TZ: Neuropsychological assessment in clinical trials of Alzheimer disease, *Alzheimer Dis Assoc Disord* 5 (suppl 1):S49-S56, 1991.

Farlow M, and others: Low cerebrospinal fluid concentrations of soluble amyloid β-protein precursor in hereditary Alzheimer's disease, *Lancet* 340:453-454, 1992.

Fillenbaum GG and others: Comparison of two screening tests in Alzheimer's disease, *Arch Neurol* 44:924-927, 1987.

Fisk AA and others: Alzheimer's disease: a five-article symposium, *Postgrad Med* 73:204-256, 1983.

Fuld PA: Psychometric differentiation of the dementias: an overview. In Reisberg B, editor: *Alzheimer's disease*, New York, 1983, Macmillan.

Fuld PA and others: Intrusions as a sign of Alzheimer's dementia: chemical and pathological verification, *Ann Neurol* 11:155-159, 1982.

Gainotti G and others: Neuropsychological markers of dementia on visual-spatial tasks: a comparison between Alzheimer's type and vascular forms of dementia, *J Clin Exper Neuropsychol* 14:239-252, 1992.

Galasko D, Corey-Bloom J, Thal LJ: Monitoring progression in Alzheimer's disease, *J Am Geriatr Soc* 39:932-941, 1991.

Golden CJ: A standardized version of Luria's neuropsychological tests. In Filskov S, Boll TJ, editors: *Handbook of clinical neuropsychology*, New York, 1981, Wiley-Interscience.

Hachinski VC and others: Cerebral blood flow in dementia, *Arch Neurol* 32:632-637, 1975.

Haley J: *Problem-solving therapy*, San Francisco, 1976, Jossey-Bass.

Harrell LE: Alzheimer's disease, *South Med J* 84:15-23, 1991.

Hart RP: and others: Digit Symbol performance in mild dementia and depression, *J Consult Clin Psychol* 55:236-238, 1987.

Hart RP and others: Rate of forgetting in dementia and depression, *J Consult Clin Psychol* 55:101-105, 1987.

Hodges JR, Salmon DP, Butters N: Semantic memory impairment in Alzheimer's disease: failure of access or degraded knowledge? *Neuropsychologia* 30:301-314, 1992.

Huber SJ and others: Cortical versus subcortical dementia: neuropsychological differences, *Arch Neurol* 43:392-394, 1986.

Katzman RD: Alzheimer's disease, *N Engl J Med 314:*964-973, 1986.

Katzman R, Jackson JE: Alzheimer disease: basic and clinical advances, *J Am Geriatr Soc* 39:516-525, 1991.

Katzman R and others: Validation of a short orientation-memory-concentration test of cognitive impairment, *Am J Psychiatry* 140:734-739, 1983.

Lesher EL, Whelihan WM: Reliability of mental status instruments administered to nursing home residents, *J Consult Clin Psychol* 54:726-727, 1987.

Luria AR: *Higher cortical functions in man*, New York, 1966, Basic Books.

Mangone CA and others: Impaired insight in Alzheimer's disease, *J Geriatr Psychiatry Neurol* 4:189-193, 1991.

Mayeaux R and others: Is "subcortical dementia" a recognizable clinical entity? *Ann Neurol* 14:278-283, 1983.

Minuchin S: *Families and family therapy*, Cambridge, Mass, 1974, Harvard University Press.

Moss MB and others: Differential patterns of memory loss among patients with Alzheimer's disease, Huntington's disease, and alcoholic Korsakoff's syndrome, *Arch Neurol* 43:239-246, 1986.

Navia BA, Jordan BD, Price RW: The AIDS dementia complex. I. Clinical features, *Ann Neurol* 19:517-524, 1986.

Navia BA, Price RW: The acquired immunodeficiency syndrome dementia complex as the presenting sole manifestation of human immunodeficiency virus infection, *Arch Neurol* 44:65-69, 1987.

Nebes RD, Brady CB: Generalized cognitive slowing and severity of dementia in Alzheimer's disease: implications for the interpretation of response-time data, *J Clin Exper Neuropsychol* 14:317-326, 1992.

Olson DH, Lavee Y, McCubbin H: Types of families and family response to stress across the family life cycle. In Aldous J, Klein DM, editors: *Social stress and family development*, New York, 1986, Guilford Press.

Reitan RM, Wolfson D: *The Halstead-Reitan neuropsychological test battery: theory and clinical interpretation*, Tucson, 1985, Neuropsychological Press.

Rosen WG and others: Pathological verification of ischemic score in differentiation of dementias, *Ann Neurol* 7:486-488, 1980.

Rouleau I and others: Quantitative and qualitative analyses of clock drawings in Alzheimer's and Huntington's disease, *Brain Cogn* 18:70-87, 1992.

Samuel WA, Henderson VW, Miller CA: Severity of dementia in Alzheimer's disease and neurofibrillary tangles in multiple brain regions, *Alzheimer Dis Assoc Disord* 5:1-11, 1991.

Shay KA and others: The clinical validity of the Mattis Dementia Rating Scale in staging Alzheimer's dementia, *J Geriatr Psychiatry Neurol* 4:18-25, 1991.

Skelton WP, Skelton NK: Alzheimer's disease: recognizing and treating a frustrating condition, *Postgrad Med* 90:33-41, 1991.

Sloan P: Clinical neuropsychology in evaluating and treating brain dysfunction, *South Med J* 77:4-6, 1984.

Solomon DP, Thal LJ, Butters N: Longitudinal evaluation of dementia of the Alzheimer type: a comparison of three standardized mental status examinations, *Neurology* 40:1225-1230, 1991.

Talland CA: Age and immediate memory span. In Talland CA, editor: *Human aging and behavior*, New York, 1968, Academic Press.

Tierney MC and others: Psychometric differentiation of dementia: replication of the findings of Storandt and coworkers, *Arch Neurol* 44:720-722, 1987.

Wsyolek ZK and others: Comparison of EEG background frequency analysis, psychologic test scores, short test of mental status, and quantitative SPECT in dementia, *J Geriatr Psychiatry Neurol* 5:22-30, 1992.

Zandi T: Changes in memory processes of dementia patients. In Zandi T, Ham RJ, editors: *New directions in understanding dementia and Alzheimer's disease*, New York, 1990, Plenum Press.

4

Brain imaging

Gary S. Figiel and Charles B. Nemeroff

With the development of sophisticated brain imaging equipment and methods, highly detailed in vivo analysis of the brain's structure and function is currently possible. Through preliminary imaging studies it has been observed that the structure and physiology of the brain in patients with Alzheimer's disease are different from those of healthy elderly control subjects and other groups of patients. It is hoped that eventually brain imaging techniques will be helpful in differentiating dementia of the Alzheimer type from normal aging and other types of dementia. Although some imaging studies have provided useful information in the examination of Alzheimer's disease, brain imaging is in its infancy, and additional work is needed to understand the potential role that new imaging techniques may play in the diagnosis of Alzheimer's disease.

This chapter discusses the brain imaging techniques of computed tomography, magnetic resonance imaging, positron emission tomography, and single photon emission computed tomography and how these techniques have been applied to the investigation of Alzheimer's disease.

COMPUTED TOMOGRAPHY

Computed tomography (CT) involves the use of x-rays to generate images of the brain's structure. The x-rays are sent through the brain and are absorbed in various amounts in different areas of the brain. A computer is used to reconstruct an image of the brain based on the x-rays that have passed through the brain.

65

In general, brain CT studies have not proved reliable for diagnosing Alzheimer's disease because there is considerable overlap between CT measurement of atrophy in healthy aging and Alzheimer's disease. Early brain CT studies found that patients with Alzheimer's disease often had increased ventricular size compared with healthy controls; however, measurements of ventricular size done through brain CT have failed to separate patients with Alzheimer's disease consistently from healthy age-matched control subjects. Other studies have reported that brain CT may separate patients with Alzheimer's disease more clearly from control subjects if the rate of ventricular enlargement is examined or if the measurements of lateral ventricular size are combined with other brain CT measurements, such as sulcal width or size of temporal lobe structures. However, these studies need to be examined further before any definitive conclusions can be made. Most brain CT studies of patients with Alzheimer's disease have reported that lateral ventricular enlargement correlates with measures of cognitive impairment. The main purpose of doing a CT scan of the brain is not to make a positive diagnosis of Alzheimer's disease but to exclude other causes of cognitive impairment. Some of these conditions, for example, benign brain tumor or subdural hematomas, may be reversible.

MAGNETIC RESONANCE IMAGING

Unlike CT, magnetic resonance imaging (MRI) does not use x-rays; instead, it involves the use of magnetic fields to generate images of the brain. The patient is placed in a strong magnetic field, which causes most of the individual's protons to align with the magnetic field. A low-frequency radiowave is then aimed at the magnet and causes the protons to realign. When the radiowave is discontinued, the protons realign with the magnetic fields. This realignment causes the emission of an electromagnetic wave. The return of the protons to their original state occurs in two phases, referred to as relaxation times. The first relaxation phase, known as T_1, is caused by the dissipation of energy to neighboring particles. The second phase, T_2, results from the small magnetic fields produced by the neighboring particles. The electromagnetic waves are then digitized to reconstruct an image of the brain.

Brain MRI offers a more detailed analysis of subcortical gray and white structures than does brain CT. These observations may be important, since subcortical gray structures, such as the hippocampus, have been implicated in the neuropathologic findings of Alzheimer's disease. Preliminary studies are being done to investigate whether quantitative brain MRI analyses of hippocampal volumes can be helpful in the diagnosis of Alzheimer's disease.

Although these preliminary brain MRI studies, in general, have supported autopsy data by noting a reduction in hippocampal volumes in patients with Alzheimer's disease, some studies are still finding that brain MRI hippocampal volume measurements incompletely separate patients with Alzheimer's disease from healthy controls. Nonetheless, brain MRI hippocampal volumetry is clearly a promising area of research in the field of dementia. One of the main advantages of MRI of the brain is that it is capable of detecting small infarcts that may not be apparent on a CT scan of the brain.

Structural changes occurring in the white matter are easily observed when T_2-weighted and proton-density MRI images are used. Such changes may be of potential importance, since some studies have suggested that structural changes in white matter occur in Alzheimer's disease. White matter hyperintensities are usually found in areas adjacent to the ventricles (periventricular) and in the deep white matter. Hyperintensities occur more commonly in people older than 60 years and are often found to be associated with atherosclerotic risk factors.

Comparisons between the prevalence of white matter hyperintensities in patients with Alzheimer's disease and in healthy controls have yielded contradictory findings. Although it does not appear that MRI white matter hyperintensities will be useful in the diagnosis of Alzheimer's disease, the presence of more severe white matter hyperintensities may predict poor neuropsychological performance in some patients with Alzheimer's disease. Some studies have examined the potential utility of the T_1 and T_2 relaxation times determined by brain MRI in diagnosing Alzheimer's disease. In general, T_1 and T_2 relaxation times are related to the water content of the brain. However, T_1 and T_2 times in control subjects often have a significant overlap with these measurements in patients with Alzheimer's disease. In addition, several investigators have suggested that increases in T_1 and T_2 relaxation times may correlate with the severity of the disease.

POSITRON EMISSION TOMOGRAPHY

Although brain MRI and brain CT studies have offered important information on brain structure, neither technique provides a functional analysis of the brain. Positron emission tomography (PET) is an analytical imaging technique that provides in vivo measurements of the anatomical distribution and ratio of specific biochemical reactions. PET uses radioactive compounds to measure the brain's functions. An injected radioactive compound emits positrons, which are measured by detectors. Based on this information, a computer constructs an image of the brain.

Glucose metabolism is most commonly studied in patients with Alzheimer's disease. Overall, PET glucose metabolism studies of patients with Alzheimer's disease have demonstrated global reductions in glucose metabolism, with most abnormalities found in the parietotemporal regions followed by the frontocortical areas.

Several PET studies have compared patients with Alzheimer's disease and patients with multiinfarct dementia. In general, the patients with Alzheimer's disease have shown regional declines, whereas those with multiinfarct dementia tended to have scattered focal defects. Longitudinal PET studies in patients with Alzheimer's disease suggest that metabolic declines can be detected before measurable declines in cognitive function are noted. As a result, future PET studies may prove to be helpful in the early diagnosis of Alzheimer's disease before the development of significant cognitive dysfunction.

SINGLE PHOTON EMISSION COMPUTED TOMOGRAPHY

Single photon emission computed tomography (SPECT) is similar to PET. Both methods involve the use of radioactive compounds. In SPECT the radioactive compounds emit photons that are measured by detectors. Computers then measure the levels of cerebral blood flow throughout the brain. The main advantage of SPECT in comparison to PET is that SPECT is less expensive. The disadvantage of SPECT versus PET is that SPECT has a lower spatial resolution than PET.

Consistent with PET studies, most SPECT studies in patients with Alzheimer's disease show bilateral decreased blood flow in the temporoparietal areas of the brain. In addition, frontocortical abnormalities appear to be present in patients with severe dementia. To date, SPECT has not been highly accurate in the diagnosis of mild Alzheimer's disease, but it has proved more accurate for diagnosing patients with moderate to severe dementia. Perhaps newer imaging techniques with more sophisticated cameras will address this problem in the future. As with the previously described imaging techniques, significant correlations between SPECT measurements of cerebral blood flow and cognitive test scores have been observed.

SUMMARY

Initial hopes that sophisticated new imaging techniques would lead to earlier, more accurate diagnosis of Alzheimer's disease have not yet been achieved. To date, the diagnosis is still based on clinical and pathological data.

The imaging techniques discussed in this chapter appear to be most accurate in differentiating patients who are severely impaired by Alzheimer's disease from healthy control subjects. However, whether brain MRI hippocampal volumetry will prove helpful in the diagnosis of mild Alzheimer's disease remains to be seen. All the techniques discussed here have demonstrated structural or functional abnormalities that correlate with neuropsychological defects, supporting these techniques as indexes of brain functions. As research continues and these imaging techniques become more accurate, it is hoped that they will play a larger role in the diagnosis of Alzheimer's disease.

BIBLIOGRAPHY

Albert MS, Lafleche G: Neuroimaging in Alzheimer's disease, *Psychiatr Clin North Am* 14:443-458, 1991.

Brun A, Gustafson L, Englund E: Subcortical pathology of Alzheimer's disease, *Adv Neurol* 51:73-77, 1990.

Clifford RJ and others: MR-based hippocampal volumetry in the diagnosis of Alzheimer's disease, *Neurology* 42:183-188, 1992.

Cummings JL, Benson DF: *Dementia: a clinical approach*, Boston, 1991, Butterworth-Heinemann.

Figiel GS and others: Subcortical hyperintensities on brain magnetic resonance imaging: a comparison between late age onset and early onset elderly depressed subjects, *Neurobiol Aging* 26:245-247, 1991.

Grady CL and others: Longitudinal study of the early neuropsychological and cerebral metabolic changes in dementia of the Alzheimer type, *J Clin Exp Neuropsychol* 10:576-596, 1988.

Harrell LE and others: The relationship of high-intensity signals on magnetic resonance images to cognitive and psychiatric state in Alzheimer's disease, *Arch Neurol* 48:1136-1140, 1991.

Kesslak JP, Nalcioglu O, Cotman CW: Quantification of magnetic resonance scans for hippocampal and parahippocampal atrophy in Alzheimer's disease, *Neurology* 41: 51-54, 1991.

Luxenberg JS and others: Rate of ventricular enlargement in dementia of the Alzheimer type correlates with rate of neuropsychological deterioration, *Neurology* 37:1135-1140, 1987.

McDonald WM and others: Brain MRI findings in early-onset Alzheimer's disease, *Biol Psychiatry* 29:799-810, 1991.

Phelps ME, Mazziotta JC, Schelbert HR: *Positron emission tomography and autoradiography,* New York, 1986, Raven Press.

Sandor T and others: Use of computerized CT analysis to discriminate between Alzheimer patients and normal control subjects, *Am J Neuroradiol* 9:1181-1187, 1988.

ALZHEIMER'S DISEASE

5
Historical perspectives

Kim Salyer

HISTORY OF SENILE DEMENTIA

Senile dementia, the loss of memory and other intellectual faculties that occurs in the elderly, was recognized in the time of Hippocrates. In the ensuing centuries this condition was thought to be simply a result of old age. Even as late as the nineteenth century, senile dementia was considered by many to be an inevitable accompaniment of aging. It was generally accepted that as individuals grew older, their mental faculties declined. Older persons became unable to remember or to communicate, and they often developed eccentric habits, such as talking to themselves or hoarding useless possessions.

Unfortunately, the diseases of the aged were considered relatively unimportant until the second half of the nineteenth century, when interest in geriatric medicine began to grow. This interest was initiated by the French, who introduced more humane treatment of the impoverished sick, elderly, and insane patients housed in their asylums. Until the end of the eighteenth century, conditions at these asylums had been decidedly inhumane.

At Bethlehem Hospital in London, commonly referred to as Bedlam (which became a synonym for chaos), the conditions were appalling. The patients were subjected to filthy living conditions, poor food, isolation, darkness, and brutal guards. Common treatments for these patients and others throughout western Europe included the use of emetics and purgatives (substances used to induce vomiting and evacuation of the bowels, respectively), bloodletting, and other procedures such as dousing the patient with ice cold water or putting him in a gyrating chair (a spinning chair that left the patient unconscious) in order to cause a shock to his system.

73

King George III of England may even have been subjected to some of these treatments. In 1788, when the king suffered from a depressive psychosis, in addition to arguing over whether he was insane or physically ill, physicians disagreed about whether he should "have his skull blistered, his intestines purged, be bled, be made to vomit, or be walked around the gardens of the royal castle while he listened to soothing music."

PATIENT CARE REFORM MOVEMENT

The leader of the movement to reform the asylums in France was Philippe Pinel, a French physician who was greatly influenced by the science of psychology, which was then a new field. Pinel became physician-in-chief at the Bicetre asylum in Paris in 1793. Before he took charge, conditions at the Bicetre asylum, where patients were kept in chains, had been as appalling as those at Bedlam. However, major changes were implemented when Pinel gained authority. Pinel ensured that the patients were treated kindly, freed them from their chains, and allowed them clean air, sunshine, and healthy food. He insisted that the staff physicians live with the insane patients in order to study their habits and personalities and to follow the progression of their illnesses. Pinel believed that if a physician had no understanding of human behavior, he was not qualified to work with the mentally ill.

During his tenure at Bicetre, Pinel studied his patients carefully, systematically described their symptoms, and determined whether those symptoms were linked to difficulties with memory, attention, or judgment. Unlike most of his predecessors, Pinel believed that mental illness was not inflicted on victims by evil spirits or other sources. Instead, he thought it was caused by adversities in their lives or by heredity.

Since many elderly people were placed in asylums because of their poverty or eccentric behavior, a large population of elderly patients was available for physicians to study. As a result, French physicians began to build up a large body of work on geriatrics, and they called for more attention to be given to the problems of the elderly. The French were soon followed by the Germans and the English. Together, physicians from the three countries developed the founding principles of modern geriatrics.

Soon the rest of society began to accept these new attitudes concerning the treatment of the elderly. However, there were a few notable exceptions. In 1874 George M. Beard, an American neurologist, concluded that the sharpness of the mind diminished as one aged. He estimated that 70% of a person's work was accomplished before age 45 and that 90% was done before age 50. In 1905 Sir William Osler repeated Beard's conclusions in a speech and joked that men should be put to sleep when they reach age 60. He was severely criticized by his peers, among them Sir James Chricton-Browne, who believed that, although there was no way to avoid the aging process, many of the ailments that accompany old age could be prevented. Like many of his contemporaries, Chricton-Browne was a proponent of more humane treatment of the elderly.

DISCOVERY OF ALZHEIMER'S DISEASE

It was in this milieu in 1906 that Alois Alzheimer (1864-1915) presented his findings on what was first called presenile dementia. Alzheimer was the son of a government officer in Marktbreit, Bavaria. He studied medicine at the universities of Würzburg, Tübingen, and Berlin and received his medical degree in 1887 from the University of Würzburg after completing a thesis on the wax-producing glands of the ear.

Alzheimer next served as an assistant at Irrenanstalt in Frankfurt am Main, where he met Franz Nissl in 1889. It was Nissl who inspired Alzheimer to study neuropathology and stimulated his interest in brain pathology research. As a young medical student, Nissl had demonstrated his flair for experimentation by winning a competition on the "Pathological Changes of Nerve Cells in the Cerebral Cortex." The resulting method, now called Nissl's stain, was considered a scientific breakthrough and a major advance in neuroanatomy and neuropathology.

Alzheimer and Nissl complemented each other perfectly. Alzheimer had meticulous research practices and strong reasoning ability, and Nissl had imagination and original ideas. For 7 years the two men worked together at the psychiatric hospital in Frankfurt. During this time they introduced new laboratory techniques, new methods of examining tissue throughout the nervous system, and new ways of handling the brain during autopsy.

In 1895 Nissl joined Emil Kraepelin, one of the founders of modern psychiatry, in Heidelburg to study the framework of psychiatric disease. Alzheimer followed in 1902 and then moved to Munich with Kraepelin in 1903. In Munich, Alzheimer and Kraepelin devoted themselves to presenting the exact clinical-anatomical relationships in psychiatric diseases.

It was while working in Munich that Alzheimer described the first case of the disease that would later bear his name. A 55-year-old woman suffering from dementia had been admitted to the psychiatric hospital in Frankfurt. Her symptoms had begun at the age of 51 with an unreasonable jealousy of her husband. As her illness progressed, the woman endured a rapid decline in memory, paranoid delusions, auditory hallucinations, and, finally, complete dementia. Within 4½ years of the onset of symptoms, the woman died at age 56.

This patient's illness was unique because of her age, the speed of the disease's progression, and the neuropathological findings. Unlike senile dementia, which begins at age 65 or older and progresses slowly, this woman's illness began at a relatively young age and progressed very rapidly.

At autopsy, Alzheimer discovered not only the senile plaques that were found to be common in the brains of people with senile dementia but also neurofibrillary tangles—thick, coiled fibers within the cytoplasm of the cerebral cortical neurons. This discovery led Alzheimer to note in his report: "On the whole, it is evident that we are dealing with a peculiar, little-known disease process."

During the next 5 years, 12 other cases of this new disease were reported. Already, the condition was being referred to by many authors as "Alzheimer's disease." This designation was in part the result of its endorsement as a separate disease by Alzheimer's mentor, Emil Kraepelin, who was the leader of the organic school of psychiatry. This school of thought held that psychiatric ailments could be traced to an organic origin. It was in direct competition with the functional school of psychiatry, which taught that psychological elements, such as an unhappy childhood, could produce mental disease. Alzheimer's discovery effectively established the organic school and Emil Kraepelin as the chief authorities on the causes of mental illness.

The most prolific of the authors who described Alzheimer's disease from 1906 to 1911 was not Alzheimer but Gaetano Perusini, an Italian physician who reported four cases in 1910 alone. Because of Perusini's efforts, many Italian authors still refer to the condition as Alzheimer-Perusini disease. Another Italian physician, Francesco Bonfiglio, reported the second case of Alzheimer's disease in 1908. His paper described in detail the neuropathological findings and included the first drawing of neurofibrillary tangles as seen under a microscope. It was not until 1911 that Alzheimer reported his second case of the disease.

Alzheimer did not make his discovery in a vacuum. His research was made possible by the work of other researchers, such as Nissl, who first produced a stain for neuronal cell bodies in 1892, and Max Bielschowsky, whose silver-based stain permitted Alzheimer to view neurofibrillary tangles. Senile plaques such as those detected by Alzheimer in the brain of his first patient were initially described by Paul Blocq and Georges Marinesco in 1892. Alterations in neurofibrils similar to those discovered by Alzheimer had been found in the brains of experimental animals before Alzheimer reported on his findings in humans. In fact, in 1845 Wilhelm Griesinger had been the first researcher to recognize presenile dementia. Even though Griesinger's book was translated into French and English, his report was overlooked. Although the disease bears Alzheimer's name, its discovery can also be credited to many other scientists whose work enabled Alzheimer to make his discovery.

After Alzheimer's discovery, many questions were still unanswered. It is likely that since the first patient reported as having Alzheimer's disease was only 51 years old and the next few cases involved patients less than 65 years of age, the initial assumption was that Alzheimer's disease predominantly affected younger people. At the turn of the century, it was thought that mental functions tended to deteriorate as an individual aged. Since different terms were needed to distinguish the impairment of mental functions that occurs in old age, known as senile dementia, from that which occurs in younger people, the term "presenile dementia" was introduced. A few cases in which the disease manifested itself in the fourth decade were reported, and these cases reinforced the concept that Alzheimer's disease should be classified as a presenile dementia. In fact, until the 1970s the diagnosis of Alzheimer's disease was restricted to patients less than 65 years of age.

However, as clinical and postmortem findings resulted in more cases being described in patients over 65 years of age, it was acknowledged that Alzheimer's disease was not confined to younger people but also was affecting older patients. Thus another term was introduced, "senile dementia of the Alzheimer's type."

For many years the debate continued in regard to whether Alzheimer's disease affecting younger people, or presenile dementia, was the same condition as senile dementia of the Alzheimer's type. Some experts raised the question of whether the disorder was one disease that could have an early onset (presenile dementia) and a late onset (senile dementia) or whether there were two different diseases that sometimes displayed the same or similar features.

In the early 1980s a consensus was reached, and it is now generally accepted that the presenile and senile types of Alzheimer's disease are actually the same. The currently accepted position is to refer to Alzheimer's disease and to note that its onset can occur early or late in life.

ALZHEIMER'S DISEASE RESEARCH

Alzheimer's disease research and the questions it raises have withstood the test of time. Almost 90 years after Alzheimer first reported on the disease, scientists still do not understand its causes and have yet to discover a cure. Because of our aging population, Alzheimer's disease is a much greater problem now than it was at the beginning of the twentieth century. Therefore, findings about this disease may be even more important now than they were at the time of their discovery. In 1900 there were only 3 million Americans aged 65 or older, and in 1989 there were more than 27 million. By the year 2050 approximately 67 million Americans will be 65 or older. Unless a cure or method of prevention is found, of those 67 million people, it is estimated that 14 million will have Alzheimer's disease. Today Alzheimer's disease is the fourth leading cause of death among adults, and the cost to Americans for the care and treatment of patients with this disease is estimated at $80 to $90 billion a year.

Because of the rapidly growing elderly population, the prevalence of the disease, and the high cost of patient care, much more attention is being given to Alzheimer's disease than in the past. This attention resulted in the formation of the Alzheimer's Disease and Related Disorders Association (ADRDA) in 1979. The ADRDA has encouraged a great deal of media attention on Alzheimer's disease, and it has acted as a source of information for the lay public. Increasing public awareness of Alzheimer's disease has resulted in the establishment of support groups for families and caregivers of patients with Alzheimer's disease and adult day care for the patients themselves.

Another benefit of public interest in Alzheimer's disease is increased funding for research, which has resulted in new research procedures. Although a cure for Alzheimer's disease has not yet been found, researchers have made considerable advances since Alzheimer first identified the disease in 1906. Whereas in the past a diagnosis of Alzheimer's disease could be made only by ruling out all other possibilities and then examining the brain at autopsy, now researchers are on the brink of being able to make a positive diagnosis before death by using brain imaging studies.

In addition to making advances in diagnostic procedures, researchers are currently experimenting with new treatments for patients with Alzheimer's disease. One reason for optimism in the area of treatment is the similarity of Alzheimer's disease to Parkinson's disease. In Parkinson's disease one neurotransmitter is missing, whereas in Alzheimer's disease five or six neurotransmitters are lacking. Since researchers have discovered several treatments for Parkinson's disease, they hope to develop similar treatments for replenishing the missing neurotransmitters in the brains of Alzheimer's patients.

These advances offer hope that a cure for Alzheimer's disease is on the horizon. Like polio, whooping cough, and other deadly diseases, Alzheimer's disease eventually may become almost obsolete.

BIBLIOGRAPHY

Alexander FG, Selesnick ST: *The history of psychiatry: an evaluation of psychiatric thought and practice from prehistoric times to the present,* New York, 1966, Harper & Row.

Alois Alzheimer, *JAMA* 208:1017-1018, 1969.

Alzheimer's Disease and Related Disorders Association: *Alzheimer's disease statistics,* Chicago, 1990, The Association.

Beach TG: The history of Alzheimer's disease: three debates, *J Hist Med* 42:327-349, 1987.

Brick K, Amaducci L, Pepeu G: *The early story of Alzheimer's disease,* New York, 1987, Raven Press.

Evans DA and others: Estimated prevalence of Alzheimer's disease, *Milbank Q* 68(2):267-289, 1990.

Kreutzberg GW: 100 years of Nissl staining, *Trends Neurosci* July:236-237, 1984.

Rocca WA, Amaducci LA: Letter to editor, *Alzheimer Dis Assoc Disord* 2:56-57, 1988.

Wisniewski HM: *Milestones in the history of Alzheimer disease research.* In Iqbal K, Wisniewski H, Winblad B, editors: *Alzheimer's disease and related disorders,* New York, 1989, Alan R Liss.

6

Etiology and pathogenesis of Alzheimer's disease: current concepts

Eleanor P. Lavretsky and Lissy F. Jarvik

The dramatic increase in life expectancy during this century, achieved primarily through the cure of infectious diseases, has enabled many people to reach an age at which degenerative diseases of the brain, particularly Alzheimer's disease, become common. Dementia, the loss of our most human qualities—reasoning, memory, and language—formerly was accepted as the natural consequence of reaching advanced old age. A grandparent who became confused and forgetful suffered from "hardening of the arteries in the brain." In the past, two etiological factors were thought to be responsible for initiating the dementing process: age and arteriosclerosis or atherosclerosis. It is now obvious that both statements are false, at least partially.

Although old age is an important risk factor for Alzheimer's disease, it is by no means the only one. In addition, dementia is not a normal or necessary consequence of aging. According to epidemiological studies done in Western countries, most individuals do not have dementia, no matter how old they are. The prevalence of dementia, from all causes, ranges from 5% to 10% among persons age 65 and older, and the rate increases exponentially as age advances. Integrative analysis of 47 surveys done in 17 countries suggests approximate rates of less than 1% for dementia in persons aged 60 to 69 years and 39% in those aged 90 to 95.

This work was supported in part by National Institute of Mental Health Research Grants MH 36205 and MH 31357 and the Department of Veterans Affairs. The opinions expressed are those of the authors and not those of the Department of Veterans Affairs.

Most studies report that Alzheimer's disease is responsible for the cognitive decline in approximately 50% of older adults with dementia (Table 6-1). It may occur in association with multiinfarct disease in an additional 18% to 24%. However, multiinfarct dementia alone comprises a relatively small portion of dementia. Thus vascular insufficiency cannot explain the majority of dementia cases.

Despite stringent clinical and research protocols, the definitive diagnosis of Alzheimer's disease still rests on histopathological confirmation, that is, the presence of characteristic neuritic plaques, neurofibrillary tangles, and granulovacuolar degeneration. Although neither neuritic plaques nor neurofibrillary tangles alone can be used to diagnose Alzheimer's disease, they have been considered pathognomonic when present together and accompanied by the appropriate clinical history. The brain of a patient with Alzheimer's disease shows marked atrophy, particularly in the frontotemporal, parietal, and hippocampal regions. These morphological changes are believed to be the anatomical basis of amnesia. Numerous other associations between abnormalities of the brain and mental impairment have also been examined. For example, loss of neurons and, more specifically, loss of synapses in the cortical association areas and the hippocampus were recently reported as being directly related to the clinical presentation of dementia. With the increased use of neuroimaging techniques, understanding of brain/behavior relationships will improve substantially.

NEURITIC PLAQUES, AMYLOID, AND GENETICS

The etiological basis of the degenerative changes in Alzheimer's disease is still unknown. However, recent discoveries indicate that understanding the genesis of neuritic or senile plaques may provide powerful clues regarding the pathogenesis of the disease. In 1907, peering through a microscope at the brain of his first patient, the German psychiatrist Alois Alzheimer prophetically wrote: "Scattered through the entire cortex, especially in the upper layers, one found miliary foci that were caused by the deposition of a *peculiar substance* in the cerebral cortex." This "peculiar substance" is known as the beta-amyloid protein. The neuritic plaque is a complex, slowly evolving structure believed to require years, if not decades, to reach maturation. It consists of a central amyloid core surrounded by abnormal neurites, altered glial cells, and cellular debris.

Table 6-1 Etiologies of dementia (expressed in percentages)

	Year	No. of Patients	DAT*	MID*	Mixed (DAT + MID) or other type*	Mass Lesion	NPH*	Alcoholic Dementia	Huntington's Disease	Creutzfeldt-Jakob Disease	Other*
Tomlinson et al.†	1970	50	50	18	18			2			12
Todorov et al.	1975	675	40	29	24			7			7
Freeman	1976	60	43	8		3	12	7	7		20
Harrison & Marsden	1977	49	44	12		5	7	9			23
Smith & Kiloh	1981	164	50	14		2	5	19	3		7
Larson et al.†	1984	107	69	4		2		4			21
Molsa et al.†	1985	58	48	19	10		2				21
Sulkava et al.	1985	141	50	39							11
Schoenberg et al.	1987	178	52	5	14	2		2			25
Wade et al.†	1987	65	59	9	15					3	14
Evans et al.	1989	113	84	3	7			2			4

From Jarvik LF, Lavretsky EP, Neshkes RE: The central nervous system: dementia and delirium in old age. In Brocklehurst JC, editor: *Textbook of geriatric medicine and gerontology*, ed 4, Edinburgh, 1992, Churchill Livingstone.
*DAT, Dementia of Alzheimer's type; *MID*, multiinfarct dementia; *NPH*, normal pressure hydrocephalus; "other" includes chronic drug toxicity, posttrauma, postsubarachnoid hemorrhage, encephalitis, syphilis, subdural hematoma, hypothyroidism, and depression.
†Autopsy study.

In 1853 Rudolf Virchow, the great German pathologist, called these deposits "amyloid," an unfortunate term because it implies that the deposits are made of a starchlike substance. In fact, chemical studies have shown that the principal constituents of the amyloid filaments are actually proteins and that various types of protein characterize the different diseases marked by the deposition of amyloid. The common thread linking these amyloidoses is the extracellular deposition of normal or mutated protein fragments, always folded in a particular three-dimensional pattern called a beta-pleated sheet. It is this feature that gives amyloid the property of apple-green birefringence in polarized light after being stained with Congo red dye.

The formation of amyloid deposits in different diseases seems to follow a common chain of events: normal protein → pathological (abnormal, mutated) protein → amyloid deposition. The sequence starts within the amyloid precursor protein, a protein molecule that is a normal body constituent. The beta-amyloid precursor protein in Alzheimer's disease is a membrane-bound glycoprotein that is present in normal neurons and nonneuronal cells. Its exact role in the adult brain is not known, but it does have a trophic function and is required to maintain both fibroblasts and hippocampal cells in tissue culture. To date, five different isoforms of amyloid precursor protein have been described, containing amino acids 563, 695, 714, 751, and 770. The gene for the amyloid protein precursor is located on chromosome 21.

Several different factors can induce the formation of an abnormal protein from the precursor molecule with subsequent amyloid deposition, including abnormal messages from mutated genes. In Alzheimer's disease the protein is the insoluble beta-amyloid protein (βAP). This protein is also found in the brain of patients with Down's syndrome, normal aged humans, and monkeys. It consists of 39 to 43 amino acid residues. How the βAP is released from its large protein precursor molecule is not completely understood and is being intensively investigated. Recent experimental data demonstrate that some cultured cells may normally produce and release soluble βAP that is essentially identical to the βAP deposited as insoluble amyloid fibrils in Alzheimer's disease. Thus it is likely that amyloid deposition in Alzheimer's disease involves pathways that normally produce extracellular βAP, and the amount of amyloid deposited depends on the rate of βAP production, the rate of its removal, and the rate at which soluble βAP forms insoluble amyloid fibrils.

Another very important question is being studied and discussed: Is the βAP toxic to nerve cells and thus a prime suspect in the degeneration noted in the brains of patients with Alzheimer's disease? If the answer is yes, as work by Harvard researcher Bruce Yankner suggests, scientists will have understood a fundamental feature of the pathological nature of Alzheimer's disease and also, perhaps, have developed an animal model for the disease. However, experiments to date have yielded equivocal results concerning this key question.

In addition to beta-amyloid, the neuritic plaques contain $alpha_1$-antichymotrypsin (ACT), an acute-phase reactant. ACT is a serine protease inhibitor, a serum glycoprotein synthesized in the liver and by astrocytes in the brain. The synthesis of ACT is positively regulated by interleukin-6 (IL-6), the primary cytokine mediator of the acute-phase response. An increased amount of ACT in some patients with Alzheimer's disease may reflect the presence of localized inflammatory reactions in the brain. It is interesting to note that IL-6 stimulates synthesis of the amyloid precursor protein and may influence amyloid formation.

As mentioned earlier, Alzheimer's disease has been associated with a mutation on chromosome 21. At the time of this writing, 375 families with Alzheimer's disease have been examined for possible gene mutations (Table 6-2). Only eight of these families have been identified as having a chromosome 21 mutation. All eight were among the 144 families in which the disease was characterized by onset at a young age. Among the eight families, three different mutant alleles were harbored. Thus the rate of occurrence is less than 5%, even for the highly selected families with the early-onset familial type of Alzheimer's disease. If all the patients with Alzheimer's disease reported so far are considered, the risk of this type of gene mutation is less than 2%. Nonetheless, the discovery of gene mutations on chromosome 21 is a significant leap forward in research of Alzheimer's disease. It has also led to another question: How does a single amino acid substitution that occurs as a result of these mutations enhance proteolysis so that the beta-amyloid fragment is released from the precursor molecule? This is the subject of current research.

A group of investigators at Duke University, headed by Dr. Allen Roses, found linkage of some cases of late-onset familial Alzheimer's disease to chromosome 19. These investigators postulate that even though early-onset familial Alzheimer's disease has been associated with a chromosome 21 abnormality, a chromosome 19 abnormality may cause late-onset familial Alzheimer's disease. Early onset of Alzheimer's disease is generally defined as occurring before age 65; late onset, occurring at age 65 or older. Most recently, chromosome 14 has been linked to Alzheimer's disease.

Table 6-2   Genetic changes in Alzheimer's disease and associated disorders

Disease	Type of Amyloid	Amyloid Precursor	Gene Location (Chromosome)	Gene Mutation	Amino Acid Substitution
Alzheimer's disease	βAP	βAPP	21	Exon 17 Codon 717	
				C to T	Valine→isoleucine
				T to G	Valine→glycine
				G to T	Valine→phenylalanine
				Codon 670/671	Lysine-methionine→ asparagine-leucine
			21	?	?
			19	?	?
			14	?	?
Down's syndrome	βAP	βAPP	21		Chromosome 21 abnormality
HCHWA					
Dutch type	βAP	βAPP	21	Exon 17 C to G	Glutamic acid→ glutamine
Icelandic type	Cystatin variant	Cystatin C			Leucine→glutamine
Prion diseases					
Creutzfeldt-Jakob disease	PrP	PrP^C	20	Codon 178	Aspartic acid→ asparagine
				Codon 200 G to A	Glutamine→lysine
				Codon 53	Octapeptide repeats of 2, 4, 5, 6, 7, 8, or 9
Gerstmann-Sträussler-Scheinker disease	PrP	PrP^C	20	Codon 102 C to T	Proline→leucine
				Codon 117 A to G	Alanine→valine
				Codon 198	Phenylalanine→serine
Familial amyloidosis, Finnish type	Amyloid protein	Gelsolin	9	Codon 187	Aspartic acid→ asparagine

βAP, Beta-amyloid protein; *βAPP*, beta-amyloid protein precursor; *PrP*, prion protein; *PrP^C*, prion protein precursor; *HCHWA*, hereditary cerebral hemorrhage with amyloidoses; *A*, adenine; *C*, cytosine; *G*, guanine; *T*, thymine.

Point mutations have also been implicated in amyloid depositions in other brain diseases, including hereditary cerebral hemorrhage with amyloidosis (HCHWA), Dutch and Icelandic types (see Table 6-2). The mutation described in Alzheimer's disease was also found in one family with clinical features of both processes—HCHWA (Dutch type) and dementia. The human prion diseases known as Creutzfeldt-Jakob disease and Gerstmann-Straüssler-Scheinker disease have been associated with mutations on chromosome 20.

Three major conclusions can be reached from this linkage. First, one specific molecular cause of Alzheimer's disease may have been identified in a very small number of families with mutations in the gene for the beta-amyloid precursor protein. Second, there may be more than one genetic locus influencing the development of Alzheimer's disease. Third, segregation and linkage data suggest a dichotomy between early-onset and late-onset forms of Alzheimer's disease.

In addition, family, twin, and survey studies have yielded strong clinical evidence for a genetic etiological basis in Alzheimer's disease. On the whole, this evidence has been interpreted as showing that approximately 50% of adult members in families with Alzheimer's disease develop the disease, a ratio expected for an autosomal dominant trait. Families with disease onset at a young age predominate in this group.

NEUROFIBRILLARY TANGLES, MICROTUBULES, AND TAU

Neurofibrillary tangles, like neuritic plaques, are not specific to Alzheimer's disease. They occur in about a dozen other chronic diseases of the human brain and in normal aging brains. The core structures of the neurofibrillary tangles, paired helical filaments, contain proteins that may be important in the pathogenesis of Alzheimer's disease, specifically tau (A-68) and ubiquitin. The major protein associated with paired helical filaments is tau, a microtubule-associated protein that exists in different isoforms. Several lines of evidence point to altered phosphorylation as a general feature of the pathological nature of Alzheimer's disease. Thus tau isoforms are excessively phosphorylated in Alzheimer's disease, probably secondary to abnormality of enzymes involved in protein phosphorylation, such as protein kinase C and casein kinase II. Abnormalities of the growth-associated protein GAP-43 have also been suggested. GAP-43 is a neuron-specific phosphoprotein involved in the regulation of phosphorylation.

A-68, another protein, or group of proteins, has a molecular weight of 68,000 dalton. This protein was detected in high concentrations in the brain of patients with Alzheimer's disease by using the antibody Alz-50. Abnormally phosphorylated tau may be unable to bind to neuronal microtubules, and as a consequence the microtubules become destabilized.

Microtubules are tiny structural components present in all cells. The microtubule system is both complex and integral to numerous cellular functions, including several functions impaired in patients with Alzheimer's disease. These impaired functions include cell division, goal-directed cell motion, and axonal transport of neurotransmitters. An impaired microtubule system could account for many of the abnormalities observed in Alzheimer's disease, including formation of neurofibrillary tangles, loss of neurons, and abnormalities in the action of nerve growth factor and cholinergic and other neurotransmitters. Microtubule impairment could also account for non-neural abnormalities. The hypothesis has been proposed that an impairment of the microtubule system, regardless of the cause, leads to impaired cellular function and that the effects accumulate with time and eventually reach threshold levels sufficient for the manifestation of the symptomatic behaviors and neuropathological changes characteristic of Alzheimer's disease. At the time of this writing, the microtubule hypothesis has been confirmed in some respects; in others, data are yet to come.

NEUROTRANSMITTERS AND NEUROTROPHIC FACTORS

The concept concerning the etiology and pathogenesis of Alzheimer's disease that has had the staunchest advocates for the longest period of time is that it is a neurotransmitter disease, specifically, a cholinergic disorder. However, most investigators now believe that the cholinergic abnormalities are secondary rather than primary factors in Alzheimer's disease. Nonetheless, the importance of the cholinergic system remains beyond dispute when it comes to memory and the other higher mental functions impaired in patients with Alzheimer's disease. There is also no dispute about the repeated observation of decreased cholinergic activity in the disease. This observation is supported by a significant loss of neurons in the nucleus basalis magnocellularis, which provides cholinergic innervation to the brain (Table 6-3). Moreover, the activity of choline acetyltransferase, the enzyme that synthesizes acetylcholine, is consistently reduced in the cerebral cortex of patients with

Table 6-3   Select cholinergic parameters in patients with and without dementia

	Nucleus Basilis Magnocellularis (Neurones in Thousands)	Choline Acetyltransferase (nmol-^{1} h-^{1} mg-^{1} protein)	
		Frontal Cortex	Hippocampus
Normal	81 ± 13	12.3 ± 3.9	14.8 ± 5.2
Alzheimer's disease	49 ± 10	6.0 ± 2.9	3.6 ± 2.7
Parkinson's disease			
Nondemented	48 ± 13	7.5 ± 2.5	8.7 ± 4.6
Demented	12 ± 5	4.6 ± 2.4	2.5 ± 3.1

From Perry EK, Irving D, Perry RH: *TINS* 14: 483, 1991.
These data (mean ± SD, 4 to 12 cases per group) indicate that neuron loss in the nucleus basalis magnocellularis does not underpin symptoms of dementia per se; in fact, these symptoms relate more closely to cholinergic enzyme reductions that are more than half of the normal levels of the enzyme.

Alzheimer's disease. In addition, deficits in the level of cholinergic activity correlate significantly with cognitive impairment. However, attempts to treat patients with Alzheimer's disease with cholinomimetic agents have generally been unsuccessful, calling into question the place of the cholinergic hypothesis in the pathogenesis of the disease.

The development of muscarinic agonists and cholinesterase inhibitors as therapeutic agents was based on the assumption that replacement of the missing acetylcholine would compensate functionally for the 40% to 70% loss of presynaptic cholinergic neurons in the brain of a patient with Alzheimer's disease. The results of therapeutic trials have been disappointing. It seems that the regulation of memory and other cognitive functions by the cholinergic system is much more complicated than previously suspected. For example, electrophysiological and other studies suggest that the cortical cholinergic system may modulate or amplify other afferent inputs rather than initiate specific behavioral functions. Thus treatments with cholinesterase inhibitors and muscarinic agonists may actually disengage the remaining presynaptic cholinergic neurons and increase the deficit rather than decrease it. It might be more promising to focus on presynaptic modulation of cholinergic activity, using, for example, potassium channel blockade.

The complexity of cholinergic involvement in Alzheimer's disease is further supported by recent data on changes in galanin receptors. Galanin-containing interneurons envelop cholinergic cell bodies and dendrites where they seem to modulate cholinergic neurotransmission. There appears to be no loss of galanin-containing neurons in the basal forebrain of patients with Alzheimer's disease; indeed, these neurons appear to hyperinnervate the remaining cholinergic neurons in the brain of affected persons.

The data on other neurotransmitters are less clear, although both noradrenergic and serotonergic denervation have been reported in patients with Alzheimer's disease who die at a relatively early age. Reduction in gamma-aminobutyric acid has also been reported, but is believed to be a result of postmortem changes rather than Alzheimer's disease itself. Attempts to correlate the other neurotransmitter deficits with the cholinergic changes and the cognitive impairment have been largely unsuccessful.

Researchers have also looked at the possible role of excitatory amino acids in Alzheimer's disease. The excitatory amino acids have been most clearly implicated in the pathogenesis of Huntington's disease and stroke. Their involvement in Alzheimer's disease has not yet been demonstrated.

There is much more evidence for the role of neurotrophic factors in Alzheimer's disease. Those factors are endogenous polypeptides apparently essential for the function and survival of neurons. Nerve growth factor is the best characterized neurotrophic factor. It seems to have specific trophic qualities for the cholinergic neurons most vulnerable to degeneration in Alzheimer's disease. It has been hypothesized that a dysfunction in neurotrophic systems is directly responsible for the neurodegeneration observed in certain diseases, including Alzheimer's disease. Although no direct evidence has been found for this hypothesis, attempts are already under way to use nerve growth factor in the treatment of the disease.

ABNORMALITIES OF TISSUES OTHER THAN BRAIN

It is important to understand that Alzheimer's disease affects both peripheral and brain tissue. Abnormalities have been reported in fibroblasts, red and white blood cells, and platelets. In addition, alterations in blood proteins have been observed. These include the accumulation of the enzyme alpha$_1$-antichymotrypsin and the presence of beta-amyloid peptide in the gut and skin of some patients with

Alzheimer's disease. Further research is needed to confirm these changes, their generality, and their role in the etiology and pathogenesis of Alzheimer's disease.

ENVIRONMENTAL RISK FACTORS

Several environmental risk factors have been reported as having a role in Alzheimer's disease, but, in general, confirmation is lacking. Among the putative environmental risk factors are myocardial infarction, prior malnutrition, alcohol consumption, and smoking; exposure to solvents, aluminum, and lead; lack of education; and sedentary life-style. Even a history of nose-picking has been suggested as a risk factor! Several of the proposed risk factors deserve more attention.

Head Trauma

The one risk factor reported independently by more than one group of investigators is head trauma. Repeated head trauma has been associated with neuropathological lesions similar to, but not identical with, those found in Alzheimer's disease. In dementia pugilistica, which is noted among professional boxers, there is an abundance of neurofibrillary tangles but few plaques. There are also septal fenestration, loss of pigment in substantia nigra, and scarring of the cerebellar tonsils—none of which is found in Alzheimer's disease. Reports vary about the frequency of head trauma in Alzheimer's disease, with some noting a definite excess in patients and others failing to obtain differences from controls.

The role of head trauma in the development of Alzheimer's disease is readily accommodated by the following conceptual framework: Since there is some evidence that the degree of dementia in Alzheimer's disease is a function of loss of synapses, any condition that reduces the number of synapses could have a role in the development of the disease. Aside from head trauma, such conditions would include normal aging with its associated neuronal losses, developmental retardation in early life with an associated reduction in synaptic connections, and deficits in formal education and other intellectual challenges to spur development of synaptic connections. All these could logically be risk factors for Alzheimer's disease. Conditions such as head trauma and periods of ischemia associated with coronary artery disease could lead not only to the death of neurons but also to the deposition of diffuse plaques. Eventually, the accumulated damage would exceed threshold values and result in the manifestation of Alzheimer's disease.

Infection

The significance of infection in the development of Alzheimer's disease is now considered to be low. It was discussed in the literature in connection with human prion diseases (Creutzfeldt-Jakob disease, Gerstmann-Straüssler-Scheinker disease, and kuru) characterized by the development of dementia and protein brain deposits similar to the beta-amyloid deposits of Alzheimer's disease. These disorders can be transmitted to animals by injecting brain extracts from deceased patients. There have also been reports of apparently accidental interhuman transmission. However, attempts to induce Alzheimer's disease in animals by injecting brain extracts from deceased patients have not been replicated, and the "infectious hypothesis" of the disease is now chiefly of historical interest.

Inorganic Compounds

Attention has also been given to inorganic compounds in the brain of patients with Alzheimer's disease. Aluminum and silicon have been found in plaques and tangles. The relevance of the aluminum accumulation is unclear. It may be secondary to incompetence of neuronal membranes and tangle formation. Once in the cell, however, aluminum may cause further damage by interfering with intracellular transport and transmission systems. Other metals, drugs, and toxins have also not been excluded as potential pathogenic factors in Alzheimer's disease.

SUMMARY

After this brief survey of current concepts of the etiology and pathogenesis of Alzheimer's disease, we come to the following four conclusions. First, Alzheimer's disease is even more complex than generally assumed. Second, a vast array of abnormalities in brain function and structure has been reported; in Alzheimer's disease many of these abnormalities require replication. Third, what we call Alzheimer's disease today is most likely a heterogeneous disorder with manifest symptoms that reflect a common final pathway. Fourth, our knowledge concerning the etiology and pathogenesis of Alzheimer's disease needs to be supported by aggressive research.

REFERENCES

Advisory Panel on Alzheimer's Disease: *Third report of the Advisory Panel on Alzheimer's Disease, 1991.* DHHS Pub No (ADM) 92-1917, Washington, DC, 1992, US Government Printing Office.

Cassel CK and others, editors: *Geriatric medicine,* New York, 1990, Springer-Verlag.

DeKosky ST, Scheft SW: Synapse loss in frontal cortex biopsies in Alzheimer's disease: correlation with cognitive severity, *Ann Neurol* 27:457-464, 1990.

Farrer LA and others: Segregation analysis reveals evidence of major gene for Alzheimer disease, *Am J Hum Genet* 48:1026-1033, 1992.

Haines JL: The genetics of Alzheimer disease: a teasing problem (invited editorial), *Am J Hum Genet* 48:1021-1025, 1991.

Jarvik LF, Lavretsky EP, Neshkes RE: The central nervous system: dementia and delirium in old age. In Brocklehurst JC, editor: *Textbook of geriatric medicine and gerontology,* ed 4, Edinburgh, 1992, Churchill Livingstone.

Jorm AE: *The epidemiology of Alzheimer's disease and related disorders,* London, 1990, Chapman & Hall.

Katzman R, Jackson JE: Alzheimer disease: basic and clinical advances, *J Am Geriatr Soc* 39:516-525, 1991.

Matsubura E and others: $Alpha_1$-antichymotrypsin as a possible marker for Alzheimer-type dementia, *Ann Neurol* 28:561-567, 1990.

Matsuyama SS, Jarvik LF: Hypothesis: microtubules, a key to Alzheimer disease, *Proc Natl Acad Sci USA* 86:8152-8156, 1989.

Neurobiology of Aging. Special issue on amyloid protein and neurotoxicity, Sept 1992.

Pericak-Vance MA and others: Linkage studies in familial Alzheimer disease: evidence for chromosome 19 linkage, *Am J Hum Genet* 48:1034-1050, 1991.

Perry EK, Irving D, Perry RH: Cholinergic controversies (letter to editor), *TINS* 14:483, 1991.

Schellenberg GD and others: Genetic linkage evidence for a familial Alzheimer's disease locus on chromosome 14, *Science* 258:668-671, 1992.

Selkoe DJ: Deciphering Alzheimer's disease: the amyloid precursor protein yields new clues, *Science* 248:1058-1060, 1990.

St. George-Hyslop PH and others: Genetic linkage studies suggest that Alzheimer disease is not a single homogeneous disorder, *Nature* 347:194-197, 1990.

Tanzi RE and others: Assessment of amyloid 6-protein precursor gene mutations in a large set of familial and sporadic Alzheimer disease cases, *Am J Hum Genet* 512:273-282, 1992.

7

Pathology of Alzheimer's disease

Michael L. Woodruff

Alzheimer's disease is clinically characterized by the progressive changes in behavior and cognitive functioning described throughout this book. However, it is also defined by a variety of pathological changes that occur in the brain. On gross inspection, one of these changes may be observed in the brain of many patients with Alzheimer's disease as shrinkage of the neocortical gyri. Observation of other neuropathological changes associated with Alzheimer's disease requires application of special stains to a cross section taken from the brain and can be seen only with the assistance of a microscope. Still other changes are only demonstrable by using biochemical methods. The purpose of this chapter is to present and discuss the neuropathological changes associated with Alzheimer's disease.

GROSS PATHOLOGY

The brains of many, but not all, victims of Alzheimer's disease reveal loss of neurons from the brain by marked shrinkage of parts of the cerebrum. This condition, known as cerebral atrophy, is manifested by narrowing of the gyri and consequent widening of the sulci (Fig. 7-1). If present, atrophy will be most noticeable in the association areas of the frontal, temporal, parietal, and occipital lobes. However, with the exception of the primary olfactory cortex, atrophy will be essentially absent from the primary motor and sensory cortical areas. Thus the atrophy associated with Alzheimer's disease is not diffusely distributed across the cortex; however, if present, it will be more severe in the cortical association regions. Even within areas where cortical atrophy is obvious, the microscopic neuropathological changes associated with Alzheimer's disease will not be uniformly present.

93

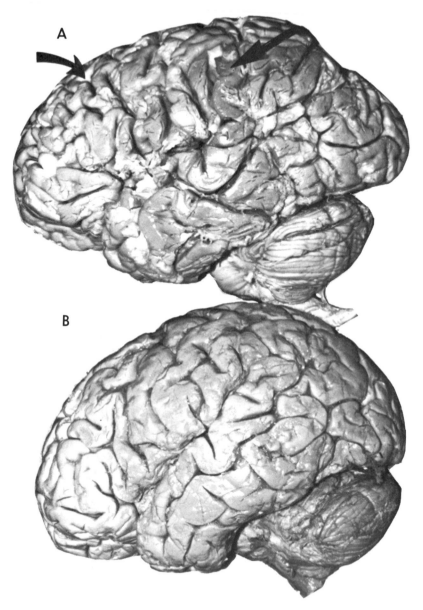

Fig. 7-1. Hemisphere from a patient diagnosed as having Alzheimer's disease (**A**) demonstrates mild neocortical atrophy when compared to the hemisphere from a normal brain (**B**). Widening of the sulci is particularly noticeable in the frontal and parietal areas (*arrows*) of the affected brain but may also be observed in the temporal lobe.

MICROSCOPIC NEUROPATHOLOGY

Because the presence and extent of cerebral atrophy are variable from one case of Alzheimer's disease to another, the neuropathological changes that aid in the diagnosis of Alzheimer's disease need to be observed through a microscope. These changes are noted as neurofibrillary tangles, neuritic (senile) plaques, Hirano bodies, and granulovacuolar degeneration (Fig. 7-2). The primary hallmark of Alzheimer's disease is the exceptionally large number of neurofibrillary tangles and neuritic plaques found in the brains of patients with Alzheimer's disease.

Hirano bodies and granulovacuolar degeneration are essentially restricted to the pyramidal neurons of the hippocampus. The cytoplasmic inclusions called Hirano bodies appear in several neurodegenerative diseases and may be stained with eosin. Granulovacuolar degeneration appears as a granule contained in a membrane-bound vacuole within the cytoplasm of hippocampal pyramidal neurons (see Fig. 7-2, *F*). The granule is probably the result of abnormalities in the neuronal cytoskeleton.

Granulovacuolar degeneration is restricted to the hippocampus, but significantly higher than normal numbers of another entity associated with abnormalities of the neuronal cytoskeleton serve as one of the truly defining neuropathological markers of Alzheimer's disease. This entity is the neurofibrillary tangle. In addition to the neocortex and the hippocampus, neurofibrillary tangles (see Fig. 7-2, *D* and *E*) occur in subcortical structures such as the anterior nuclei of the thalamus, the noradrenergic locus ceruleus, the serotonergic raphe nuclei, the cholinergic basal nucleus of Meynert, and the amygdala. Neurofibrillary tangles may be visualized in the light microscope with silver stains. They may also be seen as associated with amyloid if stained with Congo red or thioflavin S. In the electron microscope the neurofibrillary tangles are seen to be composed of twisted filaments arranged in pairs called paired helical filaments. Neurofibrillary tangles were formerly thought to be composed of the polypeptides of neurofilaments. However, more recent experiments using molecular biochemical procedures and antibodies raised against isolated paired helical filaments indicate that they are made of accumulations of a microtubule phosphoprotein called tau.

The second microscopic hallmark of Alzheimer's disease is the neuritic, or senile, plaque (see Fig. 7-2). As used here, the term "neurite" refers to any unmyelinated neuronal process and includes dendrites and axon terminals. A long-established plaque may be several hundred

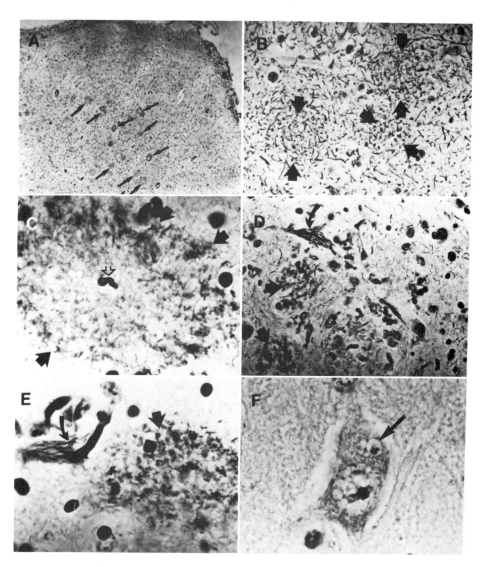

Fig. 7-2. Example of the distribution of senile plaques from the neocortex of a patient in whom Alzheimer's disease has been diagnosed is shown in **A**. This silver-stained tissue demonstrates that the plaques are not spread evenly throughout the cortical layers but are concentrated in layer III. Higher power photomicrographs indicate the appearance of individual plaques (*arrows*), including core material (*open arrow* in **C**). Neurofibrillary tangles (*curved arrows* in **D** and **E**) often may be found in the same area as plaques (*short arrows* in **D** and **E**). Granulovacuolar degeneration appears in hippocampal pyramidal neurons in Alzheimer's disease (*arrow* in **F**) and in other degenerative neurological diseases. This degeneration takes the form of a clear area (vacuole) containing a solid granule. In this type of neuron these elements are immediately adjacent to the cell's nucleus.

micrometers in diameter. Several different components constitute any given plaque. These include a core of extracellular amyloid (see Fig. 7-2, *C*), dystrophic neurites, reactive astrocytic processes, and microglia. Neurochemical analysis reveals that a plaque may contain a variety of neurotransmitters and neuromodulators. The precise complement of these neurochemicals varies from plaque to plaque and probably reflects the content of the neurites, particularly axon terminals contained within the plaque.

Although a significant increase in the number of senile plaques and neurofibrillary tangles found in the brain of a person with Alzheimer's disease as compared to that of an elderly individual without dementia is the defining neuropathological hallmark of Alzheimer's disease, plaques and tangles are not evenly distributed throughout the brain of affected individuals.

HISTOLOGICAL PATTERN OF NEUROPATHOLOGY

As described in Chapter 1, the neurons of the neocortex are arranged in six layers. The layers are designated by Roman numerals, beginning with layer I at the brain's surface. The neurons of each layer have relatively separate connections and functions. The severity of loss of neurons in Alzheimer's disease is not equal across these layers, even in regions of the neocortex such as the entorhinal cortex of the medial temporal lobe, which are severely affected by the disease; nor are plaques and tangles uniformly distributed.

The entorhinal cortex comprises the anterior third of the parahippocampal gyrus overlying the hippocampus and is the origin of neocortical input to the hippocampus. The hippocampus and brain areas associated with it are of particular interest in a discussion of Alzheimer's disease. Degeneration within the entorhinal cortex and degeneration of structures that provide input to it or receive its output are probably responsible for the memory deficits associated with Alzheimer's disease.

Neurofibrillary tangles, senile plaques, and neuron loss frequently occur within the hippocampus and the entorhinal cortex in Alzheimer's disease. However, these neuropathological counterparts of the disease are not generalized throughout the structures. Detailed study of the location of neurofibrillary tangles and neuritic plaques within the hippocampus and entorhinal cortex has revealed that layer II of the entorhinal cortex exhibits a very large number of neurofibrillary tangles and that neuron loss is more severe in these regions than in other parts of the entorhinal cortex. The neurons of layer II give rise to the perforant pathway, which is the major avenue of input to the hippocampus from the neocortex. The axons of this path terminate within the hippocampus primarily on the dendrites of granule cells of the dentate gyrus. In Alzheimer's disease a large number of neuritic plaques are located within this terminal zone. The granule cell neurons show few neurofibrillary tangles, and the pyramidal cells of the hippocampus that receive input from the dentate granule cells demonstrate few pathological signs associated with Alzheimer's disease. However, the parts of the hippocampus that provide its output demonstrate a great number of neurofibrillary tangles. Finally, the target of hippocampal output to the neocortex, layer IV of the entorhinal cortex, contains many neuritic plaques. Neuron layers III, V, and VI of the entorhinal cortex show very few plaques and tangles.

The neuropathological condition associated with Alzheimer's disease selectively attacks only the input and output of the hippocampus. Such selectivity has also been noted in areas of association neocortex affected by Alzheimer's disease where accumulation of plaques and tangles is far more significant in layers III and V than in the other layers. The conclusion to be reached from these anatomical observations is that many of the clinical changes associated with Alzheimer's disease may not be caused by a ubiquitous neuropathological condition, but by a disconnection of functional neurons from other areas with which they normally communicate. Moreover, knowledge of the restricted distribution of neuropathological correlates of Alzheimer's disease must be taken into account in the process of developing hypotheses concerning the pathogenesis of the disease.

NEUROTRANSMITTER LOSS

Various indicators of the activity level and amount of norepinephrine show that this neurotransmitter is reduced in the neocortex of persons with Alzheimer's disease. Further, this reduction appears to correlate with the presence of neurofibrillary tangles in neurons of the locus ceruleus. It seems likely that loss of cortical norepinephrine contributes to the overall decline in cognitive ability in persons with Alzheimer's disease, but the precise contribution to intellectual function of the norepinephrine-containing axons that go from the locus ceruleus to synapse on neocortical neurons is not known.

Some evidence indicates a reduction in cortical activity and content of the neurotransmitter serotonin. However, such changes have not been consistently reported, and a correlation between the loss of serotonergic projections and a pathological condition of the neurons in the raphe nuclei that are the source of the serotonin in the cortex has not been found.

Most peptides found in cortex are thought to be associated with interneurons, and many of these have been studied in the brain of patients with Alzheimer's disease. Although no changes in somatostatin-containing neurons were found in subcortical structures, a substantial reduction in the number of somatostatinergic neurons has been found throughout the cortex of persons with Alzheimer's disease, with the most significant reductions observed in the temporal, frontal, and occipital lobes. This finding suggests a loss of cortical local circuit interneurons in Alzheimer's disease. It is also known that glucose hypometabolism and density of neurofibrillary tangles and neuritic plaques correlate with decreased somatostatin levels. However, the precise contribution of this loss to the clinical symptom complex is not known, and administration of the somatostatin analog octreotide fails to have beneficial clinical effects in patients with Alzheimer's disease.

In addition, some evidence suggests that the amount of cortical substance P, neuropeptide Y, and corticotropin-releasing neurons may be decreased in Alzheimer's disease. These observations have been disputed and need to be confirmed. However, there is no doubt that the number of neurons using the excitatory amino acid transmitters such as glutamate and aspartate is reduced in Alzheimer's disease. The excitatory amino acids presumably serve as transmitters in the corticocortical association pathways and corticofugal pathways such as the perforant pathway. Thus loss of these transmitters reflects loss of the neurons that give rise to these pathways.

The most familiar neurochemical deficit in Alzheimer's disease involves the cholinergic innervation of the cortex. Two enzyme markers, acetylcholinesterase and choline acetyltransferse, are normally used for evaluation of the status of the cholinergic system. There is a significant decline in choline acetyltransferse activity in Alzheimer's disease, whereas histochemical staining for acetylcholinesterase indicates a significant reduction of cholinergic neurons in the nucleus basalis of Meynert. Many, but not all, of the neurons in the nucleus basalis are cholinergic, and these supply the axons of the ascending cholinergic system that innervates the entire cerebral mantle. Loss of this system is thought to be at least partially responsible for the memory impairments associated with Alzheimer's disease. However, many noncholinergic systems are involved in Alzheimer's disease, and, even within the nucleus basalis, neurons that are noncholinergic demonstrate neurofibrillary tangles. Therefore the theory that the cholinergic deficit in Alzheimer's disease is the causal, or even primary, event in the disease needs further testing.

However, the results of recent research indicate that acetycholine may be involved in the genesis of Alzheimer's disease, but in an unexpected way, not entirely predictable from the observation of reduced cholinergic activity in the brains of patients with Alzheimer's disease. Nitsch and his colleagues have demonstrated that activation of two of the four types of cholinergic muscarinic receptors can lead to increased release of beta-amyloid protein (βAP) from cell membranes. The possible role of βAP as a causative agent in the genesis of Alzheimer's disease is discussed in Chapter 6.

REFERENCES

Ball MJ, Lo P: Granulovacuolar degeneration in the aging brain and in dementia, *J Neuropathol Exper Neurol* 36:474-487, 1977.

Beal MF and others: Widespread reduction of somatostatin-like immunoreactivity in the cerebral cortex in Alzheimer's disease, *Ann Neurol* 20:489-495, 1986.

Bowen DM: Neurotransmitters in Alzheimer's disease, *Age* 11:104-110, 1988.

Curcio CA, Kemper T: Nucleus raphe dorsalis in dementia of the Alzheimer type: neurofibrillary changes and neuronal packing density, *J Neuropathol Exper Neurol* 43:359-368, 1984.

Davies P, Malone AJF: Selective loss of central cholinergic neurons in Alzheimer's disease, *Lancet* 2:1403, 1976.

Gibson PH, Tomlinson BE: Numbers of Hirano bodies in hippocampus of normal and demented people with Alzheimer's disease, *J Neurol Sci* 33:199-206, 1977.

Goldman JE: The association of actin with Hirano bodies, *J Neuropathol Exper Neurol* 42:146-152, 1983.

Hirano A: Pathology of amyotropic lateral sclerosis. In Gajdusek DC, Gibbs CJ, Alpers M, editors: Slow, latent and temperate virus infections, *National Institute of Neurological Diseases and Blindness Monograph*, No. 2, 1965, pp. 23-27.

Hyman BT, Van Hoesen GW: Hippocampal and entorhinal cellular pathology in Alzheimer's disease. In Chan-Palay V, Kohler C, editors: *The hippocampus: new vistas*, New York, 1989, Alan R. Liss.

Hyman BT and others: Alzheimer's disease: cell-specific pathology isolates the hippocampal formation, *Science* 225:1168-1170, 1984.

Mouradian MM and others: Somatostatin replacement therapy for Alzheimer dementia, *Ann Neurol* 30:610-613, 1991.

Nakima N, Kosik KS, Selkoe DJ: Recognition of Alzheimer paired helical filaments by monoclonal neurofilament antibodies is due to crossreaction with tau protein, *Proc Natl Acad Sci USA* 84:3415-3419, 1987.

Nitsch RM and others: Release of Alzheimer amyloid precursor derivatives stimulated by activation of muscarinic acetylcholine receptors, *Science* 258:304-307, 1992.

Palmer AM and others: Catecholamineric neurones assessed antemortem in Alzheimer's disease, *Brain Research* 414:365-375, 1987.

Perry EK and others: Neurochemical activities in human temporal lobe related to aging and Alzheimer type changes, *Neurobiol Aging* 2:251-256, 1981.

Price DL and others: Aggregation of tubulin in neurons in Alzheimer's disease, *J Neuropathol Exper Neurol* 44:366, 1985.

Rasool CG, Svedsen CN, Selkoe DJ: Neurofibrillary degeneration of cholinergic and non-cholinergic neurons of the basal forebrain in Alzheimer's disease, *Ann Neurol* 20:482-488, 1986.

Scoville WB, Milner B: Loss of recent memory after bilateral hippocampal lesions, *J Neurol Neurosurg Psychiatry* 20:11-21, 1957.

Selkoe DJ: The molecular pathology of Alzheimer's disease, *Neuron* 6:487-498, 1991.

Selkoe DJ and others: Isolation of low-molecular-weight proteins from amyloid plaque fibers in Alzheimer's disease, *J Neurochem* 146:1820-1834, 1986.

Squire LR, Amaral DG, Press GA: Magnetic resonance imaging of the hippocampal formation and mammillary nuclei distinguish medial temporal lobe and diencephalic amnesia, *J Neurosci* 10:3106-3117, 1990.

Struble RG and others: Hippocampal lesions in dominantly inherited Alzheimer's disease, *J Neuropathol Exper Neurol* 50:82-94, 1991.

Tagliauini G and others: Preamyloid deposits in the cerebral cortex of patients with Alzheimer's disease and nondemented individuals, *Neurosci Lett* 93:191-196, 1988.

Tamminga CA, Foster NL, Chase TN: Reduced brain somatostatin levels in Alzheimer's disease, *N Engl J Med* 313:1294-1295, 1985.

Terry RD: The fine structure of neurofibrillary tangles in Alzheimer's disease, *J Neuropathol Exper Neurol* 22:629-641, 1963.

Trojanowski JQ and others: Human olfactory epithelium in normal aging, Alzheimer's disease, and other neurodegenerative disorders, *J Compar Neurol* 310:365-376, 1991.

Van Hoesen GW, Hyman BT, Damasio AR: Cell-specific pathology in neural systems of the temporal lobe in Alzheimer's disease, *Prog Brain Res* 70:361-375, 1986.

Whitehouse PJ and others: Alzheimer's disease and senile dementia: loss of neurons in the basal forebrain, *Science* 215:1237-1239, 1982.

8

Clinical presentation

Ronald C. Hamdy

In 1907 Dr. Alois Alzheimer described one of the first cases of the disease that now bears his name. Alzheimer, a physician in a German asylum, had noticed that one woman's condition seemed quite different from that of most of the other patients.

The woman was only 51 years old. Her main problems were a very poor memory and a tendency to get lost in the asylum. She was not violent or aggressive, but she needed to be confined because she was unable to look after herself. Alzheimer noted that she had some language impairment, including difficulty finding the right words, and that her comprehension was also impaired. When he examined the patient, Alzheimer could not identify any neurological deficit. Her motor power was good, sensations were normal, and all tendon reflexes were present and within normal limits. The patient's gait and coordination were unremarkable.

Alzheimer followed up on the patient for about 4½ years, until she died after a gradual but relentless deterioration. He performed a postmortem examination and found that her brain was much smaller than the average brain of people of the same sex and age. He also noticed that the ventricles (cavities normally present in the brain) were dilated and much larger than he had expected. It was as if the brain had shrunk and atrophied. A microscopic examination revealed a reduced number of brain cells and numerous neurofibrillary tangles and senile plaques. These findings constitute the characteristic features of Alzheimer's disease.

CLINICAL SYMPTOMS
Memory Deficit

Memory impairment is the hallmark of Alzheimer's disease. However, it is by no means the only characteristic feature, nor is it the most important. Indeed, many conditions apart from Alzheimer's disease can lead to memory impairment. In Alzheimer's disease the memory impairment is associated with evidence of cognitive deficit and impaired judgment, and it has an insidious onset.

Memory has three different modalities: immediate memory (remembering for a few seconds), short-term memory (remembering for a few minutes or hours), and long-term memory (remembering for a few years). Early in Alzheimer's disease, short-term memory is impaired but long-term memory is preserved. Immediate memory is also affected, but this change is probably secondary to a short attention span. The main problem for patients with this disease is the short-term memory impairment, which interferes with their social and professional activities. Learning and recalling new information, both verbal and visuospatial, are gradually reduced.

It is important to differentiate the memory impairment of Alzheimer's disease from that sometimes noted in normal people, which is often called "benign forgetfulness," "benign, senescent forgetfulness," or "age-associated memory impairment." Learning and recalling new information also may decline in normal old age.

The main difference between memory impairment in Alzheimer's disease and benign forgetfulness is that the former is undiscriminating and interferes with the patient's social and professional activities. Benign forgetfulness, on the other hand, usually is sporadic, limited to trivial matters, and does not significantly interfere with the patient's life, apart from causing frustration and irritation (e.g., when a person cannot remember where the keys were left). Unlike memory impairment associated with Alzheimer's disease, that seen in benign forgetfulness usually can be remedied fairly easily, for example, by concentrating and trying to remember or by keeping written records. In Alzheimer's disease, although patients initially may try to overcome their problem by writing down what they want to remember, sooner or later the memory deficit is such that they may forget to check their written record. Patients with Alzheimer's disease have difficulties encoding material to be recalled. Unlike patients with benign forgetfulness, they are not helped by including the target material in stories, by providing a semantic connection between words to be remembered, or by cueing.

Obviously, the degree of impairment necessary to interfere with a patient's social and professional life depends a great deal on the person's activities. This situation can be demonstrated best by comparing two patients of the same age, a housewife and a professional.

The housewife lives with her husband and is dependent on him because she has been crippled with osteoarthritis for many years. She does not need to pay bills or shop. She does some cooking, but her husband makes most of the decisions and does most of the housework. By the time that this woman's memory impairment affects her day-to-day activities, it will be severe. On the other hand, any degree of memory deficit experienced by the professional interferes with that person's professional life. Physicians, pharmacists, attorneys, or accountants, for instance, may find it very difficult to pursue their professional activities with any memory deficit. Even though the degree of mental impairment may be mild, it is constant and sufficient to interfere with the person's professional life and thus must be considered part of a dementia process rather than benign forgetfulness. Whether this process is secondary to Alzheimer's disease or not depends on the rest of the patient's clinical picture and laboratory investigations.

Early in the course of Alzheimer's disease, patients usually are aware of their memory deficit and may make notes to remember important things. Later they may become frightened and apprehensive about their memory problems and may feel depressed and discouraged. As the disease progresses, patients lose insight into their memory deficit and no longer are aware of it. At this point patients must be protected from themselves. For instance, they may try to enter into new business ventures or invest their assets with disastrous results. They may prepare a meal and forget that the stove is on, or they may try to drive, oblivious to the fact that they are becoming lost or are making dangerous errors in judgment.

Inability to Acquire and Process New Information

One of the earliest manifestations of Alzheimer's disease is the inability to acquire and retain new information and to integrate it with previously acquired knowledge. This problem is partly the result of short-term memory impairment and can be readily observed in the difficulty the patient has in keeping abreast of recent developments in his or her profession and an inability to discuss current events. These difficulties often lead the patient to withdraw from discussions revolving around these topics and to appear to have lost interest in them.

Often the first indication that something is wrong occurs when the patient needs to develop new skills at work. For instance, when computerization is introduced in the office or the individual's job is reorganized, he may be unable to adapt to these changes. Consequently his colleagues may think that he is getting old and set in his ways. At this stage the patient may elect to take early retirement or may be assigned a more routine, less demanding job. At this early stage, patients also may appear to have a change in personality. For instance, the keen bridge player may start declining invitations to play the game and may make excuses for not joining his partners. Similarly a golfer may ask a partner to keep the score, or an avid reader may find books "less interesting." At this stage the patient may stop cooking or knitting because of an inability to integrate and process new information.

A sudden change in a person's environment can trigger an episode of severe confusion. The individual suddenly finds himself in a strange place and is unable to remember how he got there. For instance, during a stay in a hotel or a visit with his children, a man may wake up in the middle of the night and be totally disoriented and confused. As a result, he becomes agitated. In the early stages of Alzheimer's disease, this type of state does not last long. With explanations and reassurance, the patient soon becomes reoriented, alert, and rational.

Language Difficulties

Language difficulties are present at the earliest stages of the disease. Initially they may be so subtle as not to be readily apparent to most observers, even professional ones, and can be detected only by neuropsychological tests (e.g., a word list generation, in which the subject is asked to list words in a specific group, such as animals, plants, or fruits beginning with the same letter). As the disease progresses, these language deficits become more marked and are readily noticed by most observers, even lay people.

Anomia, the inability to find the right word, is a characteristic feature of Alzheimer's disease. At first the patient usually is aware of these deficits and may try to make up for them by using sentences to describe the object he cannot name (paraphrasia). Thus in the very early stages of Alzheimer's disease, the patient's speech becomes picturesque and interesting as he attempts to overcome the problems of anomia. In the early stages of the disease, the anomia is confined to objects that the patient does not come into contact with on a regular basis. As the condition worsens, however, anomia also includes common objects. The patient recognizes these objects but is unable to recall their name. For instance, when shown a key, the patient recognizes it, knows what it is used for, and can use it, but he cannot think of the word "key." It is interesting that in Alzheimer's original description his patient was unable to recall the word "jug" and instead said "pourer." Rather than referring to the "milk jug," she said "milk pourer."

As the disease progresses, agnosia sets in. Agnosia is more serious than anomia because, in addition to being unable to name an object, the person cannot identify it. For instance, he may not recognize a key; he may think it is a spoon and try to eat soup with it. Alternatively the patient may think that a knife is a comb and may attempt to comb his hair with the knife. On a more personal level, patients may not recognize people they have not seen for a long time. For example, they may confuse their grandchildren with their children or their children with their siblings. As the disease progresses, patients may not recognize their spouse or other close relatives and often accuse them of being intruders. This development is a traumatic experience for the caregivers. One of my patients thought that her only son was her husband. She regularly made sexual advances to him and demanded that they sleep together. This situation was very distressing to the son, who developed severe depression and even contemplated suicide.

As the agnosia becomes more extensive, the patient cannot use sensory information to recognize objects or people. With time, the anomia also becomes more noticeable, and the paraphrasia becomes less related to the target word and more rambling. At this stage conversation becomes very difficult. This situation is worsened by the patient's inability to concentrate for normal periods. Often words and themes related to previous discussions and unrelated to the present conversation intrude. As a result, the listener is unable to follow any coherent train of thought.

Aphasia develops later. This impairment in language prevents the patient from understanding what he hears, from following instructions, and from communicating needs (e.g., the need to go to the toilet or being in pain). This situation is distressing to the patient and trying to the caregivers, who now must guess what the patient's needs are. As the disease progresses, spontaneous speech deteriorates. The patient tends to repeat words and questions (echolalia) without making any effort to answer the questions. With further deterioration the patient repeats one word (paralalia) or the first syllable of a word (logoconia) again and again. In the advanced stage of the disease, speech becomes unintelligible, and eventually complete mutism occurs.

Impaired Visuospatial Skills and Apraxia

Apraxia, the inability to carry out purposeful movements and actions despite intact motor and sensory systems, is evident early in the course of Alzheimer's disease, but patients and relatives often do not connect it with the disease. In the early stages, for instance, a patient may be unable to lace his shoes but still be able to put on loafers or boots. He may attribute this inability to tie the laces to "lack of practice." In fact, the impairment represents an early stage of apraxia.

The patient may be unable to adjust the controls of the video recorder and the television set simultaneously, although he may still be able to adjust each independently. In other words, the more complex or technical skills, particularly those recently acquired or requiring integration of various stimuli, are lost early in the process. The "automatic" actions, such as eating, walking, dressing, and undressing, tend to be preserved until the late stages. This discrepancy exists because the complex and technical skills are controlled mainly by the cerebral cortex, whereas the control of automatic actions is relegated to the basal ganglia.

Impaired visuospatial skills may be the reason a patient becomes lost in familiar surroundings or while driving a car. In the latter instance, however, the inability to integrate new information and to make rational decisions also plays an important part.

Apraxia often becomes a source of frustration: minor tasks that the patient once performed easily become major tasks involving almost insurmountable obstacles. The patient does not understand what is happening or how or why he is losing control over his environment. This situation often leads to discouragement and depression. For instance, when asked to set the table, the patient is faced with so many choices (knives, forks, spoons, plates, glasses) and so many alternative positions for the items that he may not be able to tackle this "complex" task. On the other hand, if given only a knife, a fork, and a plate, he may be able to cope with this limited choice and arrange them adequately on the table.

As the disease progresses, simply getting dressed becomes an impossible task. The patient may see his shirt and recognize the front, back, left, and right sides, but he is unable to translate these stimuli and coordinate his movements accordingly to put the right sleeve of his shirt on his right arm while keeping the top part of the shirt up and its front on his chest.

Poor Judgment

Sooner or later the patient's ability to use correct judgment deteriorates. This development is often the point at which relatives recognize the disease. They no longer consider the person odd or eccentric but realize that something is seriously wrong. This situation occurs when the patient pays the same bill twice, does not pay some bills, or cannot balance his checkbook. Difficulty in managing finances is one of the most common reasons relatives insist that a person seek medical attention and is often the first indication of cognitive deficit. The inability to manage one's finances is one of the most common presenting symptoms of Alzheimer's disease.

Poor judgment also may be reflected when the patient makes a large donation to a charity after watching a television commercial sponsored by a charitable organization or after speaking to unscrupulous representatives of such an organization. Sometimes the patient may start buying unnecessary items or giving extravagant gifts.

Self-Neglect

Another degree of mental impairment is reached when, in addition to impaired memory and impaired judgment, the patient shows evidence of carelessness, particularly self-neglect. One of the earliest manifestations is that patients stop taking pride in the impression they make. This very useful sign can be appreciated by looking at the patient's general appearance. For instance, if a patient makes no attempt to comb her hair and if her dress is stained or torn, in the absence of physical incapacitation, the caregiver can assume that self-neglect is present.

In hospitals and nursing homes this carelessness and self-neglect can be recognized easily by asking the patient to get up from her chair and take a few steps. If after standing up the patient adjusts her clothes before walking or makes sure that her hospital gown is properly closed and that her genital area is not exposed, then she is aware of her body image and cares about the impression she projects in public. A patient with Alzheimer's disease, when asked to stand up and walk, may do so without realizing that her hospital gown is wide open at the back. She would probably walk the length of the room without making any effort to cover her back and without showing any signs of embarrassment; in fact, she is not aware of and does not care about the image she projects in public.

Personality Changes

Changes in personality are often seen in patients with Alzheimer's disease, and they can be severe. These changes include self-centeredness, withdrawal, increased passivity, and agitation. At least half of the patients with this condition develop delusions of persecution, including infidelity and fear of theft or harm.

Mood changes also have been described in patients with Alzheimer's disease. These changes are manifested by loss of interest, loss of energy, and depressed mood in the early stages, although insight is retained.

Behavioral Problems

Aberrant behavior is almost always distressing to both caregivers and patients. Such behavior may include stubbornness, resistance to care, suspicion of others, use of abusive language, acting in response to delusions or hallucinations, rummaging through other people's rooms, "stealing," hiding articles, urinating in inappropriate places, and angry outbursts ("catastrophic reactions") precipitated by apparently trivial events.

These abnormal behavioral patterns often are the reason that caregivers seek institutionalization for the patient. Ironically, these same behaviors frequently are the reason nursing homes refuse to admit patients with Alzheimer's disease, on the grounds that such behavior would disrupt the harmony of the institution, could be offensive and dangerous to other residents, and could lead to litigation. Because of this aberrant behavior, patients with Alzheimer's disease often are prescribed potent sedatives and tranquilizers and are physically restrained.

Restlessness, aimless wandering, and reversal of the sleep/wake cycle are often seen in patients with Alzheimer's disease and frequently put the patient at risk of self-injury.

Patients with this condition sometimes engage in asocial sexual behavior, such as masturbating in front of others. Although this is distressing to caregivers, especially the patient's children, there is no evidence that patients with dementia pose a sexual threat to others.

Physical Deterioration

Most patients with Alzheimer's disease remain physically well until the late stages of the disease. They gradually become more unsteady, may experience repeated falls, and tend to spend more time sitting in a chair or lying in bed. As time goes by, they develop generalized muscle rigidity. Later they become bedridden, assume the fetal position, and often become incontinent of urine and feces. Grasping and sucking reflexes are often seen in the late stages of the disease. Seizures and myoclonus affect about 10% of the patients in late-stage disease. The three most common causes of death in these patients are pneumonia, urinary tract infection, and infected decubitus ulcers.

CLINICAL STAGES

At present, Alzheimer's disease is an irreversible, gradually progressive condition associated with relentless deterioration. In the earliest stage the patient may exhibit only minimal memory impairment and cognitive deficit. In the last stage the patient is commonly bedridden in the fetal position, doubly incontinent, and mute. Several classifications have been developed for categorizing patients according to stage. Although these classifications are useful for determining the level of care a patient needs and for comparing groups of patients with one another, they are not truly useful as prognostic indicators because of the great variability in the rate of deterioration exhibited by different patients. However, usually the younger the patient is when the disease manifests itself, the faster will be its rate of progression. Similarly, when there is a strong family history of Alzheimer's disease, the rate of progress tends to be more rapid than if no such history exists.

The two classifications most widely used involve three stages and seven stages. It is important to realize that both classifications are arbitrary and that there is a great deal of overlap among the various stages. Furthermore, not all patients go through all these stages. It also must be emphasized that a rapid rate of deterioration is often caused by other diseases or factors (see Chapter 10).

Alzheimer's disease has a very insidious onset and a slow, relentless progress. One of the best indicators of these two aspects of the disease is the inability of the patient's relatives to agree on a specific date when the symptoms started to manifest themselves. For instance, the patient's daughter may think it was last Christmas, whereas his wife may believe that the patient's condition started to deteriorate much earlier. In contrast to strokes of multiinfarct dementia, no one can pinpoint an exact date or time when the disease manifested itself or the patient's condition suddenly deteriorated.

For practical purposes, the three-stage classification is preferred because the characteristic features of each stage are easier to recognize and the needs of the patient in each stage are so different.

Stage 1

Stage 1, which lasts between 1 and 3 years, is characterized by the following signs:

- Poor recent memory
- Impaired acquisition of new information
- Mild anomia
- Minimal visuospatial impairment
- Personality change

The patient may appear "normal" to people who do not know him. However, the patient's immediate contacts know that there has been a change in his behavior, personality, and intellectual functioning. This stage is a difficult period because the patient still has some insight into his condition and yet cannot understand or cope with the complexity of his situation. At times the patient may rebel and refuse to accept the implications of his condition; at other times he may realize that he is fighting a losing battle and become depressed and irritable or withdraw into apathy.

This stage can be particularly taxing for the patient's family. On one hand, they understand and appreciate the patient's actions; on the other, they question the validity of his judgment and yet do not want to appear to question or doubt his integrity, intentions, and ability to look after his family. Such a situation may require professional intervention to safeguard the family's financial assets.

A particularly difficult problem concerns the patient's ability to drive a motor vehicle. Driving is a symbol of independence and may be the person's only means of transportation. However, while driving, the patient may make serious mistakes that could endanger himself or others. In addition to having poor judgment, many patients with Alzheimer's disease have a slow reaction time and may be easily distracted, both of which make driving hazardous.

Toward the end of stage 1, memory impairment and impaired ability to make rational decisions often cause the patient to become lost even in familiar surroundings. This development is another trau-

Table 8-1 Stages of Alzheimer's disease

	Duration (yr)	Characteristics
Stage 1	1-3	Poor recent memory
		Impaired acquisition of new information
		Mild anomia
		Minimal visuospatial impairment
		Personality change
Stage 2	2-10	Profound memory loss
		Significant impairment of other cognitive parameters
		Severe impairment of judgment
Stage 3	8-12	Severe impairment of all cognitive functions
		Physical impairment: unsteadiness, repeated falls, reduced mobility
		Loss of ability to care for oneself

matic and stressful experience for the patient's relatives. For example, a man goes to a store one block away to buy something, and 2 hours later he has not returned. Five hours later the police call his wife to tell her that they have found her husband a few miles away.

It is understandable that a patient's relatives may be reluctant to take away his sense of initiative and independence by confining him indoors. Yet, whenever he leaves home, they worry that he may become lost, be mugged, or be involved in an accident. Often the relatives resort to writing their address and phone number on a card and leaving it in one of the patient's pockets.

Patients with Alzheimer's disease can become lost because they may not recognize familiar signs. Since they do not know where they are, they start to panic. When they panic, their judgment becomes even more impaired and they may not be able to retrace their steps. Although stress may sharpen a normal person's mental abilities, in a patient with dementia, it can lead to severe confusion.

In the first stage of Alzheimer's disease, the clinical examination is essentially within normal limits, although some patients have a reduced sense of smell. Although the computed tomography (CT) scan, the magnetic resonance imaging scan, and the electroencephalogram (EEG) are usually essentially normal, single photon emission tomography is often abnormal (see Chapter 4).

Stage 2

Stage 2 lasts between 2 and 10 years and is characterized by the following signs:
- Profound memory loss, both remote and recent
- Significant impairment of other cognitive parameters, as evidenced by two or more of these symptoms: anomia, agnosia, apraxia, and aphasia
- Severe impairment of judgment

In stage 2 the anomia and agnosia become much more pronounced and interfere with the patient's daily activities. These signs can be recognized by people who are meeting the patient for the first time. Later in this stage the patient may develop significant apraxia, which leaves him unable to perform simple tasks such as feeding or washing himself, even though he has no muscle weakness or coordination difficulties.

At this stage patients with Alzheimer's disease tend to become very restless. They often are seen pacing the room or walking outside as if constantly searching for something. They do not like to stay in one place and want to keep moving.

The patient's personality, which in the first stage was variable, now is mostly apathetic. The individual has no insight into his condition and does not seem bothered by his relatives' distress over it. This lack of insight is exemplified by the patient's denial of problems with his memory despite evidence of profound memory loss. If confronted with the fact that his memory is poor, the patient usually makes some excuse, such as that he was not really paying attention, that he is getting old, or that he has other things to remember and cannot be bothered with such details.

The patient may make "near misses." For instance, when asked which day of the week it is, he may say that the day is Monday (rather than Tuesday). When corrected, he may question the relevance of today being Tuesday rather than Monday. If an examiner asks him to remember three or four objects, he may question the importance of being able to do so. In contrast, patients suffering from depression readily acknowledge problems with their memory; rather than making near misses, they refuse to cooperate with an examiner.

In stage 2, a CT scan usually shows evidence of brain atrophy an ventricular dilation. The EEG also may be abnormal and may shov generalized slowing of the waves.

Stage 3

Stage 3, which lasts between 8 and 12 years, is notable for th following features:
- Severe impairment of all cognitive functions
- Physical impairment involving unsteadiness, repeated falls, re duced mobility
- Total loss of ability to care for oneself

Gross intellectual impairment is obvious at this stage. For exam ple, a patient may not recognize his wife and children and may confus them with his parents. Complete disorientation to time, place, an other individuals is evident, and the patient cannot cope with his basi needs. As the condition progresses, complete mutism may occur an motor deficits may become apparent. The patient may develop gen eralized muscular rigidity, and his mobility may be grossly reduced

In contrast to stage 2, in which the patient wandered constantly he now spends most of the time sitting in a chair or lying in bed. Ar attitude of generalized flexion gradually is adopted, with the patien lying curled up in bed. Eventually the patient assumes the fetal posi tion. At this stage urinary (and sometimes fecal) incontinence may develop. The CT scan shows gross atrophy and ventricular dilation and the EEG shows slow waves.

Staging of Patients

In general, stages proceed according to a pattern. In the first stage memory is impaired, but other cognitive deficits are minimal and easily overlooked. In the second stage there is also evidence of gross deficits in other cognitive fields. In the third stage, besides the severe intellectual deterioration, physical deficits become apparent.

CAUSE OF DEATH

The usual cause of death is not Alzheimer's disease itself. Instead, it is septicemia that is a complication of pneumonia, urinary tract infection, or infected decubitus ulcers. Decubitus ulcers are very likely to develop unless pressure areas are given special care.

Although Alzheimer's disease is characteristically irreversible and slowly progressive, it often is punctuated by sudden bouts of reversible deterioration caused by other diseases or factors apart from Alzheimer's disease (see Chapter 10).

BIBLIOGRAPHY

Bennett DA, Evans DA: Alzheimer's disease, *Dis Mon* 38:1-64, 1992.

Bucht G, Sandman PO: Nutritional aspects of dementia, especially Alzheimer's disease, *Age Ageing* 19(4):S32-S36, 1990.

Donnelly RE, Karlinsky H: The impact of Alzheimer's disease on driving ability: a review, *J Geriatr Psychiatry Neurol* 3(2):67-72, 1990.

Fabiszewski KJ: Alzheimer's disease: overview and progression, *J Adv Med Surg Nurs* 1:1-17, 1989.

Galasko D, Corey-Bloom J, Thal LJ: Monitoring progression in Alzheimer's disease, *J Am Geriatr Soc* 39:932-941, 1991.

Gauthier L, Gauthier S: Assessment of functional changes in Alzheimer's disease, *Neuroepidemiology* 9:183-188, 1990.

Heston LL: Alzheimer's disease: the end of the beginning? *Psychol Med* 20:7-10, 1990.

Katzman R, Jackson JE: Alzheimer disease: basic and clinical advances, *J Am Geriatr Soc* 39:516-525, 1991.

Kluger A, Ferris SH: Scales for the assessment of Alzheimer's disease, *Psychiatr Clin North Am* 14:309-326, 1991.

Larson EB, Kukull WA, Katzman RL: Cognitive impairment: dementia and Alzheimer's disease, *Annu Rev Public Health* 13:431-449, 1992.

Lecso PA: Murder-suicide in Alzheimer's disease, *J Am Geriatr Soc* 37:167-168, 1989.

Lee VK: Language changes and Alzheimer's disease: a literature review, *J Gerontol Nurs* 17(1):16-20, 1991.

Lehmann HD: The puzzle of Alzheimer's disease (AD), *Med Hypotheses* 38:5-10, 1992.

Maas ML, Buckwalter KC: Alzheimer's disease, *Annu Rev Nurs Res* 9:19-55, 1991.

Mendez MF, Tomsak RL, Remler B: Disorders of the visual system in Alzheimer's disease, *J Clin Neuro Ophthalmol* 10:62-69, 1990.

Mohr E, Mann UM, Chase TN: Subgroups in Alzheimer's disease: fact or fiction? *Psychiatr J Univ Ottawa* 15:203-206, 1990.

Morris JC, Rubin EH: Clinical diagnosis and course of Alzheimer's disease, *Psychiatr Clin North Am* 14:223-236, 1991.

Nebes RD: Semantic memory in Alzheimer's disease, *Psychol Bull* 106:377-394, 1989.

Reisberg B and others: The stage-specific temporal course of Alzheimer's disease: functional and behavioral concomitants based upon cross-sectional and longitudinal observation, *Prog Clin Biol Res* 317:23-41, 1989.

Ship JA: Oral health of patients with Alzheimer's disease, *J Am Dent Assoc* 123:53-58, 1992.

St George-Hyslop PH and others: Familial Alzheimer's disease: progress and problems, *Neurobiol Aging* 10:417-425, 1989.

Swartz KP and others: Does the melody linger on? Music cognition in Alzheimer's disease, *Semin Neurol* 9:152-158, 1989.

Teri L, Wagner A: Alzheimer's disease and depression, *J Consult Clin Psychol* 60:379-391, 1992.

Vitiello MV, Poceta JS, Prinz PN: Sleep in Alzheimer's disease and other dementing disorders, *Can J Psychol* 45:221-239, 1991.

Vitiello MV, Prinz PN: Alzheimer's disease: sleep and sleep/wake patterns, *Clin Geriatr Med* 5:289-299, 1989.

9

Clinical diagnosis

James M. Turnbull

From 1990 to 1992, more than 250 articles dealing with the subject of diagnosis in Alzheimer's disease appeared in scientific journals. Despite tremendous scientific interest and research, the diagnosis of this disease remains a clinical one before death. There are no specific antemortem markers for it.

In 1984 a work group on the diagnosis of Alzheimer's disease was established by the National Institute of Neurological and Communicative Disorders and Strokes (NINCDS) and the Alzheimer's Disease and Related Disorders Association (ADRDA). The clinical criteria for the diagnosis of probable, possible, and definite Alzheimer's disease were outlined. The diagnosis of probable Alzheimer's disease, it was stated, could be made with confidence if the dementia has a typical insidious onset with progression and no other systemic or brain diseases that could account for the progressive memory and other cognitive deficits are present. Using the criteria for probable Alzheimer's disease, Burns and his colleagues at the Institute of Psychiatry in London were able to predict accurately (as confirmed by autopsy) the presence of the disease in 88% of 50 patients. The diagnosis of definite Alzheimer's disease requires histopathological confirmation at the time of autopsy.

Among the disorders that must be excluded are major depression, Parkinson's disease, multiinfarct dementia, drug intoxication, thyroid disease, vitamin B_{12} deficiency, subdural hematoma, occult hydrocephalus, Huntington's disease, brain tumors, and chronic infections of the nervous system. The criteria for clinical diagnosis of Alzheimer's disease are shown in the box on p. 118.

The information needed to make the clinical diagnosis depends on the patient's medical history; neurological, psychiatric, and clinical examinations; neuropsychological tests; and laboratory studies.

CRITERIA FOR CLINICAL DIAGNOSIS OF ALZHEIMER'S DISEASE

1. The criteria for the clinical diagnosis of *probable* Alzheimer's disease include:
   - Dementia established by clinical examination and documented by the Mini Mental Test, Blessed Dementia Scale, or some similar examination and confirmed by neuropsychological tests
   - Deficits in two or more areas of recognition
   - Progressive worsening of memory and other cognitive functions
   - No disturbance of consciousness
   - Onset between ages 40 and 90, most often after age 65
   - Absence of systemic disorders or other brain diseases that in and of themselves could account for the progressive deficits in memory and cognition
2. The diagnosis of *probable* Alzheimer's disease is supported by:
   - Progressive deterioration of specific cognitive functions, such as language (aphasia), motor skills (apraxia), and perception (agnosia)
   - Impaired activities of daily living and altered patterns of behavior
   - Family history of similar disorders, particularly if confirmed neuropathologically
   - Laboratory results of normal lumbar puncture as evaluated by standard techniques
   - Normal pattern of nonspecific changes in EEG, such as increased slow-wave activity
   - Evidence of cerebral atrophy on CT scan with progression documented by serial observation
3. Other clinical features consistent with the diagnosis of *probable* Alzheimer's disease, after exclusion of causes of dementia and other than Alzheimer's disease, include:
   - Plateaus in the course of progress of the illness
   - Associated symptoms of depression; insomnia; incontinence; delusions; illusions; hallucinations; catastrophic verbal, emotional, or physical outbursts; sexual disorders; and weight loss
   - Other neurological abnormalities in some patients, especially with more advanced disease and including motor signs such as increased muscle tone, myoclonus, or gait disorder
   - Seizures in advanced disease
   - CT scan normal for age
4. Features that make the diagnosis of *probable* Alzheimer's disease uncertain or unlikely include:
   - Sudden, apoplectic onset
   - Focal neurological findings such as hemiparesis, sensory loss, visual field deficits
   - Incoordination early in the course of the illness
   - Seizures or gait disturbances at the onset of, or very early in, the course of the illness

Modified from McKhann G and others: *Neurology* 34:939-943, 1984.

MEDICAL HISTORY

It is paramount that information about the patient's medical history be obtained not only from the patient but also from a collateral who knows the person well. This approach is essential to establish a history that demonstrates that the person has progressively deteriorated and to identify tasks that the patient can no longer perform adequately (e.g., those requiring sequential steps). The history may disclose difficulties that the person has with memory, problems with activities of daily living, alterations in mood, delusions, and illusions. The collateral will often be able to identify the fact that the affected individual forgets appointments and errands or is unable to find his way to an accustomed destination. They may report that the person is unable to use money and instruments of daily living such as the telephone. Other difficulties, as described throughout this book, will often be present.

Probably the most important part of the clinical examination is the mental status testing. This testing includes assessment of orientation, registration, attention, calculation, recent recall, comprehension, reading and writing, and the ability to draw or copy designs. Quantitative aids to the clinical examination include the Mini Mental State Examination (see box on p. 120), the Blessed Dementia Scale (see box on p. 121), the Functional Dementia Scale (see box on p. 122), or the Hachinski Ischemic Scale (see box on p. 123) for estimating the likelihood of multiinfarct dementia. The psychiatric evaluation excludes various psychiatric disorders such as major depression, bipolar disorder, and schizophrenia.

The physical examination concentrates on examination of the sensory and motor systems in order to exclude other neurological disorders such as Parkinson's disease and Huntington's disease.

DIFFERENTIAL DIAGNOSIS

The differential diagnosis of Alzheimer's disease can be remembered by using the mnemonic DEMENTIA.

D—Drugs and Alcohol

In the evaluation of a person who is confused and suffering from memory loss, the first consideration should be any drugs that the individual is taking. One drug that frequently is overlooked in the elderly is alcohol. A significant number of people, particularly men, become alcoholic after they retire. These individuals may have been

MINI-MENTAL STATUS EXAMINATION

Examiner_____   Date_____

Instructions: Check items answered correctly. Write incorrect or unusual answers in space provided. If necessary, urge patient once to complete task.

Introduction to patient: "I would like to ask you a few questions. Some you will find very easy and others may be very hard. Just do your best."

1. What day of the week is this? _____
2. What month? _____
3. What day of the month? _____
4. What year? _____
5. What place is this? _____
6. Repeat these numbers: 8, 7, 2. _____
7. Say them backwards. _____
8. Repeat these numbers: 6, 3, 7, 1. _____
9. Listen to these numbers: 6, 9, 4. Count 1 through 10 out loud, then repeat 6, 9, 4. (Help if needed. Then use numbers 5, 7, 3). _____
10. Listen to these numbers: 8, 1, 4, 3. Count 1 through 10 out loud, then repeat 8, 1, 4, 3. _____
11. Beginning with Sunday, say the days of the week backwards. _____
12. 9 + 3 is: _____
13. Add 6 (to the previous answer or "to 12"). _____
14. Take away 5 ("from 18"). Repeat these words after me and remember them. I will ask for them later: Hat, Car, Tree, Twenty-six. _____

15. The opposite of fast is slow. The opposite of up is: _____
16. The opposite of large is: _____
17. The opposite of hard is: _____
18. An orange and a banana are both fruits. Red and blue are both: _____
19. A penny and a dime are both: _____
20. What were those words I asked you to remember? (Hat) _____
21. (Car) _____
22. (Tree) _____
23. (Twenty-six) _____
24. Take away 7 from 100. Then take away 7 from what is left and keep going −100 − 7 is: _____
25. Minus 7 _____
26. Minus 7 (write down answers: check correct subtraction of 7) _____
27. Minus 7 _____
28. Minus 7 _____
29. Minus 7 _____
30. Minus 7 _____
TOTAL CORRECT (maximum score is 30). _____

Patient's occupation (previous, if not employed)_____

Education _____ Age_____

Circle estimated intelligence (based on education, occupation, and history, not on test score)

Below average   Average   Above average

Patient was: Cooperative_____
Uncooperative _____ Depressed_____
Lethargic _____ Other_____

Medical diagnosis:_____

Modified from Jacobs et al.: *Ann Intern Med* 86:40, 1977.

BLESSED DEMENTIA SCALE

1. Inability to perform household tasks
2. Inability to cope with small sums of money
3. Inability to remember short lists of items
4. Inability to find way outdoors
5. Inability to find way about familiar streets
6. Inability to interpret surroundings
7. Inability to recall recent events
8. Tendency to dwell in the past
9. Eating:
   Messily, with spoon only
   Simple solids, such as biscuits (2 points)
   Has to be fed (3 points)
10. Dressing:
    Occasionally misplaced buttons, etc.
    Wrong sequence, forgets items (2 points)
    Unable to dress (3 points)
11. Sphincter control:
    Occasional wet bed
    Frequent wet bed (2 points)
    Doubly incontinent (3 points)
12. Increased rigidity
13. Increased egocentricity
14. Impairment of regard for feelings of others
15. Coarsening of affect
16. Impairment of emotional control
17. Hilarity in inappropriate situations
18. Diminished emotional responsiveness
19. Sexual misdemeanor (de novo in old age)
20. Hobbies relinquished
21. Diminished initiative or growing apathy
22. Purposeless hyperactivity

TOTAL SCORE_____

Scores range from 0 to 27. The higher the score, the greater the degree of dementia. Each item scores 1 except the items noted. A second part is the Information Score and contains items testing orientation and memory.

Modified from *Br J Psychiatry* 114:808, 1968. In Gallo JJ, Reichel W, Anderson L: Handbook of geriatric assessment, Rockville, Md, 1988, Aspen Publishers.

FUNCTIONAL DEMENTIA SCALE

1. Has difficulty in completing simple tasks on own, such as dressing, bathing, arithmetic
2. Spends time either sitting or in apparently purposeless activity
3. Wanders at night or needs to be restrained to prevent wandering
4. Hears things that are not there
5. Requires supervision or assistance in eating
6. Loses things
7. Appearance is disorderly if left to own devices
8. Moans
9. Cannot control bowel function
10. Threatens to harm others
11. Cannot control bladder function
12. Needs to be watched so does not injure self, such as by careless smoking, leaving the stove on, falling
13. Destructive of materials within reach, such as breaks furniture, throws food trays, tears up magazines
14. Shouts or yells
15. Accuses others of doing him or her bodily harm or stealing possessions when you are sure the accusations are not true
16. Is unaware of limitations imposed by illness
17. Becomes confused and does not know where he or she is
18. Has trouble remembering
19. Has sudden changes of mood, such as gets upset, angered, or cries easily
20. If left alone, wanders aimlessly during the day or needs to be restrained to prevent wandering
    Each item is rated by the caregiver as follows: none or little of the time, some of the time, a good part of the time, or most or all of the time.

Modified from Moore J et al: *J Fam Pract* 16:503, 1983. In Gallo JJ, Reichel W, Anderson L: *Handbook of geriatric assessment*, Rockville, Md, 1988, Aspen Publishers.

drinkers who had stopped drinking because they were afraid they would not be able to keep to their work schedule, or they may have drunk excessively on Friday or Saturday nights. Now that they do not need to go to work, they may start drinking earlier and earlier in the day. Some people adopt this behavior partly to drive away the symptoms of depression. However, over time, alcohol aggravates depression. Another reason people drink excessively after retirement is boredom. Depression and boredom are two real problems for many

---

HACHINSKI ISCHEMIC SCALE

1. Abrupt onset (2)
2. Stepwise deterioration (1)
3. Fluctuating course (2)
4. Nocturnal confusion (1)
5. Relative preservation of personality (1)
6. Depression (1)
7. Somatic complaints (1)
8. Emotional incontinence (1)
9. History of hypertension (1)
10. History of strokes (2)
11. Evidence of associated atherosclerosis (1)
12. Focal neurological symptoms (2)
13. Focal neurological signs (2)
    The score for each feature is noted in parentheses. A score of greater than 7 suggests a vascular component to the dementia.

Modified from *Arch Neurol* 32:634, 1975. In Gallo JJ, Reichel W, Anderson L: *Handbook of geriatric assessment*, Rockville, Md, 1988, Aspen Publishers

individuals who have not planned for retirement. Thus a history of the patient's use of alcohol is always important. Since patients often deny drinking excessively, relatives should be asked about indirect evidence, such as empty bottles found in the garbage can or bottles hidden around the house.

Most of the other drugs a patient might be taking are either prescribed or bought over the counter. Over-the-counter drugs frequently are not included in the drug history because many elderly people do not consider such drugs medication. Yet the elderly are the largest single group of purchasers of such drugs, which include sleeping pills, laxatives, antihistamines, tonics, and antacids.

Many prescribed drugs cause confusion in the elderly. Particular offenders are psychoactive medications (drugs that affect the mind), such as neuroleptic drugs, benzodiazepines, antidepressants, lithium, and hypnotic drugs. Such drugs have a prolonged action, especially in older patients because of the impaired functioning of their liver and kidneys. There also is evidence that the brain of older individuals is more sensitive to these drugs.

In a great number of nursing homes, many residents take tranquilizers, although this practice often is for the convenience of the staff rather than for the benefit of the resident. For example, many residents may have watched late-night television before entering the nursing home; however, institutional rules demand that residents retire at 9 PM. The medication is prescribed to ensure that residents will be ready to retire at this hour, as well as for other reasons. The ensuing sedation produces a state referred to as "mashed potato syndrome," so called because the resident is taking so many neuroleptic drugs that when lunch is served, the person falls face first into his mashed potatoes.

In one case a man was referred to a geriatric outreach program because two women had seen him standing naked on the balcony of an apartment building at 2 PM in midwinter. The women complained that he was a "flasher." The social worker and the physician who went to the apartment to investigate found an 80-year-old man sitting in almost total darkness with all the shades drawn. His medicine cabinet revealed that he was taking amitriptyline (Elavil), imipramine (Tofranil), haloperidol (Haldol), thioridazine (Mellaril), promazine (Sparine, which has been removed from the market), chlorpromazine (Thorazine), and diazepam (Valium).

The physician put all the drugs on the kitchen table and asked, "Now, Mr. Jones, which of these medications do you take?" Mr. Jones replied, "It depends on how I feel." The physician then asked, "Which ones did you take today?" The patient replied, "I took one of these, but I don't remember. I think I took two of the other ones because they work really good and help me, and I took one of the blue ones." The label on one of the containers revealed that the prescription had been written by a physician who had been dead for 5 years and was dead at the time the prescription was refilled. The prescription read, "Valium 5 mg q.i.d., ad lib," meaning that the prescription could be refilled an unlimited number of times, even after the physician's death.

Mr. Jones had seen several physicians since his doctor had died, but he had never been asked what medications he was taking or what drugs he had at home. He had never been instructed to throw away the old medication when a new one was added. This man's confusion was cured by discontinuing all his medication.

It is also important to remember that some elderly patients borrow drugs from their neighbors. A 75-year-old man was seen in psychiatric consultation in a local hospital because of confusion that had begun in the previous 5 days. He was unable to answer questions, was confused and delusional, and looked very ill. He was totally disoriented. Despite an intensive workup, which included a computed tomographic (CT) scan of the head, lumbar puncture, and electroencephalogram (EEG), no cause could be found for his delirium. The patient was thought to have Alzheimer's disease, and a psychiatric consultation was requested. While this consultation was taking place, a neighbor who knew the patient well entered the room and was asked what she thought had happened to him. She said that the patient had been borrowing pills from her "for swelling of the ankles." Because one pill did not work, he had taken two and ended up taking three a day. It was discovered that the patient had borrowed a form of digitalis and was suffering from digitalis toxicity.

Many elderly people never throw away old medications because they are so expensive. Consequently, as in the case of Mr. Jones, these individuals may still be using medications that were prescribed months or years earlier without informing their current physician. Elderly patients should be encouraged to show their physicians all the medications they are taking, including over-the-counter drugs, and physicians should be diligent in questioning patients about their medications.

E—Eyes and Ears

Some people appear confused because they cannot hear or see well. Out of self-consciousness they often pretend that they can hear and may answer questions with totally irrelevant responses, thus giving the impression of having dementia. Also, some elderly people may be too vain to wear a hearing aid, and they may need to be confronted with the reality of their hearing problem to be convinced of their need for such an aid.

One such person was a psychiatrist in his eighties who was a close friend of mine. He did not want anyone to know he could not hear, yet whenever anyone had a conversation with him, particularly in a restaurant or other noisy place, he could not understand what was being said unless the speaker shouted. One day I said to him, "Everybody thinks you have Alzheimer's disease. You appear demented simply because you won't wear your hearing aid." From that time on, he wore the hearing aid.

The other sensory area that is affected by aging is eyesight. When people start losing their vision, they may bump into things while walking across a room, making them appear to be confused. This problem is discussed further in Chapter 10.

M—Metabolic and Endocrine Disease and Nutritional Deficiencies

Patients with uncontrolled diabetes mellitus and hypothyroidism often display confusional states. Diabetes mellitus can become uncontrolled for a number of reasons, including infection, dietary indiscretion, failure to take necessary medication, and use of sugar-containing medicines such as cough syrups.

Any imbalance in serum electrolytes may be manifested as impaired mental functioning. Such an imbalance can be precipitated by a bout of diarrhea or by medications such as diuretic drugs and lithium, an agent used to correct mood disorders that is notorious for producing delirium through electrolyte disturbance.

Elderly people commonly do not eat wholesome meals and are likely to suffer from numerous nutritional deficiencies. Patients with such deficiencies display confusion and other signs of dementia. Patients who have had bowel surgery are particularly at risk for nutritional deficiencies. It is sometimes difficult to obtain a history of such surgery because the patient may have forgotten the relevant information, and records may not be readily available. Some patients may be starving and suffering from ketosis.

E—Emotional Disorders

Paranoid disorders and mood disorders are the two most common forms of psychiatric illness in the elderly that may be confused with Alzheimer's disease. Elderly individuals have a higher incidence of paranoid disorders than younger people. Depression, which is common in the elderly, can be confused with Alzheimer's disease because it does not manifest itself in the classic manner. Elderly patients who are depressed frequently have a list of somatic complaints and demonstrate emotional withdrawal or apparent confusion. The diagnosis of depression is made because of the abruptness of onset, lack of animation in the patient, loss of appetite, and insomnia.

N—Neurological Disease

Multiinfarct dementia is the second most common cause of dementia in older people. Unlike Alzheimer's disease, it is abrupt in onset and progresses in a stepwise fashion rather than in a steady decline. Hydrocephalus, usually found in newborns, can occur among the elderly, although only rarely (1% to 2% of dementias). This condition is associated with a clinical triad consisting of rigid gait, urinary incontinence, and impaired mental functions. The early diagnosis is important because the condition is reversible. Parkinson's disease, which generally manifests itself by affecting motor functions, can also be associated with impaired mental function.

T—Tumors and Trauma

Two of the greatest advances in medical technology in the past 20 years were CT scanning and magnetic resonance imaging (MRI). Although these methods are not very helpful in the diagnosis of early Alzheimer's disease, they do aid in diagnosing traumatic injury and tumors of the brain.

I—Infection

Elderly people often appear to be confused when they have an infection, and the clinical picture may be further obscured if the individual does not have an elevated temperature. The two most common infections in the elderly that produce a dementia-like picture are pneumonia and urinary tract infections, which are discussed in Chapter 10. In the last decade it has also been recognized that patients with AIDS often develop a dementia as part of the illness.

A—Arteriosclerosis

Arteriosclerosis can lead to heart failure and insufficient blood supply to the heart or the brain. The patient sometimes has bouts of confusion and heart failure and almost always experiences depression. These symptoms may masquerade a pseudodementia. Arteriosclerosis may also be responsible for strokes. If the stroke is massive and affects the motor area of the brain, the patient will have paralysis. Lesser strokes, on the other hand, may not be noticed until so many have occurred and sufficient brain tissue has been destroyed that a dementia results. This condition is called multiinfarct dementia.

MENTAL STATUS EXAMINATION

After the medical history, the next most important component of a patient evaluation is a mental status examination. The major purpose of this examination is to exclude other possible mental disorders. Like the differential diagnosis, the mental status examination has a handy mnemonic: AMSIT.

The "A" stands for appearance, general behavior, and speech. The patient's appearance may point to impaired mental function. For example, a person who comes to the physician's office wearing three pairs of pants, has most of the buttons on his shirt undone, has not knotted his tie, and has soup stains down the front of his suit is not likely to have normal mental functions. Behavior is commonly easy to judge: Does the person sit still? Is he agitated? Does he keep moving around? During a combined interview, the patient's behavior toward the caregiver and the examiner is a useful indicator of brain function. Some patients are mute throughout the interview, yet they appear to understand what is happening. Others may lash out at the caregiver or appear to have no interest whatsoever in the proceedings.

"M" is for mood, with sadness or elation, the two ends of the spectrum, of particular interest. Sometimes a person's relatives may believe that he has Alzheimer's disease if he is very excited, talks rapidly, cannot seem to get his words out fast enough, and is elated. However, such a condition is more likely to be a bipolar disorder than a dementia.

"S" stands for sensorium and refers to the person's orientation to time, place, and people. A person loses sensorium in the reverse order in which it was learned. A child first learns to recognize his parents and other significant people, then where he lives, and lastly how to tell time. These skills are lost in reverse order, and therefore disorientation to time is the first to manifest itself.

The "I" represents intellectual functioning. The Mini Mental Status Examination is a valuable tool for rapid evaluation of intellectual functioning. It consists of 30 questions, some that test sensorium and others that test arithmetic, abstract thinking, and memory. With a literate patient who has a high school education, a score of less than 24 is highly suggestive of impaired intellectual functions. The test also indicates the severity of the disease.

"T" stands for thinking processes. Patients with Alzheimer's disease demonstrate changes in almost all the categories included under this section. Early in the disease most patients have difficulty focusing on a goal and often are circumstantial or tangential in their thinking; that is, when asked questions, they tend to give answers that may contain many extraneous details but do not directly answer the question. Later in the course of the disease, much of a patient's thinking is illogical or incoherent or both.

As a rule, delusions and hallucinations do not occur until Alzheimer's disease is fairly advanced. The hallucinations frequently are visual and sometimes frightening, such as "seeing" smoke or flames when none exist. The delusions often focus on strangers being in the house or people from the past coming to visit, and they occur because the patient does not recognize familiar objects or people. Abstracting ability almost always is affected fairly early in the disease. The patient with Alzheimer's disease gives concrete responses when asked proverbs or when asked to state what is familiar about common objects. Social judgment frequently is impaired, and insight is almost always absent.

LABORATORY TESTS

A diagnostic accuracy of approximately 80% can be achieved through the purely clinical portions of the examinations; the addition of laboratory tests increases this rate to about 90%. The following tests are recommended (see also the glossary):

CT scan of the brain
Chest x-ray film
Comprehensive biochemical screening (autoanalysis of the blood)
Blood count and vitamin B_{12} level
Thyroid function tests
Electrocardiogram (ECG)
Human immunodeficiency syndrome (AIDS) virus test

Additional tests that may be useful in some instances include the following:

Electroencephalogram (EEG)
Lumbar puncture
MRI of the brain
Positron emission tomography (PET) scan of the brain

Occasionally, a patient must be referred for psychological testing. Neuropsychologists can be particularly helpful in differentiating Alzheimer's disease from other brain disorders that cannot be distinguished by either laboratory tests or the usual clinical measures. A group of tests known as the Halstead-Reitan Battery is especially helpful in making such distinctions. Tests of this type are discussed further in Chapter 3.

SUMMARY

The diagnosis of Alzheimer's disease currently is in a state of flux. Traditionally, this diagnosis has been made on clinical grounds with supporting laboratory data. However, some of the new techniques, such as positron emission tomography and single photon emission computed tomography, which are currently available only in large centers, may prove valuable in the future. It is also likely that a specific protein is involved in Alzheimer's disease and that this protein is present in the cerebrospinal fluid. In the near future it may be possible to assay this abnormal protein routinely.

BIBLIOGRAPHY

American Psychiatric Association: *Diagnostic and statistical manual of mental disorders,* ed III-R, Washington, DC, 1987, The Association.

Burns A and others: Accuracy of clinical diagnosis of Alzheimer's disease, *Br Med J* 301:1026, 1990.

Cummings JL: Clinical diagnosis of Alzheimer's disease. In Cummings JL, editor: *Dementia: a clinical approach,* Stoneham, Mass, 1983, Butterworth.

McKhann G and others: Clinical diagnosis of Alzheimer's disease: report of the NINCDS-ADRDA Work Group, *Neurology* 34:939-944, 1984.

Siu A: Screening for dementia and investigating its causes, *Ann Intern Med* 115:122-132, 1991.

10

Factors that aggravate Alzheimer's disease

Ronald C. Hamdy and Larry Hudgins

A generalized deterioration in functional activities of daily living is expected in patients with Alzheimer's disease. Progressive decline and gradual loss of higher cortical cognitive functions commonly spearhead the deterioration. However, in some patients the slope of declining function and disability may accelerate. When this process occurs, reversible causes should be sought and actively treated because often the underlying Alzheimer's disease process is not the cause of this sudden physical and/or mental deterioration. In many instances some other specific disease is responsible. Therefore it is important to detect the presence of any factor that worsens the patient's mental and/or physical state since many such factors are reversible if treated early. If not detected in time, they may lead to further irreversible deterioration.

A person's mental functions are controlled by the brain, which is made up of many nerve cells, or neurons. Brain functioning depends on the number of brain cells, their integrity, and the efficiency of the blood circulation. Since neurons have no nutrition stores, they depend entirely on the circulation to provide them with adequate quantities of glucose, oxygen, and various other nutrients. Similarly, an efficient circulation removes from the brain any waste or toxic substances that have been formed by the brain cells through their metabolic activity.

Therefore if the blood circulation is ineffective, not only will the nerve cells be deprived of various nutrients but also various waste or toxic substances will accumulate in or around the nerve cells. The nerve cells cannot function properly under these conditions, and the patient's mental impairment may worsen. For instance, the patient may become confused, lethargic, apathetic, and drowsy, or he may

131

become irritable, violent, and aggressive. Since patients with Alzheimer's disease already have a reduced number of brain cells, they are particularly vulnerable to several factors that may interfere with the functions of the remaining nerve cells. In healthy older individuals these factors may not lead to any deterioration of the mental functions, but they may be of sufficient magnitude to affect patients with Alzheimer's disease. These factors include (1) sudden reduction in the number of neurons, (2) sudden decrease in the blood supply to the brain, (3) diminished quality of blood reaching the brain, (4) altered sensory perceptions, (5) drugs, and (6) other influences.

SUDDEN REDUCTION IN NUMBER OF NEURONS

To function properly, the brain must have a minimum number of healthy cells. In Alzheimer's disease brain cells progressively die. If the number of neurons is also suddenly reduced, the patient's mental state may deteriorate abruptly. Several conditions may be responsible for this loss of neurons, including strokes, subdural hematomas, and space-occupying lesions in the skull.

Strokes

When a patient suffers a stroke, or cerebrovascular accident, the blood supply to part of the brain is suddenly interrupted and the brain cells in that area die. Strokes have three main causes:

- A thrombus, or blood clot, which forms inside the blood vessel and usually complicates abnormalities in the blood vessels themselves, such as arteriosclerosis or a stenotic (narrowed) lesion
- An embolus, which is part of a blood clot that becomes detached and circulates with the bloodstream until it becomes impacted in one of the small arteries
- A hemorrhage, which occurs when a blood vessel ruptures; in this situation, not only is the blood flow to the involved area of the brain interrupted, but also blood accumulates in the brain, compressing and destroying neighboring brain cells

In approximately two thirds of patients older than 65 years who suffer strokes, the cause of the stroke is a thrombus. In the other one third, the stroke is the result of an embolus. Cerebral hemorrhages are rare in old age.

The signs of a stroke depend on its severity and which part of the brain is affected. Massive strokes, particularly those affecting the motor functions, have a dramatic presentation, with the patient developing speech difficulties or paralysis of an arm or leg. Lesser strokes may not cause paralysis and therefore may go unnoticed. Such strokes may interfere only marginally with a patient's mental functions until so many have occurred and so much brain tissue has been destroyed that the patient's mental functions become severely impaired. This condition is the underlying process of multiinfarct dementia. Although currently little can be done once a stroke has occurred, several therapeutic measures can be taken to prevent additional strokes, such as taking low-dose aspirin and controlling hypertension.

Subdural Hematomas

A subdural hematoma is a hemorrhage that occurs inside the skull but outside the brain. Characteristically, subdural hematomas complicate head injuries. In most instances the trauma itself is relatively minor, such as a fall in the bathtub. Since the manifestations often are not obvious until a few days or even weeks later, by then the patient or caregivers may have forgotten all about it. Even if the trauma is severe enough to render the patient unconscious, he usually recovers consciousness and may appear normal for a few days or weeks before subtle changes develop. In contrast, patients with Alzheimer's disease may have a much more dramatic presentation. Immediately after the injury, the patient may not appear any worse than usual, but a few days or weeks later the symptoms usually are severe and may include a significant change in personality, apathy, lethargy, irritability, aggressiveness, and even violence.

The time gap between trauma and impairment of mental functions occurs because the initial hemorrhage is limited in size or because the bleeding stops. With time, however, the hemorrhage turns into a blood clot, which starts to draw fluid from the surrounding tissues (by osmosis) and grows larger. As the clot enlarges, pressure is exerted on the brain tissue and symptoms develop.

Space-Occupying Lesions in Skull

Unlike most other cavities in the body, the skull, or cranial cavity, has a constant volume that is largely occupied by the brain. If a patient develops a brain abscess or metastases (secondary cancer growths) in the brain, these space-occupying lesions can grow only at the expense of the brain, which first becomes compressed and later may be destroyed. Patients with Alzheimer's disease, who already have a reduced number of brain cells, are particularly vulnerable to space-occupying lesions in the skull.

SUDDEN DECREASE IN BLOOD SUPPLY TO BRAIN

As previously mentioned, the brain depends completely on the blood circulation for the oxygen, glucose, and other nutrients it needs. Even though enough neurons may be present for the brain to function at a certain level, mental functions can deteriorate as the cerebral blood flow is reduced. Although the brain represents only approximately 2% of a person's body weight, it receives about 15% of the quantity of blood pumped by the heart and uses about 25% of the total inhaled oxygen. *Any* compromise in the blood flow to the brain is poorly tolerated in patients with Alzheimer's dementia, whose primary normal neuron reserve is already compromised.

Circulation of blood throughout the body is maintained by the heart. The quantity of blood pumped by the heart in 1 minute is known as the cardiac output. A number of conditions can reduce the cardiac output, including myocardial infarctions and arrhythmias.

Myocardial Infarction

In myocardial infarction, part of the heart muscle is deprived of its blood supply and therefore it dies. If the area destroyed is large enough, the overall function of the heart may be disrupted and the amount of blood pumped during each contraction will be reduced. The effect of this reduction may be magnified if the heart rate is changed (see following discussion of arrhythmias). As a result, the heart will not be able to maintain an adequate cardiac output, leading to a decrease in the amount of blood that reaches various parts of the body, including the brain. If this condition arises in a patient with Alzheimer's disease, whose brain functions are already jeopardized, the patient's mental functions are likely to deteriorate considerably.

In contrast to the classic picture that develops in younger people, the elderly may suffer a myocardial infarction without having any chest pain. This condition is known as a "silent myocardial infarction." In the elderly the only sign of myocardial infarction may be a bout of confusion, dizziness, or a fall.

Arrhythmias

Elderly people are much more vulnerable to the effects of a change in heart rhythms, known as an arrhythmia, than are younger persons.

At rest, the heart of an older person beats approximately 65 times a minute, slightly faster than one beat per second. The heart functions in cycles, with each cycle consisting of a contraction (systole), during which the blood in the heart is forcefully ejected into the arteries, and a period of relaxation (diastole), during which blood returns to the heart through the veins. Systole is an active process, and diastole is generally a passive one that allows the heart muscles to relax and prepare for the next contraction. In normal healthy people, the amount of blood ejected during systole is the same as that received by the heart during diastole.

When the heart rate increases (tachycardia), both the systolic and the diastolic periods are shortened. At high rates, however, the diastolic period tends to be shortened even more than the systolic period. This change interferes with the amount of blood that fills the heart during diastole and in turn reduces the amount of blood pumped when the heart contracts. In an attempt to maintain a constant cardiac output, the heart beats even faster. At these very high rates, the cardiac output cannot be maintained and may actually fall because of the markedly reduced diastolic period.

Alternatively, an exceedingly slow heart rate (bradycardia), usually associated with complete heart block and heart rates less than 40 to 50 beats per minute, may compromise the cerebral blood flow to the point that the patient suffers episodes of syncope (fainting). If this situation occurs, a permanent cardiac pacing device may be necessary.

DIMINISHED QUALITY OF BLOOD REACHING BRAIN

Since the brain depends entirely on the blood for the oxygen and nutrients it needs to function properly, it is easy to see how, even if the number of brain cells is adequate and the blood flow (circulation) is effective, mental functions may become impaired if the quality of the blood reaching the brain is not adequate. Because patients with Alzheimer's disease already have a reduced number of brain cells, they are particularly vulnerable to any such change, which may be caused by reduced oxygenation of the blood, reduced blood glucose, or toxic compounds in the bloodstream.

Hypoxemia

As the blood passes through the lungs, the hemoglobin molecules in the red blood corpuscles take up oxygen. The oxygenated blood returns to the heart, which pumps it to other parts of the body, including the brain. If the blood is not oxygenated adequately in the lungs, less oxygen will be carried to the rest of the body, and less oxygen will reach the brain. This state of reduced oxygenation of the blood is called hypoxemia.

Blood oxygenation in the lungs may be inadequate for a number of reasons, including respiratory tract infections (pneumonias), pulmonary embolisms (small pieces of blood clots in the lungs), chronic obstructive airway diseases (asthma and emphysema), pulmonary neoplasia (cancer of the lungs), pleural effusions (accumulation of fluid between the lungs and the chest wall), and pneumothorax (accumulation of air between the lungs and the chest wall). Patients with Alzheimer's disease, particularly those in an advanced stage, may have neurological dysfunction that interferes with the swallowing reflex and leads to aspiration of the posterior pharyngeal or gastric contents into the lungs. In such patients the gag reflex is often lost, sensation is decreased, the swallowing muscles are often weak, and the cough reflex is inefficient or absent. As a result, aspiration and pneumonia will develop in the lowermost dependent parts of the lung and will result in rapid physical and mental deterioration of the patient.

Anemia also can decrease the amount of oxygen circulating with the blood. Because the number of red blood cells and the total quantity of circulating hemoglobin are reduced in persons with anemia, the amount of oxygen that can be carried by the blood also is reduced.

Hypoglycemia

Since brain cells have no glucose stores, a sudden reduction in the blood glucose level leaves them unable to function properly, resulting in impaired mental functions. Hypoglycemia, or reduced blood glucose level, commonly occurs when a patient receives an overdose of insulin or when he receives a normal dose but skips a meal. Less frequently, orally administered hypoglycemic agents used to control diabetes mellitus may induce hypoglycemia. Sustained hypoglycemia results in further brain cell death.

Toxic Substances in Bloodstream

Even during normal functioning, the body produces many potentially toxic substances that are usually of no concern because they are changed to less toxic compounds or eliminated from the body. If the organs that transform or eliminate these substances (primarily the kidneys and liver) are impaired, the toxic compounds accumulate.

Impaired renal function

One of the main functions of the kidneys is to rid the body of many toxic substances, especially the water-soluble ones, by excreting them in the urine. If the kidneys do not work properly, these toxic substances accumulate. Since renal functions are usually reduced in older persons, excess toxic metabolites, such as blood urea, cannot be fully excreted, and they will accumulate in the blood. Although all parts of the body are exposed to these toxic metabolites, the brain is particularly sensitive to them, and changes in sensorium usually occur with confusion, somnolence, and, occasionally, seizure. Several factors can cause renal impairment, including drugs, particularly antihypertensive agents, nonsteroidal antiinflammatory agents, analgesics, and some antibiotics; dehydration, a not uncommon condition, especially in older patients whose sense of thirst often appears to be blunted; infections; and obstruction to the flow of urine as occurs in prostatic hypertrophy.

Impaired hepatic function

Whereas the kidneys eliminate water-soluble compounds by excreting them in the urine, the liver eliminates water-insoluble or fat-soluble toxic compounds by excreting them with bile or by conjugating them with compounds that make them water soluble so that they can be excreted later by the kidneys. Alcohol abuse is one cause of impaired hepatic function. However, hepatic impairment also may be caused by certain drugs, especially those metabolized (broken down) in the liver, such as most tranquilizers, sedatives, and other compounds that act on the central nervous system.

Infection

If a patient develops an infection, regardless of its location, toxic compounds are likely to accumulate in the body, circulate with the bloodstream, and reach the brain, possibly interfering with the brain's functioning. This situation may produce an acute confusional state in the patient. If the infection is located in the chest, not only do toxic products accumulate but the amount of oxygen in the blood often is also diminished since the lung congestion that complicate such infections interferes with the free passage of oxygen molecules Chest infections are notorious for producing confusional states in eld erly people. Although individuals who do not have Alzheimer's disease sometimes become confused as a result of chest infections, the confu sion tends to be much more severe in patients with the disease.

Chest infections frequently are difficult to diagnose in older peo ple because most of the characteristic symptoms and signs seen in younger adults are absent. Such signs include fever, tachycardia (rapid heart rate), cough with expectoration of sputum, and the char acteristic findings detected during the clinical examination and through x-ray films.

An older person who has a chest infection may not have a fever because often the temperature-regulating center in the brain does not function properly in old age and is less sensitive than in youth. This situation may be one reason why elderly people are more likely to develop hypothermia. Similarly, an increased heart rate may not be observed if some disorder in the heart's conduction tissue prevents it from increasing its rate. Cough and expectoration of sputum may be absent if the patient is dehydrated. Alternatively, cough and expecto ration of sputum may have been present for a long time if the patient has a chronic obstructive airway disease. Similarly, the characteristic physical findings may be obscured by dehydration, kyphosis, and ky phoscoliosis. The last two conditions may also mask the characteristic radiological features of chest infection.

One of the most important signs in the diagnosis of chest infec tions in old age is an increased respiratory rate. Unfortunately, this sign is often overlooked, and, when considered, it is often approxi mated. Yet a rapid respiratory rate may be the only sign of a chest infection in an older person. It is ironic that this single sign usually is the one that is given the least importance during the clinical exami nation and subsequent observation of the patient.

Subacute bacterial endocarditis is another cause of confusion and impaired mental functioning in old age, especially in patients with Alzheimer's disease. In this condition the heart valves are infected and the heart may be unable to maintain an adequate circulation. In addition, bacteria and their toxic products circulate with the blood producing bacteremia or toxemia, and further interfere with the patient's mental functions. Subacute bacterial endocarditis is insidious in onset and progresses slowly. The diagnosis usually is not made until fairly late, when the disease has become well established.

ALTERED PERCEPTION OF ENVIRONMENT

The normal individual receives sensory input from the environment, processes the information, and develops a logical plan of action. To react appropriately to any situation, a person must be able to perceive and understand several messages received from the environment. For example, a normal person who wakes up at 2 AM will not begin to prepare breakfast for the whole household. If he does not know what time it is, he will check a clock, realize the time, and try to go back to sleep. Even if no clock is available, he might guess that it is too early to get out of bed, let alone fix breakfast. If, on the other hand, his vision is poor, he may not be able to read the time on the clock accurately and may think that it is time to get up. A person's perceptions can be altered by impaired vision and hearing, a sudden change in surroundings, and pain and discomfort.

Impaired Vision

In most instances vision is the prime factor that determines a person's behavior. For example, if a person notices black particles in his food while eating, his immediate reaction depends on what he thinks the particles are. This reaction is mainly governed by his visual acuity and his ability to correlate what is actually seen with past visual experiences. Similarly, a person's reaction to someone who knocks on the door and identifies himself as a sales representative will be governed largely by the customer's perception of the salesman and whether he "looks honest." On a more basic level, finding one's way to a restroom, for example, depends largely on visual acuity.

If the light rays that enter the eyes are abnormally distorted, as may happen with cataracts and glaucoma, the patient's perception of objects may be erroneous and may lead him to "see" things that are not really there, that is, to have illusions. This situation is particularly likely to happen if the patient is not fully conscious, as may occur if he has received sedative or hypnotic preparations or if he awakens in the middle of the night or is confused for any other reason.

It is important to realize that elderly people often have reduced visual and auditory acuity. It has been estimated that about 1.4 million people in the United States suffer from severe visual impairment. Of these, approximately 990,000 are older than 65 years. The three main diseases responsible for diminished vision are glaucoma, cataracts, and senile macular degeneration of the retina. In addition, the curvature of the cornea becomes less smooth and more irregular in old age, a condition known as astigmatism, and frequently light that enters the eye may be refracted by deposits in the cornea, which are increasingly present in old age.

Although many elderly people wear eyeglasses, these glasses are frequently inadequate. It is recommended that older people have their eyeglasses checked at regular intervals of 2 or 3 years or whenever their eyesight seems to have deteriorated. Many people in nursing homes or other institutions wear glasses that are covered with a layer of dust, which further interferes with their visual acuity. It should be the responsibility of the caregivers, attendants, and supervisors to ensure that the patient's glasses are kept clean.

Impaired Hearing

Any deterioration in a patient's hearing may interfere with his conversational ability. Since the patient may misinterpret questions, he is likely to give inappropriate answers. Furthermore, if the patient experiences buzzing in his ears (because of wax or other diseases), he may be under the impression that someone is talking to him. If his eyesight is also poor, he may think that a shadow is a person talking to him.

As an individual ages, visual and auditory acuity gradually deteriorate. If the patient also has a sudden decline in eyesight or hearing, he may become or appear to have become confused or disoriented and to have impaired mental functions. The individual thus may not be able to perceive his environment accurately and may make errors of judgment. Therefore, before the patient's mental functions are assessed, it is important to make sure that he can hear adequately and that there is no significant hearing loss. Otherwise, the results of the test may be false. Some improvement may occur with hearing aids, as indicated by audiometric testing. In addition, a common problem is excessive cerumen in the external canal. This cerumen buildup may become impacted and may be difficult to remove with irrigation alone. However, once the wax has been removed, a remarkable improvement in hearing may be noted.

Sudden Change in Surroundings

A sudden change in surroundings can be confusing to older people, especially those suffering from Alzheimer's disease. Such confusion frequently occurs when a patient is first admitted to a nursing home or other similar institution, where the patient may not recognize any of his surroundings. This situation is particularly likely when a patient wakes up at night and finds himself in a strange environment. During the day he may recognize his environment, but in the dark, after just awakening, he may not remember at once that he is in a new situation. This type of confusion may also be noted when a patient with Alzheimer's disease is taken away from his familiar environment to spend a few days with a relative.

Pain and Discomfort

In a patient who is confused, pain and discomfort may significantly increase the person's degree of confusion and may impair his mental functions. For example, the patient may be unable to understand or describe his pain or discomfort.

Common causes of discomfort include a full bladder, urinary incontinence, a full rectum, constipation, fecal incontinence, and decubitus ulcers. Hunger and thirst also are uncomfortable sensations, as are being too hot or too cold and lying on crumpled sheets or foreign objects such as food debris. Pain can be caused by a number of diseases (e.g., osteoarthritis), leg cramps, and infections.

DRUGS

Nowhere in medicine is the first tenet of the field—Primum non nocere (first do no harm)—more apt than in geriatrics. In regard to medications, practitioners are cautioned to always use the least effective dose practical. Since elderly patients are very sensitive to medications, adverse drug reactions occur often.

In addition, prescribed medications can aggravate mental impairment. Drugs that act on the central nervous system, such as hypnotics, sedatives, tranquilizers, antihistamines, and cold remedies, are particular offenders. There is considerable evidence that older people are much more susceptible to the effects of these drugs than younger patients are, largely because an older person's body cannot eliminate the drug as quickly, through either excretion by the kidneys or breakdown by the liver. Therefore it is important that these drugs be given in the smallest effective dose. If necessary, the dosage can be adjusted according to the patient's response. Also, short-duration drugs are preferable since older patients tend to metabolize and excrete drugs more slowly than normal.

Many over-the-counter drugs contain compounds that can sedate a patient. Besides sleeping preparations, such drugs include many cold remedies, antiallergic medications, and even some antacids and antidiarrhetic mixtures. If these drugs are given to the patient in large doses or in conjunction with other medications, drug overdose may result and the patient's confusional state may worsen.

It must also be remembered that alcohol is a potent sedative and that it often potentiates the action of many other drugs. Drinking an excessive amount of alcohol may cause discomfort by increasing the volume of urine produced, thereby distending the bladder, and by precipitating dehydration.

Many other drugs may interfere with a patient's mental activities, for example, by altering the blood electrolytes (diuretics), precipitating anemia (drugs that irritate the gastrointestinal mucosa), inducing heart failure, precipitating cardiac irregularities, and reducing the blood pressure or the blood glucose level.

Because drug-induced confusion and impaired mental function are so common in old age, it is paramount that the physician be aware of all medications that the patient is taking, whether prescribed, bought over the counter, or borrowed from others.

OTHER INFLUENCES
Physical Restraints

Physical restraints are often used to control patients who demonstrate abnormal behavior and to prevent patients from injuring themselves. Restraints are necessary for only a very small number of patients, and they generally are overused. Injudicious use of restraints aggravates a patient's irritability, frustration, and confusion. Physical restraints are discussed further in Chapters 18 and 19.

Sleep Deprivation

Sleep deprivation is a known and common cause of confusion, not only in older patients with Alzheimer's disease but in any age group. This problem and its effects are further discussed in Chapter 10.

Coexisting Medical Conditions

Many diseases can cause a confusional state, particularly in elderly people. Some of these diseases were described earlier in this chapter. Others were dealt with in Chapter 10. It is important to ensure that no medical condition is responsible for a patient's deteriorating mental state before the assumption is made that the deterioration is secondary to Alzheimer's disease.

Because patients with Alzheimer's disease may suffer from other diseases that can considerably worsen their mental and physical impairment, caregivers must be aware of this fact and need to report any sudden deterioration to the physician, who will try to identify the cause. Often the cause is reversible, and the patient's condition may improve once the disorder has been identified and treated. Alzheimer's disease progresses slowly and insidiously and seldom is the cause of sudden deterioration in a patient's condition.

BIBLIOGRAPHY

Johnson JC: Delirium in the elderly, *Emerg Med Clin North Am* 8(2):255-265, 1990.

Klein-Schwartz W, Oderda GM: Poisoning in the elderly: epidemiological, clinical, and management considerations, *Drugs Aging* 1(1):67-89, 1991.

McDougall GJ: A review of screening instruments for assessing cognition and mental status in older adults, *Nurse Pract* 15(11):18-28, 1990.

Moran MG, Thompson TL II: Changes in the aging brain as they affect psychotropics: a review, *Int J Psychiatry Med* 19(2):137-144, 1988.

Orticio LP: Confusion and the patient on an intensive topical ocular antibiotic regimen: a case analysis, *J Ophthalmic Nurs Technol* 9(4):145-151, 1990.

Rasin JH: Confusion, *Nurs Clin North Am* 25(4):909-918, 1990.

Rasmussen BH, Creason NS: Nurses' perception of the phenomenon confusion in elderly hospitalized patients, *Vard Nord Utveckl Forsk* 11(1):5-12, 1991.

Scott RB, Mitchell MC: Aging, alcohol, and the liver, *J Am Geriatr Soc* 36(3):255-265, 1988.

Stewart RB, Hale WE: Acute confusional states in older adults and the role of polypharmacy, *Annu Rev Public Health* 13:415-430, 1992.

Straatsma BR and others: Aging-related cataract: laboratory investigation and clinical management, *Ann Intern Med* 102(1):82-92, 1985.

Tess MM: Acute confusional states in critically ill patients: a review, *J Neurosci Nurs* 23(6):398-402, 1991.

Thompson L, Wood C, Wallhagen M: Geriatric acute myocardial infarction: a challenge to recognition, prompt diagnosis, and appropriate care, *Crit Care Nurs Clin North Am* 4(2):291-299, 1992.

Tyers AG: Aging and the ocular adnexa: a review, *J R Soc Med* 75(11):900-902, 1982.

Veith RC, Raskind MA: The neurobiology of aging: does it predispose to depression? *Neurobiol Aging* 9(1):101-117, 1988.

Walsh DA: Aging and visual information processing: potential implications for everyday seeing, Part I, *J Am Optom Assoc* 59(4):301-306, 1988.

Whalley LJ, Bradnock J: Treatment of the classical manifestations of dementia and confusion, *Br Med Bull* 46(1):169-180, 1990.

11

Other dementias

Ronald C. Hamdy, James M. Turnbull, and Daniel Merrick

The term "dementia" refers to the loss of previously attained cognitive abilities. This condition is sufficiently severe to produce social or occupational impairment. The disturbances involved always include memory impairment, loss of abstract thinking, poor judgment, and alterations in higher cortical functioning. Sometimes a personality change is also involved.

Dementia is not synonymous with benign senescent forgetfulness, which is very common in old age and affects recent memory. Although the latter is a source of frustration, it does not significantly interfere with the individual's professional or social activities because it tends to affect only trivial matters (or what the individual considers trivial). Furthermore, patients with benign forgetfulness usually can remember what was forgotten by using certain strategies, such as writing lists or leaving notes in conspicuous places. In contrast, patients with dementia may write lists for themselves, but they often forget to check them or cannot remember where they left the list. Furthermore, whereas individuals with benign forgetfulness are acutely aware of their memory deficit, those with dementia (except those in the early stages of the disease) have no insight into their memory deficit and often blame others for their problems.

In addition to the memory deficit interfering with the patient's daily activities, certain other features must be present before a diagnosis of dementia can be made. These criteria have been outlined in the *Diagnostic and Statistical Manual of Mental Disorders*, Third Edition, Revised (DSM III-R) and include impaired abstract thinking, impaired judgment, or other disturbances of higher cortical (mental) functions such as aphasia, apraxia, or agnosia. The Mini Mental State Examination is a valuable tool for the evaluation of cognitive function

145

in alert patients. It consists of 30 questions that test memory, orientation, sensorium, ability to do simple mathematical calculations, and abstract thinking. A score of less than 24 in a literate patient with a high school education is highly suggestive of significant cognitive deficit.

CORTICAL AND SUBCORTICAL DEMENTIAS

Dementia can result from damage to the brain cortex or to subcortical structures. Although memory is impaired in both cortical and subcortical dementias, the associated features are different. In cortical dementias, for instance, cognitive functions such as language, ability to do mathematical calculations, and perceptions are severely impaired. In subcortical dementias, on the other hand, patients often exhibit flattening of affect, disturbances of arousal, motivation, and mood, and a significant slowing of cognition and information processing, which is sometimes referred to as "bradyphrenia." Some features of subcortical dementias may be seen in cortical dementias and are probably secondary to damaged projections to and from the cortex.

Cortical Dementias

Although Alzheimer's disease is the most common cortical dementia, attention also needs to be given to Pick's disease.

A rare disease, Pick's disease is characterized by cortical atrophy localized to the frontal and temporal lobes. It has a similar course as Alzheimer's disease but tends to affect younger patients and women more frequently than men. In the early stages of the disease, signs of frontal and temporal lobe involvement are evident. These signs include changes in personality, disinhibition, inappropriate social and sexual conduct, and lack of foresight—features that are not common in Alzheimer's disease. Later in Pick's disease patients may become euphoric or apathetic. Nonfluent aphasia is often present and gradually progresses to mutism. Speech comprehension is usually spared. Prominent grasp and sucking reflexes are present. In late stages of the disease rigidity and dystonia are often noted.

Some physicians think it is important to diagnose Pick's disease because it is often inherited as a dominant trait. The brain of a patient affected by Pick's disease exhibits a sharp demarcation between the atrophic and the normal parts of the cortex, an observation that can be easily made without the use of a microscope. The atrophic changes are not limited to the cortex but extend to the subcortical structures, including the caudate nucleus, putamen, thalamus, substantia nigra, and descending frontopontine fiber system. The microscopic features, which are characteristic of the disease, consist of fibrillary deposits within the cytoplasm of the neurons and Pick's bodies composed of densely packed spherical aggregates.

Vascular Dementias

Vascular dementia, the second most common cause of dementia in patients over the age of 65 years, is responsible for 8% to 20% of all dementia cases. It is caused by an interference with the blood flow to the brain. Although the overall prevalence of vascular dementia is decreasing, there are some geographical variations, with a higher prevalence in countries where the incidence of cardiovascular and cerebrovascular diseases remains high, such as Finland and Japan. Approximately 20% of patients with dementia have both Alzheimer's disease and vascular dementia. Several types of vascular dementia have been identified and are discussed in the following sections.

Multiinfarct dementia

The most common type of vascular dementia is multiinfarct dementia. As its name implies, this condition is the result of multiple cerebral infarcts that have destroyed enough brain tissue to interfere with the patient's mental functions. It is not caused by chronic diffuse cerebral ischemia. The onset of multiinfarct dementia is usually sudden and is often associated with evidence of neurological deficit, such as paralysis or paresis of an arm or leg or dysphasia. The course of the disease characteristically progresses in steps. With each stroke experienced, the patient's condition suddenly deteriorates and then stabilizes or may even improve slightly until another stroke occurs. About 20% of patients with multiinfarct dementia, however, have an insidious onset and gradual deterioration. Most patients also have evidence of arteriosclerosis and factors predisposing them to the development of thromboembolic strokes, such as hypertension, cigarette smoking, hypercholesterolemia, diabetes mellitus, carotid artery stenosis, cardiac disorders, and, especially, atrial fibrillation. Somatic complaints, emotional lability, depression, relative preservation of the personality, and nocturnal confusion tend to be more common in vascular dementias but are not diagnostic. The Hachinski Ischemic Scale is useful in differentiating multiinfarct dementia from Alzheimer's disease (see Chapter 9). A score of seven or more on the 10 items is suggestive of MID, whereas a score of four or less is suggestive of Alzheimer's disease. Computed tomography (CT) or magnetic resonance imaging (MRI) of the brain often reveals multiple hypodensities, brain atrophy, and occasionally ventricular dilation. It must be emphasized, however, that brain mass is a poor indicator of brain function and therefore the presence of generalized atrophy noted on a CT scan is not an indication of dementia.

Lacunar dementias

Strokes are not always associated with clinical evidence of neurological deficits because the stroke may affect a "silent" area of the brain, or it may be so small that its immediate impact is not noticeable. Nevertheless, when several small strokes have occurred, the resulting loss of brain tissue may interfere with the patient's cognitive functions. Such deterioration is the basis of the lacunar dementias. The lacunae result from small infarcts, ranging from 2 to 15 mm in diameter. When the infarcted brain tissue becomes absorbed, small lacunae remain. These lacunae usually result from hypertensive damage to small penetrating arteries in the brain. Although CT scans often show evidence of multiple small hypodensities, many small lacunae may not be detected by CT scan because of either their small size or their location. MRI, a more sensitive method, can identify small lacunae, even in the brainstem and pons, that are not easily visualized by CT scanning.

Other vascular dementias

Binswanger's disease is associated with diffuse loss of subcortical white matter and ventricular dilatation. Features of subcortical dementias are evident on this disease. The condition tends to manifest itself at a relatively young age, 50 to 65 years. Hypertension is a central feature of this dementia. However, unlike multiinfarct dementia, major strokes are not frequent in Binswanger's disease. The CT scan usually shows extensive periventricular densities extending deep into the white matter.

Cerebral amyloid angiopathy is another type of vascular dementia. It is characterized by the presence of amyloid in the media and adventitia of the cerebral arterioles.

Dementias Associated with Neurological Disorders

A number of neurological disorders are associated with dementia. These include space-occupying lesions (subdural hematomas, primary and secondary tumors), paraneoplastic encephalitis, carcinomatous meningitis, progressive supranuclear palsy (Steele-Richardson-Olszewski syndrome), Shy-Drager syndrome, motor neuron disease, multiple sclerosis, pugilistic dementia, brain anoxia, encephalitis, Huntington's chorea, hydrocephalus, and Parkinson's disease. Only the common disorders are briefly discussed in the following sections.

Hydrocephalus

The triad of dementia, gait disorder resulting from increased muscle rigidity, and urinary incontinence should raise the suspicion of normal- or low-pressure hydrocephalus. Signs of increased intracranial pressure are usually absent. A CT scan demonstrates enlargement of the ventricles. Injection of a radioactive material into the cerebrospinal fluid followed by brain scanning will reveal the pattern of cerebrospinal fluid flow. It is, nevertheless, difficult to identify patients who would benefit from surgery. An improvement of cognitive and psychomotor functions lasting for a few hours after the removal of 40 to 50 ml of cerebrospinal fluid is suggestive of a good prognosis following surgery. However, postoperative complications are significant and include strokes, subdural hematomas, and shunt malfunction.

Parkinson's disease

Parkinson's disease usually manifests itself in middle or late life. It has an insidious onset and a slow progression rate. Although intellectual deterioration is not part of the classic features of Parkinson's disease, dementia is being recognized as a late manifestation of the disease, with as many as one third of patients eventually being afflicted. The dementia process also has an insidious onset and slow progression rate and may be heralded by disorientation at night. In advanced stages patients may have vivid auditory and visual hallucinations that are sometimes worsened by therapy. As many as half of the patients with Parkinson's disease develop depression, which often responds to appropriate therapy. Anticholinergic drugs, sometimes used in the treatment of Parkinson's disease, may induce confusional states and visual and sensory hallucinations, particularly in older patients, even in the absence of dementia. If dementia is present, these drugs may worsen that condition.

Subdural hematomas

Subdural hematomas can lead to mental impairment and are precipitated by trauma to the head. Characteristically, the trauma is slight and the patient neither loses consciousness nor experiences any significant immediate posttraumatic effect. A few days or even weeks later, however, he may start developing evidence of mental impairment. By that time, often the patient and caregivers may have forgotten all about the slight trauma that the patient experienced. A subdural hematoma should be suspected with a fairly abrupt onset and progressive course. Headaches are not uncommon. A CT scan will reveal the presence of the hematoma, which, if surgically removed in a timely manner, is associated with a good prognosis.

Space-occupying lesions

Primary or metastatic brain tumors may be associated with dementia, particularly if they are slow-growing and situated deep in the white matter, the frontal lobe, or the midline. Symptoms of elevated intracranial pressure, such as headaches, are not always present, and there may be no evidence of focal neurological deficits, except for the grasp or sucking reflex. Most of these lesions can be diagnosed by CT scanning or MRI. Occasionally, cancer may induce dementia through an inflammation of the brain. In these conditions the cerebrospinal fluid is abnormal.

Dementias Associated with Chronic Infection

Many chronic infections affect the brain and can lead to dementia. These include conditions that, when treated, may reverse or prevent the progression of dementia. Examples include syphilis, tuberculosis, slow viruses, and some fungal and protozoal infections.

Human immunodeficiency virus (HIV) infection is a rare cause of dementia in older people, but it should be considered if the rate of progress is rapid and the patient has risk factors for the development of HIV infection. Although this type of dementia is part of the acquired immunodeficiency (AIDS) complex, it may occasionally be the first manifestation of the disease. The clinical features appearing early in the disease include forgetfulness, loss of concentration, and slow thought processes. Loss of balance and generalized weakness are present in many patients. Some patients may show behavioral changes, including apathy, depression, and withdrawal. Late in the disease process other symptoms, such as ataxia, tremors, frontal release signs, and seizures, develop.

Creutzfeldt-Jakob disease, a rare condition caused by a slow viral infection, affects approximately 1 in 1 million people. The initial symptoms are vague and include headaches, dizziness, fatigue, and impaired judgment. Memory loss tends to progress rapidly and is accompanied by aphasia, apraxia, and agnosia in approximately one third of the cases. Extrapyramidal signs, such as rigidity, tremors, and dysarthria, are present in about 60% of cases. Cortical blindness and seizures occur in approximately 40% and 9% of cases, respectively. The importance of diagnosing Creutzfeldt-Jakob disease is that it is potentially transmissible. Pathologists who perform autopsies and surgeons should be warned of this danger so that they can take appropriate protective measures.

Depression

Dementia frequently coexists with clinical depression. In some cases depression is so severe that it is mistaken for dementia. The term "depression" is used to denote a clinically significant disorder marked by a depressed mood or anhedonia. Other characteristics are sleep disturbance, possible weight change, and intermittent observable psychomotor agitation or retardation. Signs also noted are fatigue, feelings of worthlessness or guilt, difficulties in concentration, and preoccupation with suicidal thoughts. These signs and symptoms must have been present for at least 2 weeks, although they may have been evident for many years by the time the patient is seen by the physician or nurse.

When depression and dementia exist together, the situation becomes more difficult. There are four possible causes of this combination:

1. The dementia and the depression may result from different causes. For example, a patient with Alzheimer's disease who has a history of major depression may develop another episode of depression.
2. The depression may be caused by the patient's reaction to an awareness of his increasing cognitive difficulties.
3. Dementia and depression may come from a single cause, as in left frontal cerebral vascular accidents.
4. Depression may produce cognitive dysfunction caused by the mood disorder itself.

The term "pseudodementia" has often been applied to depression that produces cognitive dysfunction related to the mood disorder itself. However, it is a misleading term and suggests diagnostic and therapeutic nihilism.

ALZHEIMER'S DISEASE AND REVERSIBLE DEPRESSION

Reitler and Hanley at the University of Washington discovered that 23% of geriatric outpatients with cognitive impairment also suffered from depression. In 85% of these patients, the depression was superimposed on a dementia. As the cognitive impairment increased the level of coexisting dementia decreased significantly. Thirty-three percent of mildly cognitively impaired patients were depressed, 23% of moderately impaired patients had depression, and only 12% of severely impaired patients were depressed.

Studies of patients with probable Alzheimer's disease who were also depressed revealed that treatment with a tricyclic antidepressant was effective in reducing the severity of the depression. Thus it would seem obvious that depression, occurring as it does in approximately 25% of patients with dementia of the Alzheimer's disease type, should be routinely looked for and treated.

DEPRESSION AND VASCULAR DEMENTIA

Patients who are recovering from a stroke and also develop a dementia are frequently described as being apathetic and having abulia. Abulia is a condition in which there is a lack of will or an inability to decide. Lesions of the frontal lobe, multiinfarct dementia, lesions of the right hemisphere, and Alzheimer's disease all may produce apathy and abulia.

It is estimated that 40% to 50% of patients who are in the acute phase of poststroke illness will have symptoms of major depression. An additional 30% of patients will develop depressive symptoms within the first 2 years after an infarction. Major depression is more common when the lesion is located in the left frontal cortex and the head of the caudate nucleus. A less severe form of depression following a stroke occurs in patients who do not have any intellectual decline. Treatment recommended for poststroke depression is electroconvulsive therapy. Such treatment should not, however, be given until a trial of a tricyclic antidepressant or a specific serotonin reuptake inhibitor has been undertaken.

SUMMARY

Dementia is one of the most devastating conditions that affects human beings because it destroys the mind. By impairing memory and interfering with the ability to make rational decisions, it prevents individuals from functioning adequately in their environment. Thus it deprives patients of their dignity and independence. Because dementia is almost completely irreversible, cannot yet be adequately treated, and is associated with a long survival period, it affects not only the patient's life but also the patient's family, caregivers, and society. Therefore every effort must be made to reach an accurate diagnosis.

Although Alzheimer's disease is the most common cause of dementia, many other types of dementia have been identified. It is important to diagnose the specific type of dementia because sometimes further deterioration can be prevented.

BIBLIOGRAPHY

Bishburg E and others: Brain lesions in patients with acquired immunodeficiency syndrome, *Arch Intern Med* 149:941-943, 1989.

Bone RC, editor: *Disease-a-month: Alzheimer's disease,* St. Louis, Jan 1992, Mosby–Year Book.

Cartlidge NEF: Transient global amnesia, *Br Med J* 302:62-63, 1991.

Emery VO, Oxman TE: Update on the dementia spectrum of depression, *Am J Psychiatry,* 149(3):305-317, 1992.

Erkinjuntti T, Sulkava R: Diagnosis of multi-infarct dementia, *Alzheimer Dis Assoc Disord* 5(2):112-121, 1991.

Erkinjuntti T and others: Dementia among medical inpatients, *Arch Intern Med* 146:1923-1926, 1986.

Fischer P, Berner P: Clinical and epidemiological aspects of dementia in the elderly, *J Neural Transm Suppl* 33:39-48, 1991.

Forette F, Boller F: Hypertension and the risk of dementia in the elderly, *Am J Med* 90(3A):14-19, 1991.

Gabuzda DH, Hirsch MS: Neurologic manifestations of infection with human immunodeficiency virus: clinical features and pathogenesis, *Ann Intern Med* 107:383-391, 1987.

Huber SJ and others: Cortical vs subcortical dementia, *Arch Neurol* 43:392-394, 1986.

Kase CS: Epidemiology of multi-infarct dementia, *Alzheimer Dis Assoc Disord* 5(2):71-76, 1991.

Korczyn AD: The clinical differential diagnosis of dementia: concept and methodology—Alzheimer's disease. *Psychiatr Clin North Am* 14:237-249, 1991.

Kramer SI, Reifler BV: Depression, dementia and reversible dementia, *Clin Geriatr Med* 8:289-296, 1992.

Loeb C and others: Dementia associated with lacunar infarction, *Stroke* 23:1225-1229, 1992.

Mahler ME, Cummings JL: Behavioral neurology of multi-infarct dementia, *Alzheimer Dis Assoc Disord* 5(2):122-130, 1991.

Nadeau SE: Multi-infarct dementia, subcortical dementia, and hydrocephalus, *South Med J* 84:S41-S52, 1991.

Reifler BV, Hanley R: Coexistence of cognitive impairment and depression in geriatric outpatients, *Am J Psychiatry* 139:623-626, 1982.

Rowland LP, editor: *Merrit's textbook of neurology,* ed 8, Philadelphia, 1989, Lea & Febiger.

Siu AL: Screening for dementia and investigating its causes, *Ann Intern Med* 84:S11-S23, 1991.

Wallin A, Blennow K: Pathogenetic basis of vascular dementia, *Alzheimer Dis Assoc Disord* 5(2):91-102, 1991.

UNIT THREE
MANAGEMENT

12

General principles of management

Warren Clark

Nursing management of the patient with Alzheimer's disease is both frustrating and rewarding. The inability of the patient to become oriented to a new setting or to learn new skills often makes his or her life a bewildering search for meaning. Ultimately the patient becomes vulnerable and dependent. Being able to accept this dependency and to foster a meaningful existence for the patient and the family can be a source of reward to caregivers.

The unique aspect of caring for the patient with Alzheimer's disease centers on the complications in delivery of care associated with severe cognitive deficits. The patient's needs can be defined by nursing diagnoses, self-care deficits, functional health parameters, or any other comprehensive approach to nursing assessment.

By the time a patient has been diagnosed as having Alzheimer's disease, his cognitive deficits are often severe. Such cognitive impairment brings about a wide array of behavioral and functional problems that may necessitate institutionalization and may require adaptations in the routines in delivery of nursing care. Hospitalization or placement in an institution itself often accelerates the patient's mental decline. The patient who has lost the ability to do any problem-solving also will not be able to learn new tasks and may not remember any recent events in his life. In addition, behaviors such as confusion, wandering, agitation, or aggression may need to be the focus of the nursing care plan. This focus differs significantly from the nursing care of the traditional patient with an acute or chronic physical illness. Furthermore, the patient with Alzheimer's disease who has concomitant physical disabilities will need a modified nursing process. Indeed, nursing assessment, planning of care, delivery of care, and evaluation of care all are affected by the patients' difficulty in processing information.

NURSING ASSESSMENT

The patient with Alzheimer's disease requires a thorough bio-psychosocial nursing assessment. If the patient does not understand the purpose of the examination, he may become frightened, suspicious, and resistive. A variety of strategies can be used to gain the patient's cooperation in the assessment phase of care delivery. Making the person comfortable is essential in gaining acceptance of the assessment. Having a relative or friend accompany the patient may increase the patient's comfort level and assist in interviewing him. Giving simple explanations of each step of the assessment and proceeding slowly from one step to the next decrease the stress for the patient. Keeping oneself in view of the patient and talking to him in a calm voice also are reassuring. Interruptions and extraneous noise should be kept to a minimum. If the patient becomes resistive at any step, attempts should be made to distract him and that step should be done later in the examination.

The patient's memory deficit will make him an unreliable informant for giving a health care history, especially of recent events. The patient may remember childhood illnesses or trauma but may forget, for instance, that he has a cardiac pacemaker. He may become frustrated with his inability to answer questions and may try to give socially appropriate but inaccurate information. Sometimes the patient will simply withdraw when faced with too great a challenge to his memory. Such situations can be avoided by first assessing the patient's ability to participate in the assessment process actively. Careful collection and review of health care records and contact with available family and friends can be used to supplement history-taking.

Many aspects of the physical assessment are complicated by memory deficit. Although the patient may be able to follow simple commands such as "breathe deeply," he may not understand the more complicated maneuvers required in a neurological assessment. Repeating directions in a simple form or demonstrating expected behavior may help with compliance. Simple inspection of the patient may be difficult if he cannot understand the reasons for removing his clothes. Sometimes asking the person to change clothes can be a pretext for a brief examination. Percussion, palpation, and auscultation can be very threatening to a patient who cannot understand the reason for invasion of his personal space. Performing these aspects of the assessment slowly and allowing the patient to inspect the equipment visually may help him feel at ease with the process.

Sensory examination is difficult because of the necessity for clear communication regarding responses to stimuli. With the patient who has Alzheimer's disease, it may be necessary to rely on the observations of staff to identify his sensory capacities.

Assessment of the patient's psychosocial functioning is critical in planning his care, especially if he is in the process of transition to an institution. The patient with Alzheimer's disease is rarely capable of discussing these higher level needs. Yet their satisfaction can be important in establishing a satisfactory quality of life in an institutional setting. Reliance on family or previous caregivers is essential for learning about the patient's capacities for self-care, style of relating to others, daily routines and habits, social interests and distractions, and methods of coping with stress.

Occasionally the patient with Alzheimer's disease may be hospitalized because of behaviors that are disturbing to the family or the community. Aggression, inappropriate sexual behaviors, wandering and becoming lost, and setting fires are examples of such behaviors. It is important to realize that in most cases such behaviors are not characteristic of the individual's behavior pattern; instead, they represent a deviation resulting from the mental deterioration associated with Alzheimer's disease. Since these behaviors are usually not continuous, assessment may involve observing the patient over a specified time to determine a baseline concerning the severity and rate of occurrence. Staff members should observe the patient to determine what factors precipitate the behaviors and what causes the patient to discontinue them. Identifying the patterns that characterize these inappropriate behaviors is the first step in formulating a treatment plan for the aberrant behavior.

The cognitive deficits associated with Alzheimer's disease make it difficult to complete an assessment in one session. Yet for the patient it is particularly important that assessment be considered a continuous process. The assessment must be incorporated into daily routines through assurance that all staff are observing the patient for signs of physical or behavioral change and that systematic assessments are attempted on a regularly scheduled basis.

PLANNING OF CARE

The cognitive deficit of the patient with Alzheimer's disease poses several challenges to the planning of nursing care. The patient should be encouraged to participate in planning, but expectations of self-care should be closely aligned with each patient's abilities. Goals should be carefully defined to prevent or to slow decline or regression but should be planned without the expectation of dramatic improvement. Goals for care can be compensatory, rehabilitative, or maintenance.

Compensatory goals, which need to be defined for all patients with Alzheimer's disease, should focus on the patient's ability to adapt to the treatment environment and vice-versa. Rehabilitative goals for the patient should not refer to a rehabilitation of the underlying cognitive dysfunction but to helping the patient achieve his maximum level of functioning in other domains. Maintenance goals focus on retention of function level and prevention of deterioration. The organization of nursing care should be based on goals in each of these spheres. It should incorporate an understanding of the patient's limitations resulting from the mental decline.

DELIVERY OF CARE

Compensatory Care

Much of the nursing care of the patient with Alzheimer's disease involves structuring the environment and activities in ways to compensate for his cognitive deficits. The patient feels more secure when routines are established and followed closely. Once the patient feels secure in a new environment, change should be kept to a minimum. If possible, a patient should stay in the same room with the same roommate throughout his stay. Consistency in staff assignment also will have a calming effect on the patient. The environment should be structured to provide cues to the location of important spaces and facilities. Signs that are easily seen and include figures illustrating the use of an area are helpful in orientation. The presence of personal items can help the patient identify an unfamiliar room as his own. Staff should be assigned so that they spend as much time as possible in the line of sight of the patient. Large clocks and bulletin boards can serve as reality anchors for the grossly confused patient.

In general, the unit environment should provide a low level of stimulation and confusion for the patient. Colors should be muted, and contrasting colors should be used to demarcate boundaries. Noise should be kept low and can be masked by the sound of music that was popular during the patient's youth. Television can be entertaining, and older shows on cable channels can provide a familiar background for the patient who has some capacity for memory. Such environmental cues can help the patient compensate for memory loss by anchoring him in a period he can remember.

Activities for the patient should be focused on making him more comfortable. When possible, these activities should be designed to allow the patient to use existing skills to perform familiar tasks. Some patients enjoy simple games, whereas others may like household activities such as dusting or cleaning objects. The patient should be encouraged to participate in activities that help him compensate for other deficits; the focus should not be task completion or productivity.

The environment of activities should be based on a careful assessment of the patient's abilities and interests. Such an assessment can be made only by providing sufficient opportunity for the patient to display these capacities. For this reason staff must be cautious not to allow the environment to become devoid of stimuli. Such sterility can accelerate the decline in cognitive ability that is already occurring.

Rehabilitative Care

Rehabilitation of the patient with Alzheimer's disease is a complicated process. By the time the patient has been institutionalized, he may have experienced other deficits. He may be malnourished and apathetic or may suffer from infections or insomnia. However, all patients with Alzheimer's disease are amenable to rehabilitation.

The patient with Alzheimer's disease frequently will have difficulty remembering to attend to basic hygiene and activities of daily living. He may forget to drink, eat, bathe, or dress adequately. The patient may become susceptible to infections and eventually progress to a generally debilitated state. When nursing staff provide careful attention to these aspects of self-care, much of the debilitation can be reversed.

In addition to the physical symptoms mentioned here, the patient may have social needs or abilities that are repressed because of apathy or withdrawal. Rebuilding relationships with family members of other nursing home residents may help to reverse this process.

Rehabilitation for problematic behaviors, such as aggression or inappropriate sexual behaviors, may be the most difficult task for caregivers (see Chapter 13). For most patients with Alzheimer's disease, these behaviors are related to decreased inhibition caused by the regression in mental abilities. Staff must recognize that these behaviors often serve to satisfy the patient's underlying needs, such as for security or affection. As the patient's condition deteriorates, these behaviors are often extinguished without any treatment. Occasionally the patient must be institutionalized for his own protection or for that of others. For some patients merely being in an institutional setting with decreased stimulation will cause the behavior to diminish. For other patients close supervision, finding alternative ways of satisfying the needs, or distraction can be effective in preventing stressful situations from escalating and leading to disturbed patient behavior. For some patients medications are effective in reducing the stress or decreasing the disturbed thinking that precipitates the behavior.

Maintenance Care

Maintenance care of the patient with Alzheimer's disease is centered around the need to support him in performing the full range of activities of daily living. This supportive care requires routine monitoring of the patient's food and fluid intake, bathing and toileting schedule, and sleep routine. The patient must be supervised to ensure that he receives adequate physical activity and rest. Activities that nursing staff generally rely on patients to perform independently must be observed in patients with Alzheimer's disease because of their cognitive deficits. Overlooking deficits in activities of daily living performance can lead to high-risk outcomes such as dehydration, bowel obstruction, infection, or agitation. Nursing care of these special issues in management is described in Chapter 19.

Good maintenance care also must focus on symptom identification. Since the patient usually is not able to describe routine physical symptoms, even pain, the nursing staff must rely on close observation to identify a patient's problems before they become unmanageable. Staff should suspect physical illness whenever a behavioral change occurs in a patient with Alzheimer's disease. Nonverbal cues such as anxiety, restlessness, or irritability can be brought on by physical discomfort. Behavioral changes also may be caused by sensory changes. Staff should monitor the patient for signs of decreased loss of visual or auditory acuity, such as a change in communication patterns, ignoring of incoming stimuli, or general withdrawal.

Infection control is important in the maintenance care of the patient with Alzheimer's disease. Poor hygiene can lead to minor wound infections or eye infections. In the patient with advanced Alzheimer's disease, difficulty in swallowing and immobility may contribute to a high incidence of pneumonia. Poor dental hygiene may reduce the patient's appetite and act as a septic focus. Immobility, incontinence, and the use of indwelling catheters can lead to urinary tract infections. Close observation of the patient during feeding, frequent ambulation, and attention to cleanliness and the integrity of skin and mucous membranes can prevent many infections in the patients with dementia. Safety is a major concern in the maintenance care of the patient with Alzheimer's disease. Falls and other high-risk incidents must be addressed by institutional policies. A detailed discussion of approaches to patient safety is presented in Chapter 18.

The issue of quality of life is very significant in the maintenance care of patients with Alzheimer's disease. Providing safe, supportive care is not sufficient for long-term treatment. Attention also must be paid to the patient's need for comfort. The routines of patient care must be adaptable to allow for individual patient preferences that promote the patient's sense of security. In addition, an effort must be made to introduce pleasurable experiences into the life of the patient. This goal can be achieved through exposure to music or entertainment, contact with familiar items, satisfaction of food preferences, or other activities. This aspect of care must be highly individualized since an activity that is viewed as pleasurable by one patient may be irritating to another. Including family members in identifying the patient's interests and satisfying his needs will give them a sense of participation in the patient's care and will lessen their sense of helplessness.

Another issue related to quality of life is the patient's appearance, an aspect of care that is noticed by family members. Keeping the patient clean and free from odors is important. Dressing him in his own clothes and keeping him well groomed promotes pride in family members as well as the caregiving staff. Close attention to these details also can be tied to a program of maintenance of skin integrity and oral hygiene.

Because so much of the maintenance care of the patient with Alzheimer's disease requires a sensitivity to subtle changes in behavior, it is most important that there be consistency in caregivers. Staff assignments should allow for individual caregivers to follow the same patients for a prolonged time. This approach to staffing can promote high-quality care and a sense of pride and reward among staff. It also can provide family members with a sense of continuity and confidence in the care that the patient is receiving.

EVALUATION OF CARE

Traditional approaches to evaluation of care may not be applicable to the care of the patient with Alzheimer's disease. Usually it is not possible to focus on evaluating the response to an acute situation or episodic care given. Often the maintenance goals for the patient with Alzheimer's disease are phrased in terms of retaining a functional level or slowing the decline. Rehabilitative goals, although often focused on progress, usually are aimed at transitory problems. The compensatory goals most frequently refer to adaptation to an environment and commonly change only when a patient's condition deteriorates.

The goals and the care oriented toward establishing a positive quality of life become very important. Frustration can be avoided if the objectives of the patient, family, and staff are focused on this aspect of care. If these goals are being met, the patient will be less frustrated, the family will be more accepting of his decline, and the staff will be better satisfied with the job they are performing.

BIBLIOGRAPHY

Gwyther L: *Care of Alzheimer's patients: a manual for nursing home staff,* Chicago, 1985, American Health Care Association and Alzheimer's Disease and Related Disorders Association.

Kuhlman GJ and others: Alzheimer's disease and family caregiving: critical synthesis of the literature and research agenda, *Nurs Res* 40:331-337, 1991.

Maas M, Buckwalter K, Hardy M: *Nursing diagnoses and interventions for the elderly,* Reading, Mass, 1991, Addison-Wesley.

Ronch J: *Alzheimer's disease: a practical guide for families and other caregivers,* New York, 1991, Continuum.

Sand B, Yeaworth R, McCabe B: Alzheimer's disease: special care units in long-term care facilities, *J Gerontol Nurs* 18:28-34, 1992.

Volicer L and others, editors: *Clinical management of Alzheimer's disease,* Rockville, Md, 1988, Aspen.

13

Management of difficult behaviors

Warren Clark and Mary M. Lancaster

Difficult behaviors associated with Alzheimer's disease often produce significant stress in the family and the community and result in institutionalization of the patient. Behaviors discussed in this chapter are not applicable to all Alzheimer's patients; indeed, some patients may never experience any of them. These behaviors usually are time-limited: as the disease progresses, they often disappear. However, when they arise, they demand special attention.

Helping patients with any of these behaviors requires good communication and careful definition of the problem. Communication should incorporate both patient and family and requires reflection and support. Communication with the patient is often not easy because of the patient's degree of cognitive impairment. A quiet environment, repetition of requests, use of touch, visual reinforcement, and use of speech patterns familiar to the patient enhance the communication process.

IDENTIFICATION OF PROBLEM

The problem-solving approach to difficult behaviors requires a clear definition of the problem and the identification of precipitating and aggravating factors. This approach may lead to specific interventions for change.

Investigating the nature of the difficult behavior can reveal whether it is the result of the challenge of "insurmountable" tasks, poor communication, or environmental stress. For the patient with Alzheimer's disease, insurmountable tasks are those that are too complicated, are no longer familiar to the patient, or require new learning. Assessment of the patient requires observation of his or her attempts to complete such tasks. For instance, difficulty in dressing, meeting daily hygiene needs, hair care, or applying makeup can be very frustrating for the patient with Alzheimer's disease.

Communication problems can result from unfamiliar language, confusing contexts, or misperceived nonverbal cues. Language may be unfamiliar because it was never known; indeed, knowing the patient's educational level is a rough key to his language skills. Since caregivers may have accents and may pronounce words differently from the patient, the patient may find it difficult to understand them. Observation and encouragement of verbal interaction are the best means of identifying the patient's current ability to use language. The context of verbal interaction can be confusing to the patient when too much is said at one time, when too many steps are combined into one statement, or when the purpose of the communication is unclear. Maintaining eye contact is almost always imperative. Nonverbal cues, such as tone of voice, physical stance, touch, and facial expression, should be congruent with the verbal and contextual communication. It should be remembered that patients with Alzheimer's disease also may be hearing-impaired.

Environmental stimuli may be confusing or distracting to a patient with Alzheimer's disease. These stimuli include too much noise or activity, poor lighting, an unfamiliar surrounding, or extremes of temperature. Both overstimulation and understimulation can increase the patient's sense of disorientation and confusion.

IDENTIFICATION OF SPECIFIC BEHAVIORS
Agitation and Restlessness

Agitation is a state of extreme restlessness or irritability often characterized by pacing, hitting, yelling, or resistiveness. This state can be produced by medications, physical discomfort, anxiety, fatigue, sleep loss, insecurity, sensory overload, sensory deprivation, or sensory distortion such as that produced by cataracts or tinnitus. Agitation also may result from impatience or irritability on the part of the caregiver.

The first approach to the agitated patient is assessment of any physical cause of discomfort or pain, such as fecal impaction, systemic or localized infection, dehydration, urinary retention, osteoarthritis, or fractures (even in the absence of obvious trauma). Attention to the possibility of hunger or thirst and ensuring adequate sleep also are important. Second, the environment should be surveyed to ensure an appropriate level of sensory stimulation and to determine the presence of any apparent irritants. Third, if task completion is thought to be the cause of the agitation, the patient should be observed while performing routine activities of daily living to identify contributing factors. Finally, regardless of whether the caregivers' stress is considered a contributing factor, inservice training should concentrate on teaching caregivers how their own emotional state affects their patients. Supportive supervision and the opportunity for discussion of frustrations may assist caregivers in this regard.

Aggression and Combativeness

True aggression and combativeness are relatively rare in patients with Alzheimer's disease. However, when such behaviors occur, they are frightening to caregivers. The patient's aggression may be verbal, consisting of cursing or threats, or physical, including grabbing, pinching, hitting, or biting. It may be directed at caregivers or other patients. Aggression may be an isolated event, or it may occur with regularity. It may be precipitated by specific activities such as bathing or delivery of medications.

Aggression may reflect long-standing personality traits, or it may be completely out of character for the patient. It can be provoked by caregivers through adherence to an overly rigid daily routine for patient care. Aggression may be an extension of the agitated behavior already described, especially when the underlying causes have not been adequately addressed and have been allowed to escalate. Patients may misinterpret routine activities as being invasive or threatening and respond aggressively out of self-defense. Physical aggression may result when patients no longer have the capacity for verbal expression of their frustrations.

All the strategies suggested for agitation and restlessness also should be applied to the care of the aggressive or combative patient. The aggressive patient always should be approached in a calm, low-key manner, and explanations of all activities should be given. Caregivers should be flexible in scheduling daily care and should allow the patient a sense of control over his body and personal space. Distraction can be an effective tool in breaking a cycle of escalating aggression. Situations known to provoke combative episodes should be avoided, and this approach should be followed by all those who care for the patient. The aggressive patient's environment, whether home or institution, should be free from readily available harmful objects. Medications can be effective in calming agitated patients and interrupting the escalation of aggression (see

---

AGGRESSION AND COMBATIVENESS

Mr. J., a 67-year-old man, was admitted to the nursing home 2 months ago because of deterioration in his family's ability to care for him. The diagnosis of Alzheimer's disease had been made 5 years previously. A widower, Mr. J. was confused in regard to the whereabouts of his wife. He wandered all day and frequently asked for his wife. The only time he was calm was during visits from his family, which occurred primarily on Sundays. Although the staff appreciated the calm that these visits brought, they noticed that Mr. J. became more agitated when the family left, following them to the door and attempting to leave with them. When staff tried to lead him away, he would become belligerent and combative. This behavior sometimes resulted in his receiving medication prn, which served primarily to make him drowsy. On one occasion a staff member was injured when she fell while trying to avoid Mr. J.'s attempt to strike her.

The clinical nurse specialist was asked to advise the staff about methods of reducing Mr. J.'s aggressive episodes. She observed the behaviors described here and interviewed his family to hear their suggestions and gain their support for an intervention. With the staff and the family, she then devised a care plan in which the family would notify the staff 15 minutes before their intended time of departure from visits. The family would plan to leave a small memento with Mr. J. at each visit. A staff member would then begin discussing the memento with him, encouraging some brief reminiscing. The family would say good-bye quietly in the visiting room, and Mr. J. would not be allowed to walk them to the door. The staff member would remain with him for approximately 10 minutes after their departure. This intervention appeared to distract the patient from his feelings of abandonment without altering the nature of the family's visits. No further incidents of combative behavior occurred, and the staff noted that Mr. J.'s efforts to find his wife gradually decreased.

Chapter 14). Since the use of physical restraints tends to increase the patient's confusion and aggressive behavior, it should be avoided in patients with Alzheimer's disease (see box above).

Catastrophic Reactions

Catastrophic reactions are disproportionate responses to the stimuli eliciting the reaction. They may be manifested by uncontrollable crying, extreme agitation, screaming, combativeness, or temper tantrums.

Catastrophic reactions occur in response to the patient's inability to handle a multitude of incoming stimuli. His decreased capacity to inhibit emotional responses contributes to an outpouring of affect in response to even minimal stimuli. These reactions can be frightening to both the patient and the caregiver. If the patient must make a choice between several options or must attend to several requests at the same time, such responses may result. Attempting tasks that are too complex or trying to respond to "why" questions also may overwhelm the patient. Even trivial incidents such as spilling a drink can trigger a catastrophic reaction.

Prevention of catastrophic reactions should be a part of the care plan for any patient prone to them. Avoiding the circumstances known to trigger these reactions usually can be achieved through careful planning. The unit environment and tasks demanded of the patient should be simplified. Distraction is most useful if the reaction is already in progress. Involvement in music- or food-related activities is frequently used for distraction. Caregivers must be cautioned not to overreact to the patient, thus increasing the potential for escalation of catastrophic reactions.

Screaming

Screaming behaviors can occur in patients with Alzheimer's disease who are very confused and have little ability to communicate. Being most disruptive to the home or treatment environment, they may include frequent repeated use of the same word or phrase. The patient's vocalization may or may not be understandable to the caregiver. Such behavior is most frequently related to visual or auditory deficits. Physical discomfort, sensory overload, fear, anxiety, boredom, or fatigue also may trigger this reaction in patients with Alzheimer's disease. Sometimes patients will react adversely to certain caregivers but not others. They may associate these individuals with bad memories from their past. Screaming may be reinforced by caregivers' responses that unintentionally reward the patient.

The nurse must assess and correct the physical problems noted here. Sensory input should be maximized through the use of hearing aids, eyeglasses, and careful use of touch. Massage and other attempts at relaxation may be helpful. Medications can be used with patients who are thought to be experiencing distortions of reality (see Chapter 14). Providing environmental stimuli such as soft music or television also may help. Contact with these patients must be maintained on a regular basis to help reduce the possibility of fear, feelings of abandonment, or loneliness. Relatives and volunteers who sit with such patients can assist greatly in reducing this type of behavior (see box on p. 170).

SCREAMING

Mr. A., a 75-year-old man, has been living in a skilled nursing facility for the past 4 years. Complicating his early Alzheimer's disease is a previous cardiovascular accident that resulted in expressive aphasia. Mrs. A. visits her husband daily at mealtimes and feeds him. She also reads to him while holding his hand until he falls asleep.

On her way to visit one day, Mrs. A. was involved in a serious accident and broke her right tibia and left hip. Mrs. A. has been in the hospital for 3 weeks and is now being transferred to a rehabilitation hospital for therapy. When Mr. A. was notified about his wife's accident, his condition began to deteriorate. He is now bedridden and is not assisting with any activities of daily living. Mr. A. also has begun yelling and screaming. These vocalizations occur for extended periods and are loud and incessant. This behavior has become very disturbing to everyone—staff, patients, and visitors. When his condition worsened, Mr. A. was moved to the front of the building in a semiprivate room. His yelling is now audible to anyone entering the building. At the request and concern of the nursing staff, the treatment team has been called together to devise a plan to address Mr. A.'s screaming behavior.

The team conducted a thorough assessment of the situation and reached the following conclusions:

1. Screaming is Mr. A.'s current method of communication, and it must be viewed by the staff as communication rather than meanness or harassment.
2. Mr. A. is reacting to the loss of his wife's visits plus numerous other physical and social losses.
3. Mr. A. has discovered that screaming brings attention, even if it is negative attention.
4. Through screaming Mr. A. is trying to exert some control over his life.
5. The screaming occurs primarily in the late afternoon, when Mr. A. needs to use the toilet, or when he is overly fatigued.
6. The previous tactics used by the staff to control Mr. A.'s screaming (e.g., telling him to stop, being firm, and stating that he would not get what he wanted by screaming) have become ineffective.

After discovering this information about the situation, the team developed and implemented the following plan:

1. No more changes are to be made in Mr. A.'s environment (e.g., his room will not be changed again).
2. Routines are to be established with Mr. A.'s input, and the *same* staff are to provide his care on a daily basis to establish consistency in his life.
3. The activities director is to work with Mr. A. to add new activities to his daily life.

Screaming—cont'd

4. A friendly visitor program is to begin for Mr. A., and it will involve the same two volunteers coming on a daily basis. The volunteers will be advised to try to establish a routine similar to the one that Mrs. A. established.
5. Mr. A. is given a bell to ring if he needs something. Otherwise, he will be checked on at least every 2 hours.
6. Staff received inservicing on the plan and were instructed to respond quickly to his bell calls but not to his yelling.

   Two months later, Mr. A. is using the bell to call for assistance. He yells out occasionally, but this behavior tends to occur when unavoidable changes are made in his routines. The staff feel very good about working together to make this change without the need to give Mr. A. sedatives.

Abnormal Eating and Drinking Behaviors

Patients with Alzheimer's disease may demonstrate overconsumption or underconsumption of food or fluids. They may be demanding regarding food intake, or they may refuse meals. Some patients may eat or drink all the time, whereas others never seem to feel thirst or hunger. Rarely, some patients will eat inedible objects such as newspapers or napkins (pica). Some patients even have been observed eating feces!

Food-related behavioral problems may be caused by dysphagia, depression, oral diseases, or appetite disturbances. Many medications also can decrease appetite. Lack of awareness of the meal schedule and an inability to use utensils are examples of difficulties the patient may have with the process of eating. The social environment of institutional living also may diminish appetite.

Assessing the patient's ability to successfully chew and swallow food is the first concern with patients who have eating disturbances. The patient's medications should be reviewed for possible appetite suppressants or stimulants. For undereaters, appetite stimulants can be tried, and "finger foods" should be available at all times. Offering one food at a time may simplify mealtime and promote intake. Making mealtime a simple, relaxed, and calm event can be helpful. Providing good mouth care decreases the likelihood of discomfort that can contribute to feeding problems. For some patients adaptive equipment may be necessary to promote independence and compliance with intake requirements. Providing on-unit snacks at the patient's

---

ABNORMAL EATING AND DRINKING BEHAVIORS

The husband of one of our patients observed that when eating in a restaurant sometimes his wife would eat everything on her plate. On other occasions, however, she would not eat anything. While searching for an explanation, he discovered that when his wife faced the wall she cleaned the plate and that when she faced the staff, other customers, or the cash register she failed to eat at all. The distractions offered by the busy restaurant produced a failure to eat.

---

demand can increase intake. Supplements also can be added to the diet for increased calories and nutrients.

For overeaters, smaller, more frequent meals should be provided throughout the day. Low-calorie snacks should replace calorie-rich ones. As already noted, distractions can help avoid confrontation about food. Providing daily exercise through walking, dancing, or wheelchair exercises can help overeaters keep their weight down (see box above).

Abnormal Sexual Behaviors

Sexual behaviors first must be defined on the basis of appropriateness. Such behaviors are determined to be inappropriate if the behavior is dysfunctional; serves no useful, healthy purpose; and does not fit within the setting or environment. Such behaviors may include masturbation, undressing, and touching in public (see box, p. 173). However, usually behaviors of a sexual nature are determined as inappropriate because they bother or embarrass the caregiver.

Because of their dementia, many patients with Alzheimer's disease lose the ability to determine the appropriate time, place, or way to express sexual needs and desires. The patient may no longer recognize his surroundings, may have lost the ability to inhibit certain actions, or may have no other available mechanism for sexual gratification. It is doubtful that patients with Alzheimer's disease display these behaviors to gain attention; instead, their sexual needs are not being met. Patients who demonstrate "inappropriate" sexual behaviors may do so because it feels good. At times the onset of such actions may be provoked by simple pruritus associated with an infection or a chronic stress condition.

Every attempt should be made on the part of family and caregivers to make the patient feel wanted, needed, and desired. Families

---

ABNORMAL SEXUAL BEHAVIORS

Mr. H., a 65-year-old man, was committed to a state psychiatric hospital after exposing himself to his 11-year-old niece in her bedroom. This behavior had happened at least two times and occurred while the niece's mother was at home. Mr. H. had been diagnosed as having Alzheimer's disease several years previously and had been cared for at home by his family. His wife worked during the day, and various family members watched Mr. H. during these times. Mr. H.'s wife had become increasingly tired and discouraged and had lost interest in sexual relations over the past year. Mr. H. had no previous history of sexually deviant behavior and seemed confused and unable to remember the incidents. His family was embarrassed, angry, and in conflict about how to respond to his aberrant behavior.

In the hospital Mr. H. had been very restless, had made sexually explicit remarks to female staff members, and was reported by his family to be increasingly confused. The treatment staff developed a plan for setting firm limits on Mr. H.'s behavior, while simultaneously allowing him privacy for masturbation, which he did about three times a week. A staff psychologist met with Mrs. H. to encourage her to discuss her feelings about the loss of her independence and support from her husband. The family was able to provide her additional support, allowing her to rest and recognizing the degree of stress she had experienced. Mrs. H. was gradually able to again express affection toward her husband. After 6 weeks of hospitalization with no episodes of exposing himself, Mr. H. began to receive day passes to go back to his home. A plan was developed to prevent him from being allowed to be alone with young children and to give him periods of privacy on a daily basis. There were no further incidents of exposure, and Mr. H. was discharged after 8 weeks of treatment.

---

must be encouraged to hold hands, touch, and kiss the patient as they always have. Family and nursing staff need to understand the unmet needs underlying the patient's abnormal behaviors. Providing a relaxing massage or going for a walk and holding the patient's hand provides the therapeutic touch that so many institutionalized elderly patients need.

Patients who masturbate in public places should be gently led from the public area to their room. Scolding these patients or trying to get them to understand will only serve to increase their "bad" feelings and agitation. For truly problematic sexual behaviors, such as intimate touching of visitors or suggestive statements, clear limits must be set without reacting to the situation. The behavior should be assessed for any antecedent causes such as visitation by the family. If such a connection is noted, visitation should take place in the patient's room; once the family leaves, the patient should be immediately involved in some activity. Undressing can be the result of physical factors such as being too warm or frustration about trying to remember how to dress and undress. Any behavioral management of inappropriate sexual display must recognize the embarrassment and disgust produced in the caregivers, who must be provided an opportunity to talk about their feelings.

Paranoid Thinking

Paranoid thinking is exhibited by mistrust and suspicion regarding certain persons or aspects of an individual's environment. In extreme cases this type of thinking can be delusional; the patient may have fixed false beliefs concerning plots to kill him, injure his family, or harm those he cares about in other ways. The patient may respond to these delusions as if they were real and thus may be a danger to himself or others.

Distortions of reality can occur with any type of dementia, or they may be a secondary effect of sensory deprivation or medications. Some of the symptoms of physical decline, such as malnutrition, dehydration, anemia, or infection, may contribute to the problem. In all such cases the decreased ability to receive and interpret stimuli leads to misinterpretations of ordinary situations.

Patients with Alzheimer's disease who experience paranoid thinking need a secure environment and consistent responses from caregivers. They should not be directly challenged about their thinking but should be offered frequent reality testing and assurance of their own security. Maintaining a well-lit environment and providing a nonthreatening milieu can help to reduce the patient's anxiety. Simple explanations of all activities should be offered, and the patient should be allowed to inquire about and examine any aspect of his care for more information. If the patient has family or friends who are able to calm his fears or distract him from paranoid thinking, their help should be enlisted in providing care. Sometimes the availability of telephone contact with a family member can be reassuring to a patient. If feasible, patients should have their hearing and vision checked periodically. Antipsychotic medications can be effective, but they should be administered with close supervision (see Chapter 14).

Depression and Apathy

Differentiating depression from dementia can be difficult (see Chapter 11). Patients with early-stage Alzheimer's disease may recog-

DEPRESSION AND APATHY

Mrs. C., an 80-year-old woman, resided at a continuing care center for 9 years following the death of her husband. She experienced signs of dementia for several years and was diagnosed with Alzheimer's disease shortly after the initial onset of symptoms. She functioned fairly well living in her own apartment until approximately 3 months ago, when her son and some friends noticed that she was becoming increasingly withdrawn and was eating less. Recently Mrs. C. had lost 7 pounds and had a recurrence of sleep disturbance similar to the type she had experienced after her husband's death. The physical examination was unremarkable. After psychiatric consultation, administration of a tricyclic antidepressant was recommended. After 3 months of treatment, including several changes in the dosage of the medication, Mrs. C. had improved only marginally.

An occupational therapist was consulted to recommend activities that might interest and stimulate Mrs. C. A plan was developed so that the patient would attend a partial day treatment program that focused on socialization and provided a lunch. Initially Mrs. C. expressed reluctance, but eventually she began to attend regularly. In addition, she was referred to a music reminiscence group conducted at the center. At these group sessions she discussed feelings stimulated by the music and was able to acknowledge some fears related to loneliness. She was then asked to join a telephone support network within the center and began to anticipate calls from her new friends. Mrs. C.'s level of participation in activities of daily living stabilized at a level that was higher than before the onset of symptoms, and her weight returned to normal. She remained on a small dose of antidepressant medication, which she felt helped her sleep better.

nize their poor prognosis and feel extremely sad and hopeless. Although suicide is rare in patients with Alzheimer's disease, certain highly publicized recent cases may reflect a growing acceptance of this act as an alternative. More common is the occurrence of a sense of hopelessness that may be shared by other family members. In patients with advanced Alzheimer's disease, depression may be associated with biochemical changes occurring in the brain. A common symptom among patients who cannot communicate their feelings effectively is a tendency to withdraw and become apathetic. This response may contribute to some of the problem behaviors described previously.

When patients with Alzheimer's disease are experiencing severe depressive symptoms, such as thoughts of death or inflicting self-harm, they should be assessed for the potential for suicide. If a psychiatric evaluation indicates that such potential is high, treatment in a psychiatric facility is indicated. However, all health care professionals caring for patients with Alzheimer's disease should try to minimize the patient's opportunity for self-harm by providing close observation and an environment with few objects that can be used as weapons. Depressed patients often respond to an environment that promotes physical comfort and the opportunity for performing simple, familiar, and meaningful tasks. Cheerful reminiscence and favorite music also can raise the patient's spirits. Antidepressant medications also may improve the patient's mood and sleep pattern (see Chapter 14).

Sleep Disturbances

Sleep patterns change as people age, but they change more noticeably in the presence of dementia. Some patients with Alzheimer's disease are awake during the nighttime hours and sleep during the daytime. Others sleep fitfully for very brief periods, giving the appearance of constant wakefulness. "Sundowning" refers to the phenomenon in which the patient appears more confused during the late afternoon and early evening hours. Typically the person becomes more agitated, confused, and restless during these hours. Although sometimes described as a sleep disturbance, this state actually may be caused by an alteration of the circadian rhythm. Both sleep/wake disturbances and sundowning affect the quality and quantity of sleep for both patient and caregivers. These behaviors can become very frustrating and tiresome for caregivers. Although the patient usually can fall asleep when the need arises, this option is not available to the caregiver.

Most older individuals experience a decrease in the length of time spent in deep, restful sleep and more periods of wakefulness during the night. To make up for this change, many older persons report increased daytime sleepiness. Persons with dementia disorders may experience the same changes, but during the periods of wakefulness at night they may become restless and confused. They may get up and begin to resume daytime activities, turning on the lights and wandering around. Other patients may have periods of wakefulness during which they demonstrate panic because they cannot recognize their nighttime surroundings. Institutionalization also can have an effect on sleep patterns because of increased noise, medications, pain, and unfamiliar surroundings.

An increased incidence of sleep/wake disturbances has been well documented in persons with dementia. However, little is known about specific neurologic changes associated with dementia that may produce these disturbances. Some factors believed to be involved in sleep disturbance and sundowning include disruption of the normal circadian cycle, lower intensity of light, and decreased environmental stimuli.

In order to help a patient reestablish normal sleep patterns, the caregiver should begin by investigating any factors that might keep the patient awake. Such factors include pain, medications, fear and insecurity, noise, and increased lighting. Eliminating any of these factors may be all that is necessary to help the person sleep. A nightlight is often useful in helping the patient with dementia feel more secure during the night.

Second, the patient's daily schedule of activity should be observed. Patients who have difficulty sleeping should be kept active during the day and not permitted to spend a good portion of the day sitting and napping. Exercise such as walking will help the patient to expend energy and be more fatigued at bedtime. For patients who are unable to walk, other exercises, such as emptying drawers, stacking newspapers, or folding clothes, may be recommended. It is very important to establish a bedtime routine or ritual so that the patient will realize when it is time to go to bed. Such a routine may involve bathing, putting on pajamas, brushing teeth, and toileting. Going through this same routine every night will help the patient recognize what is expected of him.

Patients should avoid the intake of any stimulant such as coffee or cigarettes near bedtime. Allowing the patient to have a light snack before bedtime also may help with sleep. Diuretics should be administered early enough in the day to avoid the need for the patient to get up several times at night to void. Providing reassurance and soft music may help to comfort the patient. Finally, if the patient continues to get up and wander at night, making sure he has a safe place to wander is imperative. Alarms can be placed on the patient's bed to alert caregivers to the fact that the patient is getting out of bed.

In the home setting caregivers must have the opportunity to obtain adequate amounts of sleep. Encouraging the caregiver to elicit the help of another person to watch the patient while he or she rests is one approach. Helping the caregiver to understand the patient's behavior and to rest whenever the patient rests is vitally important. Sleep medications and tranquilizers should be used judiciously and only under the direct supervision of a physician. Caregivers need to be educated regarding the side effects of these medications.

SLEEP DISTURBANCES

Mrs. W., a 72-year-old widow, moved in with her daughter, Joyce, approximately 6 months ago after a hospitalization for pneumonia. Diagnosed as having Alzheimer's disease 8 years earlier, Mrs. W. appears to have been in the second stage for approximately 4½ years. Her level of confusion and disorientation increased significantly when she entered the hospital, and her condition has remained about the same.

Joyce has come to the local Alzheimer's support group for help because, as she puts it, "Mom becomes like another person after supper. She doesn't recognize me, she disrupts everything, and nothing seems to calm her down until she falls asleep. She always seems so much better in the morning." The group members, many of whom have been through the same type of experience, begin to discuss the problem with Joyce.

The group facilitator initiates the conversation by asking Joyce to describe a typical day. During the discussion, it is discovered that Mrs. W. is not provided the opportunity for a nap in the early afternoon but she does sleep well at night. Joyce also comments on how hungry her mother seems to be at suppertime. In addition, it seems that Mrs. W.'s behavior became worse in October, when the time changed.

The facilitator explained to Joyce that her mother appears to be manifesting "sundowning." An explanation of this behavior, with some general information and guidelines, is given, and a plan is devised to assist Mrs. W. with functioning in the late afternoon and early evening. This plan is as follows:

1. To avoid extreme fatigue, Mrs. W. will take a 1-hour nap at 1 PM. Joyce is cautioned not to allow her mother to sleep too long since a long nap may interfere with nighttime sleep.
2. To help relieve the apparent hunger and possible low glucose level, Joyce is to provide her mother with a high-carbohydrate snack at 4 PM.
3. To maintain the same level of illumination in the house, Joyce will turn on the lights 2 hours before sundown. She also will close the curtains 1 hour before sundown so that her mother might not notice the changing light level outside.
4. Joyce will try to engage her mother in a low-stimulation (quiet) activity immediately after supper.

After 2 months Joyce reported that although her mother still exhibited increased confusion at nighttime, the frequency and the degree of confusion and disruption had decreased significantly. She also commented that she was very thankful that this improvement was accomplished without medication.

Helping the patient who is experiencing sundowning usually requires manipulating the patient's environment. Adequate levels of light must be maintained. Closing curtains to eliminate the possibility of seeing the darkness and turning on overhead lights in the late afternoon and evening can help. Exercise during the day is also recommended. Involving the patient in social activities or using techniques of distraction can help the patient remain focused. However, the amount of stimulation must be monitored closely to avoid overstimulating the patient and thereby increasing his confusion and restlessness. The patient should receive orientation cues throughout the day. Allowing the patient a short nap during the early afternoon may eliminate the possibility that he will become overtired. Physical restraints are known to increase the patient's confusion and restlessness, and so they should be avoided. Providing close supervision of the patient is necessary if he experiences sundowning. Finally, psychotropic medications may help to calm the patient if other measures prove futile. These medications should be used in small doses (see box on p. 178).

Repetitious Behaviors

Repetitious behaviors occur on a continuous basis and generally serve no functional purpose. Most of the time these behaviors are benign, posing no danger to the patient or the caregiver. However, they can be very annoying and may cause a great deal of frustration for caregivers. Some examples of repetitious behaviors frequently encountered are questioning, following the caregiver, or performing one task over and over again.

Patients in the later stages of Alzheimer's disease have significant memory loss. Many of the activities the patient engages in may be caused by the fact that he cannot remember having completed the task. The patient also may not remember that he has just been given the answer to a question. Constant questioning about the whereabouts of a certain person or continually following a caregiver may be a demonstration of the patient's concern or insecurity. Repeatedly performing a task may result from boredom, the inability to carry a task to completion, or an attempt on the part of the patient to feel as if he is helping the caregiver. Some medications can cause the patient to have "nervous" energy that is expended through repetitive actions or may be a side effect.

In dealing with repetitious behaviors, the primary emphasis is on helping caregivers understand that the patient is not behaving in a certain way just to annoy them. Caregivers need to know that the behaviors commonly occur and are part of the dementia process. If the patient is showing signs of fear or insecurity, it is helpful to try to determine the cause of these feelings. Providing reassurance through a calm manner and the use of touch can be helpful. Distracting the patient with a favorite activity may help to break the pattern of the behavior. Sometimes ignoring the behavior or questioning will stop the behavior because no reinforcement is provided. If the behavior is benign, such as folding and unfolding clothes, there is no reason to attempt to stop the behavior. However, if the behavior is causing a problem (e.g., constantly moving or hiding objects or watering plants), the patient should be encouraged to substitute a less problem-prone task.

Memory aids such as clocks, calendars, and notes can help to orient the patient to surroundings and events. It may be necessary to provide the patient with the information he is seeking as often as he asks. Engaging the patient in simple conversation may satisfy his need for interaction. Using television, music, or videotapes appropriate for the patient's cognitive ability may provide a distraction for the patient. Finally, giving the patient a chore that he is still able to perform will add a sense of control to the patient's life and bolster his self-esteem.

SUMMARY

Dealing successfully with problematic behaviors requires collaboration among caregivers (both family members and health professionals), creative thinking, and problem-solving techniques. Although not every patient with Alzheimer's disease will experience any of the behaviors discussed here, most will experience at least one or two. Since these behaviors often cannot be attributed to a specific cause, a complete investigation of the circumstances surrounding the behaviors is necessary. Health professionals play a major role in assisting family caregivers to understand the patient's behaviors and the effects those behaviors are having on their lives. Providing a family caregiver with this understanding and possible interventions to use can help give the individual a sense of control over problem situations and relieve some of the stress associated with caring for someone with Alzheimer's disease.

BIBLIOGRAPHY

Alessi CA: Managing the behavioral problems of dementia in the home, *Clin Geriatr Med* 7:787-801, 1991.

Beck C, Heacock P: Nursing interventions for patients with Alzheimer's disease, *Nurs Clin North Am* 23:95-124, 1988.

Chrisman M and others: Agitated behavior in the cognitively impaired elderly, *J Gerontol Nurs* 17(12):9-13, 1991.

Evans LK: The sundown syndrome: a nursing management problem. In Chenitz WC, Stone JT, Salisbury SA, editors: *Clinical gerontological nursing: a guide to advanced practice*, Philadelphia, 1991.

Feldt KS, Ryden MB: Aggressive behavior: educating nursing assistants, *J Gerontol Nurs* 18(5):3-12, 1992.

Gall K, Petersen T, Riesch SK: Night life: nocturnal behaviors patterns among hospitalized elderly, *J Gerontol Nurs* 16(10):31-35, 1990.

Kikuta SC: Clinically managing disruptive behavior on the ward, *J Gerontol Nurs* 17(8):4-7, 1991.

Maletta GJ: Treatment of behavioral symptomatology of Alzheimer's disease, with emphasis on aggression: current clinical approaches, *Int Psychogeriatr* 4(suppl 1): 117-130, 1992.

Robinson A, Spencer B, White L: *Understanding difficult behaviors*, Ann Arbor, 1989, Geriatric Education Center of Michigan.

Salisbury SA, Stone JT: Managing behavioral problems. In Chenitz WC, Stone JT, Salisbury SA, editors: *Clinical gerontological nursing: a guide to advanced practice*, Philadelphia, 1991, WB Saunders.

Schneider LS, Sobin PB: Non-neuroleptic treatment of behavioral symptoms and agitation in Alzheimer's disease and other dementia, *Psychopharmacol Bull* 28: 71-79, 1992.

Vitiello MV, Bliwise DL, Prinz PN: Sleep in Alzheimer's disease and the sundown syndrome, *Neurology* 42(7 suppl 6):83-93, 1992.

Volicer L and others, editors: *Clinical management of Alzheimer's disease*, Rockville, Md, 1988, Aspen.

Wooten V: Sleep disorders in geriatric patients, *Clin Geriatr Med* 8:427-439, 1992.

14

Psychopharmacology in dementia

James M. Turnbull

The diagnosis of Alzheimer's disease is more dependent on intellectual impairment and memory loss than on behavioral change. However, it is the behavioral disturbances that greatly affect the quality of life not only for the patient but also for the family and the caregivers. These behavioral changes, described in detail in other chapters of this book, include agitation, wandering, screaming, aggression, violence, and inappropriate sexual acting-out.

A close relationship exists between depression and dementia, one that is classically illustrated by the most tragic of Shakespeare's characters, King Lear. The early stages of Alzheimer's disease are frequently associated with the characteristic signs and symptoms of a mood disorder, including anhedonia (loss of pleasure in things that were formally enjoyed), insomnia, low mood, crying spells, hopelessness, change in appetite, lethargy, and thoughts of suicide. The frequency of depressive disorders in patients with dementia may be as high as 20%.

Pharmacotherapy of behavioral disturbances and depression is both appropriate and in some cases life-saving, but it is also fraught with danger. The physiological changes that take place with aging affect the pharmacokinetics and pharmacodynamics of drugs. Most patients older than 75 are taking more than one medication, which leads to problems with compliance, drug-drug interactions, and iatrogenic illness. Frequently, a close look at the combination of drugs a patient is taking is the key to explaining the appearance of new symptoms. Since drug metabolism takes place in the liver, which may have reduced perfusion, it is important to choose drugs that (1) have low hepatotoxicity and (2) have simple metabolic profiles (i.e., are inactivated by a one-step process rather than two or more steps).

Therefore haloperidol is preferred over thioridazine; desipramine, over imipramine; and oxazepam, over diazepam.

Renal function and perfusion also decline with age, and drugs such as lithium, nortriptyline, and fluoxetine, in which renal excretion is an important elimination route, are likely to have a prolonged effect. The pharmacodynamics of medications also alters with age because of a decrease in the number of receptors and in neurotransmitter levels. Target organs, particularly the brain, also undergo structural changes.

Two important steps should precede the prescription of any psychoactive drug to a patient with dementia. The first step is a thorough assessment of the problem, including the differential diagnosis (see Chapter 9). The second step is to evaluate what nonpharmacological management has already been attempted.

ANTIPSYCHOTICS

Neuroleptic drugs are almost exclusively used for the treatment of psychotic disorders in younger patients, for example, conditions such as schizophrenia, bipolar disorder, delusional disorder, and psychotic depression. In the geriatric population the set of indications for neuroleptics tends to be broader and less well defined. Therefore strict Omnibus Budget Reconciliation Act (OBRA) guidelines have been developed for the use of these drugs in nursing homes. The major drugs included in this category are listed in Table 14-1. In almost all cases the starting dose is half that of the dose for younger adults.

There are several indications for the use of neuroleptics in the patient with dementia. Aggression, restlessness, delusions, hallucinations, and some forms of inappropriate sexual behavior are more responsive to this class of drugs than symptoms such as persistent wandering or screaming.

Since neuroleptics are of equal efficacy (with the possible exception of clozapine), the choice of drug depends on the side effect profile. High-potency, low-dose drugs, such as pimozide and fluphenazine, are likely to produce extrapyramidal side effects. Low-potency, high-dose drugs, such as chlorpromazine and thioridazine, are strongly sedating and anticholinergic, and they produce orthostatic hypotension. Drugs in the middle range of potency, such as thiothixene and perphenazine, are often selected. Despite numerous studies on treatment, there are no clear guidelines regarding the length of treatment. It is

Table 14-1 Selected antipsychotic drugs

Class/Generic Name	Trade Name	Dose Equivalent (mg)	Usual Daily Oral Adult Dose (mg)	Single Parenteral Adult Dose (mg)	Usual Daily Oral Dose (mg) Over Age 65	Frequency
Phenothiazines						
Chlorpromazine	Thorazine	100	200-600	25-100	50-200	bid*
Thioridazine	Mellaril	100	200-600	N/A	50-200	bid
Mesoridazine	Serentil	50	150	25-175	25-100	bid
Trifluoperazine	Stelazine	5	5-10	1-2	2-10	od†
Fluphenazine HCl	Permitil, Prolixin	1	2.5-10	2-5	1-3	od
Perphenazine	Trilafon	9	16-64	5-10	4-16	bid
Thioxanthenes						
Chlorprothixene	Taractan	40	75-200	75-200	25-75	bid
Thiothixene	Navane	4	6-30	4	2-10	bid
Butyrophenone						
Haloperidol	Haldol	1	2-12	2-5	0.5-5	bid
Dibenzoxazepine						
Loxapine	Loxitane	10	20	12.5-50	5-10	bid
Indole derivative						
Molindone	Moban	5	15-60	N/A	5-15	bid
Diphenylbutylpiperidine						
Pimozide	Orap	N/A	2-10	N/A	2-4	bid
Dibenzodiazepine						
Clozapine	Clozaril	N/A	200-900	N/A	N/A	bid

*Twice a day.
†Every day.

advisable to provide drug "holidays" at regular intervals. Such drug-free periods provide information about the need to continue administration of neuroleptics. Symptoms often remit spontaneously as a result of environmental changes or progression of the dementia. Regular review should also include administration of the Abnormal Involuntary Movement Scale (AIMS) test (Fig. 14-1).

The following side effects have been noted for antipsychotic drugs:

1. Anticholinergic effects, including dry mouth, constipation, impairment of erectile functioning, urinary delay or obstruction, tachycardia, impaired sweating, and delusions, are possible.
2. Antiadrenergic effects, particularly orthostatic hypotension, may occur.
3. Extrapyramidal effects, consisting of dystonia, parkinsonian symptoms and signs (rigidity, tremor, shuffling gait, pill-rolling of finger), akathisia, akinesia, and, most serious, tardive dyskinesia are sometimes noted. Akathisia is particularly troublesome. It is manifested by restlessness, muscle cramps, jitteriness, pacing, and "inner anxiety." Frequently, patients who develop akathisia will be unwilling to continue taking the drug.
4. Other less common but serious side effects that may occur are agranulocytosis, epileptic seizures, cholestatic jaundice, photosensitivity, alterations in cardiac conduction, and neuroleptic malignant syndrome.

Some noncompliant patients with a demonstrated need for a neuroleptic drug may require intramuscular depot medication. The commonly used ones are haloperidol decanoate (given monthly) and fluphenazine decanoate (given every 14 days).

ANXIOLYTICS AND HYPNOTICS

The benzodiazepines have almost entirely replaced barbiturates and meprobamate in the treatment of anxiety and insomnia. Other drugs used for these purposes include antihistamines (particularly hydroxyzine) and beta-blockers (propranolol).

Buspirone is particularly well tolerated by the anxious, elderly patient with dementia, but, like all anxiolytic agents, it is not as effective in controlling agitation as the neuroleptics.

Benzodiazepines are generally divided into three groups: short-acting, intermediate-acting, and long-acting. The long-acting agents (diazepam, chlordiazepoxide, and flurazepam) accumulate in elderly

	Abnormal Involuntary Movement Scale (AIMS)				
	Patient's name _____ Rater _____ Date _____				
	Instructions: Read the examination procedure (opposite page) before making rating.				
	Movement ratings: Rate highest severity observed. Rate movements that occur upon activation one less than those observed spontaneously.				
Facial and oral movements	1. Muscles of facial expressions: include movements of forehead, eyebrows, periorbital area, cheeks. Note frowning, blinking, smiling, and grimacing. Circle one				
	0 None	1 Minimal, may be extreme normal	2 Mild	3 Moderate	4 Severe
	2. Lips and perioral area: include puckering, pouting, and smacking.				
	0	1	2	3	4
	3. Jaw: include biting, clenching, chewing, mouth opening, and lateral movement.				
	0	1	2	3	4
	4. Tongue: rate only increase in movement both in and out of mouth, not inability to sustain movement.				
	0	1	2	3	4
Extremity movements	5. Upper (arms, wrists, hands, fingers): include choreic movements (rapid, objectively purposeless, irregular, spontaneous) and athetoid movements (slow, irregular, complex, serpentine). Do not include tremor (repetitive, regular, rhythmic).				
	0	1	2	3	4
	6. Lower (legs, knees, ankles, toes): include lateral knee movement, foot tapping, heel dropping, foot squirming, and inversion and eversion of the foot.				
	0	1	2	3	4
Trunk movements	7. Neck, shoulders, hips: include rocking, twisting, squirming, and pelvic gyrations.				
	0	1	2	3	4
Global judgments	8. Severity of abnormal movements.				
	0 None, normal	1 Minimal	2 Mild	3 Moderate	4 Severe
	9. Incapacitation due to abnormal movements: Rate as in item 8.				
	0	1	2	3	4
	10. Patient's awareness of abnormal movements. Rate only patient's report.				
	0 No awareness	1 Aware, no distress	2 Aware, mild distress	3 Aware, moderate distress	4 Aware, severe distress
Dental status	11. Current porblems with teeth and/or dentures?			0 No	1 Yes
	12. Does patient usually wear dentures?			0 No	1 Yes

Fig. 14-1. Form for scoring the Abnormal Involuntary Movement Scale. (From Department of Health and Human Services, National Institute of Mental Health, Washington, DC.)

individuals and increase the risk of toxicity. Drugs that are more rapidly eliminated, such as alprazolam, lorazepam, and triazolam, are preferable.

Clonazepam is a unique member of this class because it stimulates serotonin production and has value in the management of aggression. This drug appears to be useful for patients who display hyperactivity, insomnia, social intrusiveness, and impulsivity. My experience suggests that clonazepam is also useful in conjunction with a low dose of a neuroleptic such as haloperidol. The side effects of benzodiazepines include sedation, worsening of cognitive impairment, transient global amnesia, ataxia, falls, and paradoxical worsening of symptoms. Propranolol has been described as decreasing aggression in individuals with dementia, but it may need to be taken for several weeks before any effect is noted. The potential side effects of propranolol include hypotension, depression, sleep disturbance, and worsening of both chronic obstructive airway disease and heart failure. This drug may also mask the signs of hypoglycemia.

ANTIDEPRESSANTS

The relationship between dementia and depression is a complex one. Short-lived dysphoria may occur as a reaction to loss of cognitive abilities, and major depressive disorders of late onset may be superimposed on Alzheimer's disease. Antidepressant drugs may be useful in either situation. The choice of antidepressant depends on four considerations:

1. Previous treatment for depression. What drug, if any, was useful?
2. Drug management of other family members. If a first-degree relative was responsive to a particular antidepressant, it is a good idea to try the same drug for this patient.
3. Other medications that the patient may be taking, including over-the-counter drugs. Because patients often do not remember their medications, it is helpful to have them bring the drugs in a bag and ask a relative who knows the patient to accompany him.
4. Possible need for psychiatric counseling. Treatment-resistant depression may require referral to a psychiatrist, particularly one familiar with psychopharmacology.

Antidepressants are of the following types: tricyclics, tetracyclics, triazolopyridines, lithium, monoamine oxidase inhibitors (MAOIs), stimulants, and serotonin reuptake inhibitors (Table 14-2). Tricyclic and tetracyclic antidepressants are all effective and useful, but these agents vary in their side effect profiles. Particularly troublesome for older individuals are the anticholinergic actions (see discussion of antipsychotics). All these drugs have a propensity to cause orthostatic hypotension, although imipramine, amitriptyline, and doxepin are more likely to cause this problem than nortriptyline. Orthostasis is particularly troublesome in older individuals because of the risk of falls. In younger patients, the medication is often given at bedtime, but in the elderly, divided doses are preferred because of the risk of hora somni (hs) loading and an associated fall when the patient arises at night to use the bathroom or answer the telephone.

Cardiac conduction may be affected by antidepressants. All drugs in this class act in a way similar to quinidine. Skin rash, liver toxicity, tinnitus, and myoclonus are all observed at times. Plasma levels of these drugs are useful when noncompliance is suspected, when no response is elicited with a therapeutic dose, or when a change in efficacy occurs after a switch to a generic brand.

Low starting doses are recommended in the elderly. Increases in dosage should continue until improvement is noted or until side effects become intolerable. Duration of treatment is often longer for older patients. After age 50 a typical depressive cycle lasts for 3 to 5 years, compared to 9 to 18 months in younger patients. MOAIs are not recommended in the depressed patient with dementia. The use of these agents is complicated by dietary and medication restrictions that are easily forgotten.

Trazodone is a useful drug in the elderly depressed patient. Although it is relatively free from anticholinergic side effects, it does produce sedation, hypotension, and dizziness.

Stimulants are rarely prescribed to any patient except children with attention deficit disorder and individuals with narcolepsy. These agents are associated with abuse and dependency. They may also be the only antidepressant drugs that work in a depressed person with dementia, particularly a person who has another complicating medical illness such as stroke or congestive heart failure.

Although it is advisable to administer the last dose of the day of a stimulant no later than 4 PM (because of the drug's tendency to produce insomnia), stimulants are remarkably free of side effects in the elderly.

Lithium is used in the treatment of bipolar disorder, but it has also been used in the elderly to enhance the action of antidepressants and to manage agitation. Since lithium is excreted via the kidney and

Table 14-2   Antidepressants: dose ranges and frequency

Class	Drug Name	Dose Range (mg/day)	Frequency
Tricyclics	Imipramine	25-300	hs*
	Desipramine	10-300	hs
	Amitriptyline	25-300	hs
	Nortriptyline	10-150	hs
	Doxepin	10-300	hs
Tetracyclics	Maprotiline	25-150	hs
MAOIs	Phenelzine	15-90	bid†
Triazolopyridine	Trazodone	50-600	tid‡
Stimulants	Dextroamphetamine	25-30	bid (not at bedtime)
	Methylphenidate	5-40	bid (not at bedtime)
Serotonin reuptake inhibitors	Fluoxetine	10-60	od§
	Sertraline	50-600	od
	Paroxetine	10-40	od
Chloropropiophenones	Bupropion	150-300	tid

*At bedtime.
†Twice a day
‡Three times a day.
§Every day.

renal clearance is reduced in older individuals, great care must be exercised both before and during treatment. Side effects include a fine tremor, nausea, headache, lassitude, and polyuria.

The most promising development in the class of antidepressant drugs in the past 5 years has been the introduction of fluoxetine, sertraline, and paroxetine, which inhibit the uptake of serotonin and thus make more serotonin available in the brain. These drugs, and others that will be introduced soon, have very favorable side effect profiles in the elderly. Not only are they minimally anticholinergic; they also are noncardiotoxic and do not produce orthostatic hypotension. Many physicians currently use these agents as the antidepressant of first choice. Although fluoxetine comes in a standard 20 mg capsule form, it is also available in a liquid form, which allows lower doses to be prescribed. Fluoxetine, sertraline, and paroxetine are more expensive than generic tricyclics or trazodone. They also produce nausea, insomnia, and sometimes diarrhea early in treatment. A more serious side effect is autonomic hyperactivity, often described by the patient as "nervous inside." Some authors have referred to this problem as "internal akathisia."

Another exciting new addition to the ranks of antidepressants is bupropion. The distribution of this drug was promptly halted in 1986, after 3 of 55 patients receiving up to 400 mg daily for bulimia developed seizures. Bupropion was later reintroduced with a warning that dosages should not exceed 300 mg daily. This agent appears to have a relatively selective action on dopamine reuptake. Bupropion has few anticholinergic actions, involves little or no sedation, and is noncardiotoxic. It is the one antidepressant least likely to produce erectile dysfunction in males and anorgasmia in females that is currently available in the United States. Most important, it is safe for use in elderly patients with dementia.

The disadvantages of bupropion are its thrice-daily dosing, its stimulant action (which may produce insomnia), and the rare but real possibility of seizure.

GENERAL CONSIDERATIONS

Compliance and drug-taking behavior are often ignored by health care professionals. Yet the following important issues of psychopharmacology need to be considered:

- New drugs are more expensive than established ones.
- Prescriptions for large amounts of antidepressants are dangerous because of the risk of overdose if the patient feels suicidal.
- Older individuals, especially those who are 75 and older, are often taking multiple drugs, some of which may have been purchased as over-the-counter medications.
- Older patients are more affected by troublesome side effects than younger, more resilient individuals.
- It is usually best to "start low and go slow," that is, to begin with a small dose of the psychoactive medication and gradually increase the dose to achieve the desired therapeutic effect.
- Coordination of the various specialists involved in the care of the patient is essential, and the nurse is in a unique position to perform this role.
- It is better to teach a patient how to induce sleep than to prescribe a sleeping pill (see box). Almost all elderly patients, with or without dementia, have sleep difficulties.

SUMMARY

To achieve the best results from psychoactive drugs in the treatment of dementia, special attention must be given to careful review.

TIPS FOR HANDLING SLEEP PROBLEMS

1. Elderly individuals should not be allowed to oversleep and then attempt to catch up on sleep. Oversleeping resets the biological time clock and causes insomnia.
2. If an elderly person awakens prematurely, the caregiver should tell him to relax and try to fall asleep again. In the early stages of Alzheimer's disease, the patient may be encouraged to get up and read, watch television, or listen to a radio turned to low volume. The patient should return to bed if he feels sleepy. In late stages of the disease, the patient should be stimulated to stay awake during the day and should be put to bed as late as possible.
3. Alcohol, cigarettes, and caffeine should be avoided in the afternoon or early evening before bedtime.
4. If the patient is a worrywart, the caregiver should encourage him to spend some time worrying in the early evening. For example, 1 hour each day can be set aside for worrying. The caregiver might say: "I really want you to worry about your kids, your grandchildren, the bills, and all the 'what ifs' you can cram into 1 hour!"
5. The elderly person should experiment with the bedroom environment, for example, making changes in lighting, air conditioning, or heating, using heavier drapes, and trying soothing music to discover what is comfortable for him.
6. A heavy meal should not be eaten within 2 hours of bedtime.
7. Regular exercise is vital for the patient with Alzheimer's disease, but it should not be scheduled too close to bedtime.
8. The patient should not nap during the day.
9. Caregivers can teach relaxation techniques, even to patients with early stages of Alzheimer's disease.
10. If none of the common techniques seems to work, help can be obtained from a sleep disorders clinic. The nearest clinic can be obtained by writing to: Association of Sleep Disorders Centers, National Office, 604 Second Street, N.W., Rochester, MN 55902.

Relatives and patients always have questions, and an atmosphere must be created that encourages the development of a rapport that fosters an understanding the disease and the drugs being used for treatment, including the side effects and potential benefits of these agents.

BIBLIOGRAPHY

Rapp MS and others: Behavioral disturbances in the demented elderly: phenomenology, pharmacotherapy and behavioral management, *Can J Psychiatry* 37:651-657, 1992.

Rosen J, Bohon S, Gershon S: Antipsychotics in the elderly, *Acta Psychiatr Scand* 82(suppl 358):170-175, 1990.

Shamoian CA: Somatic therapies in geriatric psychiatry. Lazarus and others, editors: In *Essentials of geriatric psychiatry*, New York, 1988, Springer-Verlag.

15

Specific drug therapy

Mark Doman

Many specific drug compounds have been investigated in the treatment of Alzheimer's disease. Neurotransmitter replacement has received the most attention. Stimulation of the brain by various agents, including nootropics, Hydergine, and narcotic antagonists, also has been attempted. Improving blood flow to and within the brain has been undertaken. Along with these methods, researchers have tried to decrease the effects of Alzheimer's disease by the removal of aluminum and heavy metals from the brain. Finally, the efficacy of vitamin supplementation has been explored. This chapter describes various therapeutic endeavors that attempt not only to treat symptoms but also to halt or even reverse the disease process itself.

CHOLINERGIC THERAPY

Alzheimer's disease has been associated with loss of cholinergic nervous activity in the brain. The markers for cholinergic activity in the brain are choline acetyltransferase (CAT) and acetylcholinesterase (AChE). These enzymes are integral factors in the production and regulation of acetylcholine, the most common neurotransmitter in the body. The levels of these markers are believed to reflect the approximate amount of cholinergic nerve activity present.

Cholinergic nerves are so named because they use acetylcholine as their transmitter. Each of these nerves is composed of single nervous cells called neurons. Acetylcholine is synthesized in the sending neuron from basic precursors. After synthesis, acetylcholine is stored in tiny packets at the far end of the neuron.

The author wishes to express his gratitude for the invaluable editorial assistance provided by Katherine Hoffman Doman in preparing this chapter.

The area between a sending neuron and a receiving neuron is called the synapse. The terms "presynaptic" and "postsynaptic" refer to the sending and receiving neurons, respectively. The acetylcholine packets wait for the neuron's firing, or depolarization of the neuron, at which time they are released by the presynaptic neuron into the synapse.

Once in the synapse, acetylcholine activates receptors on the postsynaptic neuron and causes depolarization of the postsynaptic neuron. This activity causes continuation of the presynaptic neuron's message. Enzymes present in the synapse, AChEs, break the acetylcholine down into inactive components, thus limiting the amount of acetylcholine in the synapse. This breakdown occurs very quickly after acetylcholine has been released. After all the acetylcholine has been broken down, the postsynaptic neuron readies itself for passage of the next message, and the fragments of acetylcholine are absorbed back into the presynaptic neuron and to be made eventually into acetylcholine again.

In Alzheimer's disease, CAT and AChE have been found to be decreased by factors of as high as 80%. The degree of loss of these markers correlates well with the severity of the dementia.

Animal studies have confirmed that induction of an acetylcholinergically deficient state, through surgery or the use of chemicals, interferes with learning and behavior. Studies of scopolamine, a centrally active cholinergic antagonist, showed that it caused brief impairment in the learning of new material but did not impair alertness. The learning impairment was relieved by the administration of an AChE. Scopolamine given to patients with Alzheimer's disease interfered even more with new learning.

All these findings have led to attempts to restore the lost acetylcholine in the hope that doing so will reverse or slow the course of Alzheimer's disease. There are four basic strategies employed: (1) augmentation of the production of acetylcholine within the presynaptic neuron, (2) enhanced release of the messenger contained within the neuron, (3) increased concentration of the messenger in the synapse by slowing the messenger's breakdown, and (4) increasing the sensitivity of the postsynaptic neuron to acetylcholine.

The first attempts to treat Alzheimer's disease involved the administration of the acetylcholine precursors choline and lecithin. It was shown that the administration of oral choline increased concentration of choline in cerebrospinal fluid. Studies performed in a double-blind fashion have failed to demonstrate any significant change in patient performance regarding memory or learning tests. It is still hoped, however, that long-term administration may at least slow the progress of the disease, and this approach is currently being investigated.

To increase the release of AChE effect in the synapse, two strategies have been used. The use of drugs that actually increase the release of the native transmitter from the presynaptic neuron has only been initiated. The first of the drugs used in this category, 4-aminopyridine, has been noted to have some benefit in one study and no benefit in a second. The second drug of this type, Dup 996, has shown encouraging results in rats and primates, but no human studies have been completed to date.

A second, much more extensively researched method in cholinergic replacement is the addition of a chemical that is similar in structure to native acetylcholine in an attempt to augment the action of the native transmitter acetylcholine and thus improve the patient's disability. The initial agent examined in this respect was arecoline. This agent reversed the scopolamine-induced learning impairments in normal volunteers. Unfortunately, several studies have shown that it has no significant effect in patients with Alzheimer's disease.

The use of nicotine bitartrate did decrease intrusion errors in Alzheimer's disease, but the side effects noted at a low dosage prevented investigation of higher dosages. These agents are all associated with rather significant side effects secondary to their primary effect of activating cholinergic neurons throughout the body. These side effects, which include excessive salivation, blurred vision, and high blood pressure, limit the amount of the drug that can be used and require frequent stoppage of medication.

In efforts to avoid these problems, the administration of cholinergic drugs through direct delivery to the ventricles of the brain has been investigated. The agent used in these trials has been bethanechol. These studies have been disappointing, with no improvement in cognitive functions noted on critical assessment. There is also some risk to the patient in having surgery for placement of the pump. However, some other cholinergic agonist may be effective with direct delivery systems.

The third strategy in cholinergic replacement is the use of an anticholinesterase agent to slow the degradation of acetylcholine in the synapse, to increase the concentration at that location, and to increase the duration of its action. This approach is the most extensively studied of all treatments for Alzheimer's disease.

The initial agent used in these investigations was physostigmine. This drug crosses the blood-brain barrier, but it has a short duration of action and must be administered by intravenous infusion. Most studies have shown improvement in some patients given physostigmine, although this improvement is not marked. Longer-term studies have demonstrated slowed deterioration in the patients receiving physostigmine in comparison to patients given placebos. The individuals receiving the most benefit have had early-stage dementia. In patients with advanced dementia, no effect was noted.

Further, the dosage of physostigmine for response must be individualized for optimal intracerebral concentration. Patients who respond show what is called an "inverted U-shaped curve," with a lack of response to low concentration and impairment of cognitive function at high concentrations. A recent study indicated some positive effects of oral physostigmine on verbal learning at longer dosage intervals than previously reported.

The difficulty of long-term intravenous treatment has prompted attempts to find orally active, long-acting cholinesterase inhibitors that will cross the blood-brain barrier in the manner of physostigmine. The compound that has been the focus of much interest and investigation in this group has been tetrahydroaminacridine (Tacrine).

Tetrahydroaminacridine has been the subject of controversy. A 1986 study that claimed remarkable improvements with this drug was investigated, and its findings and methods were questioned. Recently completed trials involving multiple centers have been concluded, and they document that, in the best of cases, there is a slight slowing of deterioration in certain patients. This slowing is minimal, however, and is associated with significant risks of liver toxicity. The Food and Drug Administration (FDA) reviewed the drug recently and determined that it will be released for general usage.

Several other investigational oral anticholinesterases show promise and are currently undergoing clinical trials. These are galanthamine, valnacrine maleate, metrifonate, huprezine A and B, and heptylphysostogmine.

OTHER NEUROTRANSMITTERS

Noradrenaline, dopamine, and serotonin, which are all non-cholinergic neurotransmitters, have also been noted to be present in abnormal concentrations within the brains of patients with Alzheimer's disease.

Dopamine is the most studied noncholinergic neurotransmitter of the three. Parkinson's disease is caused by with deficiency of this transmitter because of the loss of the neuronal cells responsible for its production. When administered to patient's with Parkinson's disease, levodopa, a dopamine precursor, reverses some of the effects of the disease. (Levodopa was the investigational drug that was the subject of the book *Awakenings* by Oliver Sacks.)

Replacement of levodopa itself has been attempted in the treatment of Alzheimer's disease. Although the first study reported an improvement in the patients involved, subsequent studies failed to corroborate these results. Current conjecture is that the initial study may have inadvertently included some patients with Parkinson's disease and their improvement skewed the study. No current trials with levadopa are under way.

Recently, a second anti-Parkinson treatment has been tested and has shown more promise. Deprenyl, a monoamine oxidase inhibitor, works in a manner analogous to the anticholinesterases. It blocks the degradation pathway for dopamine, serotonin, and norepinephrine. Studies have not clearly defined the usefulness of this agent since some find no benefit and others report positive results. This agent is awaiting a larger clinical trial to define its appropriateness in the treatment of Alzheimer's disease.

Other methods of augmenting the nondopamine monoamine neurotransmitters have been tried. Two alpha-2 adrenoreceptor agonists, clonidine and guanfacine, were noted to improve memory testing in one animal study. Studies of the use of these agents for other dementing illnesses, such as Korsakoff's psychosis, show some promise. However, when tested on patients suffering from Alzheimer's disease, clonidine and guanfacine have failed to show value.

Serotonin is another noncholinergic neurotransmitter that appears in decreased concentrations in the brain of patients with Alzheimer's disease. Efforts to increase this transmitter have also been attempted. These trials have involved the use of citalopram, alaproclate, and zimelidine, but, unfortunately, these agents have not demonstrated beneficial effects.

Of the investigational agents mentioned here, deprenyl currently seems most likely to prove beneficial in the treatment of Alzheimer's disease. The other agents have essentially been proven ineffectual. Although deprenyl shows promise at this time, much research remains to be done before its usefulness can be proven.

NOOTROPICS

The term "nootropic" was created from the root words "noos" (mind) and "tropein" (forward). It refers to a class of chemicals that helps to correct the decline of learning and behavior in patients with dementia by generally increasing metabolic activity within the neuron. These agents are related to gamma-aminobutyric acid (GABA), but apparently they have no effect on GABA receptors. They were originally defined as not having specific activity at any location or system within the brain. Thus their action is uncertain, although some researchers are beginning to think that these agents aid the release of acetylcholine from the hippocampal region of the brain.

The effectiveness of these agents in animal models has been good, but results of follow-up studies in humans with dementia have been much less impressive. The first of these agents was piracetam. In the early studies, which were not well controlled, it appeared that piracetam was effective in generally improving patients with Alzheimer's disease, although it did not improve cognitive test scores. Later, more tightly controlled studies produced conflicting results as to whether the agent has significant positive effects.

Animal studies have shown significant improvements in subjects when a combination of piracetam and lecithin (an acetylcholine precursor) is used. At least two studies have shown significant improvements in some of the patients tested but no change in others. This difference implies that there may be certain individuals who would benefit from this therapy but that it does not have a significant effect on every patient. On the basis of improvement in these limited populations, several countries that have less stringent requirements for drug release than the United States have allowed the distribution of this drug.

Aniracetam was the second of this class to be investigated. This agent was considered to have significant potential in animal studies. Early studies of small groups of patients with dementia (not specifically patients with Alzheimer's disease) reported some effect when this agent was used, but a larger study using placebo controls for patients with Alzheimer's disease failed to show any benefit.

Oxiracetam is the newest drug of this class to be developed. Its influence on patients with dementia has been studied and has shown some positive results. The benefits appear to be associated mainly with alcoholic or multiinfarct dementia. The largest trial of patients with Alzheimer's disease demonstrated no significant improvements.

Investigation of the effect of oxiracetam on the other types of dementia continues.

This class of drugs has not proven a definite benefit to patients with Alzheimer's disease. Although there may be a subset of patients who would benefit from these agents (especially when combined with lecithin), at this point nootropic therapy is unproven and cannot be recommended to individuals except for those who wish to participate in research protocols.

HYDERGINE

Hydergine until recently was the only drug approved for the treatment of dementia of the Alzheimer's type. This medication is a combination of four ergoloid mesylates. Despite the length of time that this medication has been both studied and used, it remains largely a mystery to clinicians.

Hydergine's mechanism of action is especially uncertain. It was initially thought to improve cerebral blood flow. With continued research, a blockade of the alpha-adrenergic and serotonergic nerves was discovered, as were effects on the dopaminergic nerves. None of these effects is currently believed to explain Hydergine's action. The current working hypothesis is that Hydergine's effects in Alzheimer's disease are secondary to the increased state of alertness produced in patients taking the drug.

The effectiveness of Hydergine has always been questioned. During 24 weeks of use, a large, well-controlled study published in 1990 showed no benefit in the use of Hydergine compared to placebo in patients with Alzheimer's disease. Earlier studies had reported either slight improvement or slowing of the loss of function in patients with dementia. It is worth noting that the dosage used in the 1990 study was only 3 mg per day, and many of the previous studies reporting Hydergine as effective involved larger dosages of the medication. Studies using larger dosages of Hydergine are ongoing, and they will help to define better this medication's place in the treatment of Alzheimer's disease.

Other ergoloid mesylates have been evaluated and are still under investigation, although none has shown a clear effectiveness in the treatment of Alzheimer's disease to date. These agents include nicergoline and acetyl-l-carnitine.

At this time, it is probably worthwhile to offer a 3- to 6-month trial of Hydergine to individual patients. During that time the patient should be carefully observed for signs of improvement. If a benefit is noted, administration of the agent should continue. If no benefit to the patient is observed, the trial should be discontinued.

NARCOTIC ANTAGONISTS

Naloxone, a drug often used clinically to reverse the effects of narcotic overdoses, has also been studied as a treatment for patients with Alzheimer's disease. During initial studies, researchers administered the drug to patients with dementia, hoping that the blockage of endogenous opiates would provide stimulation that would effect improvement in their cognition and behavior.

Several early studies reported some improvement in the patients to whom naloxone was administered, but larger, more tightly controlled studies failed to confirm these results. The later studies indicated that naloxone caused restlessness, irritability, and some hostility without offering improvement in cognition.

Based on the later, more substantial studies, naloxone is considered to be ineffective in the treatment of Alzheimer's disease.

NIMODIPINE

Nimodipine, a calcium channel blocker similar to those widely used in the treatment of hypertension, acts selectively on brain vasculature, causing dilatation of the vessels without lowering systemic blood pressure. It has also been shown to be capable of blocking experimentally induced constriction of brain vasculature. This effect is responsible for the FDA's current indication of nimodipine for the prevention of reflex vasospasm seen in subarachnoid hemorrhage. Although the use of nimodipine results in dilatation of the blood vessels, this change increases circulation but does not cause increased oxygen uptake by the brain.

The effect of nimodipine on blood flow is certainly important, but this agent may also have a second, even more important effect. The accumulation of calcium ions in large nonphysiological concentrations has been noted within neurons in aging persons and in those with dementia. This accumulation is believed to produce damage within the nerve cell, which may lead to cell death. Nimodipine has been shown to protect against this occurrence, most probably by blocking neuronal calcium channels.

Nimodipine's possible benefits regarding dementia and decreased cognitive function are still being defined. This agent may enhance learning in rabbits and has improved learning and memory in elderly rats. Nimodipine has been noted to offer some protection against strokes in certain high-risk rat populations. In tests on patients with cerebrovascular disorders, nimodipine has improved memory and learning. It has also been reported that the drug helps some patients who have chronic organic brain syndrome.

Another report asserts that nimodipine slowed deterioration in patients with Alzheimer's disease over a period of 3 months. Further testing is continuing, and there is hope that nimodipine will offer some beneficial effects in patients with Alzheimer's disease.

CHELATION

Examination of the brain in patients with Alzheimer's disease has shown increased aluminum concentrations when compared to those of normal subjects. Aluminum concentrations in the brain are also noted to be increased in patients who have dementia associated with end-stage renal failure. It is still unknown, however, whether the increased aluminum concentration is the result or the cause of the changes seen in patients with Alzheimer's disease. Against the claim that aluminum is the causative agent for Alzheimer's disease are the facts that the normal human kidney is a very efficient eliminator of excess body aluminum and that patients with Alzheimer's disease do not possess elevated aluminum levels elsewhere in the body. Also, aluminum is a very common metal that exists naturally in the earth's crust. Because of its commonality, it would not be improbable for it to collect in areas of neuronal damage.

In an effort to improve the course of patients with Alzheimer's disease, two agents have been investigated as a means of removing aluminum from the body. They are EDTA and, more recently, desferrioxamine. A 1991 Canadian study reported that desferrioxamine retarded the decline of patient's living skills over a 2-year period. Methodological concerns regarding the study's measurement apparatus, which is unique to this study, the lack of placebo control, and the lack of change of the aluminum levels in patients pose significant questions about the reliability of this study's findings. In addition, desferrioxamine is quite expensive and is in very short supply because of difficulties in its production. The bulk of this agent produced is used up by the treatment of iron overload states such as thalassemia, for which this drug is approved and proven effective. Of further concern is the toxicity of the chelating agents.

Chelation therapies have long been offered to treat a variety of illnesses, including, but limited to, cardiac disorders, aging, and senility. No clearly beneficial effects have been proven, except in chelation's universally accepted role for the treatment of metal poisonings or metal overload states such as thalassemia. The negative effects of these agents, however, are well known. Side effects, which can be severe or life-threatening, include renal tubular necrosis, hypocalcemia, hypotension, tachyarrhythmias, chills, fever, erythema, severe pain at the site of the injection, allergic reactions, and loss of zinc (which can cause acute psychiatric complications). Patients and their families must be cautioned against using unproven and potentially harmful therapies in desperate attempts for improvement of this disease.

VITAMIN SUPPLEMENTS

The idea that Alzheimer's disease is a nutritional deficiency is an attractive one because then the following possibilities would exist:
1. Alzheimer's disease would be completely preventable.
2. The disease would be treatable.
3. Treatment could be done by individuals without the need for physicians or pharmacists.
4. The American life-style could be blamed for causing another illness.

The fact that some dementias can be caused and reversed by specific nutritional deficiencies, such as thiamine and vitamin B_{12}, offers hope for this theory.

The differentiation of a dementia caused by a vitamin-deficient state from Alzheimer's disease is generally not difficult. Thiamine deficiency tends to occur only in severe alcoholics and is responsible for alcohol dementia, more specifically Wernicke's encephalitis and Korsakoff's psychosis. These conditions can be easily differentiated from classic Alzheimer's disease. A second well-known vitamin-deficiency state that sometimes causes dementia, B_{12} deficiency, is easily diagnosed on the basis of blood testing. It should be noted that neither of these conditions results from casual dietary neglect. The average alcoholic who develops thiamine deficiency exists on a diet that is little more than alcohol. Vitamin B_{12} deficiency, also known as pernicious anemia, is caused by physiological abnormalities within the digestive system that are long standing and generally not correctable.

A preliminary study in 1988 considered the possibility that high-dose supplementation with either of the more commonly mentioned candidates for vitamin treatment, thiamine and niacin, was beneficial. On testing, this study found some improvement in the patients receiving thiamine, although no behavioral changes were noted. This study needs to be followed up by large placebo-controlled and double-blind studies to confirm or deny the usefulness of these supplements.

SUMMARY

Over the years many agents have been used in the treatment of dementia. Most of these agents produced some positive response when initially tested on small groups. Later, when the factors of chance, wishful thinking, and placebo effects were controlled, the benefits of these agents seemed to diminish, if not vanish entirely. The old saying, "Enthusiastic studies are rarely controlled, and controlled studies are rarely enthusiastic" certainly applies in these situations.

"Great discoveries" in the treatment of Alzheimer's disease are often reported, but they seem to disappear. This phenomenon is a result of the tendency of the press to announce "breakthroughs" prematurely. Certainly, new developments in the treatment of such a prevalent and devastating disease are important news. However, all too often, the early reports that such press announcements are based on come from small studies that have not been carefully controlled.

The factor of chance is confounding to studies in several possible ways. Those who care for patients with Alzheimer's disease know that they have both "good" periods and "bad" ones. Any one patient may improve or decline over a given period, not because of an intervention but because of chance.

For example, a patient with Alzheimer's disease may initially be tested at his normal functional level. When a retest is done, that patient may be experiencing a "good" day and may be at his highest possible performance. This type of occurrence might cause researchers to interpret the study as a success.

The reverse situation occurs more commonly. A patient with Alzheimer's disease tested in a study might perform poorly because of an illness or the newness of the testing situation, or he may simply be experiencing a "bad" day. Once he recovers from the illness or becomes more familiar with the test or the testing environment, his normal abilities might be demonstrated.

The placebo effect must also be controlled in a sound study. It is well known that when patients are given a nonactive compound and told it is medication, they may think that they are experiencing a beneficial effect. They may even report having side effects. Such a response occurs in roughly one third of the cases in which a nonactive compound, or placebo, is administered. This type of effect, however, is not limited to inactive substances. Active medication is frequently credited with improvements for conditions on which it actually has no effect. This fact often causes flaws in early studies on treatments of Alzheimer's disease.

Obviously, there are agents that have completely measurable effects that cannot be attributed to the placebo effect—for example, antibiotics. Unfortunately, Alzheimer's research has a considerably less measurable endpoint, and the expectations of the patients, caregivers, and researchers in studies can unduly influence the "improvements" that are reported.

Even the most objective cognitive or behavioral testing is easily susceptible to the placebo effect. After all, what aspect of human performance is not affected by the emotional state of the person tested? The method for correction of this effect is called placebo control.

Placebo-controlled studies involve two patient groups. In one group a "medication" is administered to all participants, although the "medication" is actually a nonactive compound. Patients in the other group receive the actual medication being tested. This approach levels the playing field. The placebo effects should balance out between the two groups, and any improvement seen in the treatment group over the placebo group can be confidently attributed to the treatment agent.

Why do flawed studies come about in the first place? This issue revolves around two factors—resources and time.

A large, well-controlled study takes remarkable amounts of money, manpower, and cooperation. These factors do not come together easily. Large studies are done primarily as a follow-up to smaller preliminary studies.

To qualify for a grant to fund a large and definitive study, the cooperation of several major medical centers is necessary and researchers must have some strongly encouraging data. They must be able to convince the potential participants that a definitive study is indicated.

A definitive study usually involves large numbers of patients, researchers, and evaluators; careful construction to control confounding factors; and the financial resources to pay for the components of the study. These resources are not committed lightly.

Although small early studies are often flawed and their results should not be too highly regarded by researchers or the press, they *do* perform an important function. Such studies provide groundwork for more comprehensive studies. Through this foundation an effective treatment for Alzheimer's disease will eventually be found.

BIBLIOGRAPHY

Cooper JK: Drug treatment of Alzheimer's disease, *Arch Intern Med* 151:245-249, 1991.

Cummings JL, Miller BL, editors: *Alzheimer's disease: treatment and long-term management,* New York, 1990, Marcel Dekker.

Davidson M, Stern RG: The treatment of cognitive impairment in Alzheimer's disease: beyond the cholinergic approach, *Psychiatr Clin North Am* 14: 461-482, 1991.

Davis KL and Tacrine Collaborative Study Group: A double-blind, placebo-controlled multicenter study of Tacrine for Alzheimer's disease, *N Engl J Med* 327:1253-1259, 1992.

Eagger SA, Levy R, Sahakian BJ: Tacrine in Alzheimer's disease, *Lancet* 337:989-992, 1991.

Gauthier S and others: Tetrahydroaminoacridine-lecithin combination treatment in patients with intermediate-stage Alzheimer's disease, *N Engl J Med* 322:1272-1276, 1990.

Harrell LE: Alzheimer's disease, *South Med J* 84:15, 32-34, 1991.

McLachlan DR and others: Intramuscular desferrioxamine in patients with Alzheimer's disease, *Lancet* 337:1304-1308, 1991.

O'Brien JT, Eagger S, Levy R: Effects of tetrahydroaminoacridine on liver function in patients with Alzheimer's disease, *Age Ageing* 20:129-131, 1991.

Sevush S, Guterman A, Villalon AV: Improved verbal learning after outpatient oral physostigmine therapy in patients with dementia of the Alzheimer type, *J Clin Psychiatry* 52:300-303, 1991.

Tariot PN and others: Naloxone and Alzheimer's disease: cognitive and behavioral effects of a range of doses, *Arch Gen Psychiatry* 43:727-732, 1986.

16

Urinary and fecal incontinence

Ronald C. Hamdy and Larry Hudgins

Urinary incontinence is the inappropriate and involuntary passage of urine. Its exact prevalence is difficult to establish because it can occur in varying degrees and the patient may deny having the problem. This condition is particularly difficult to determine in patients with Alzheimer's disease.

Although the underlying dementia may be responsible for some of the incontinence, other conditions are present that are treatable and reversible. Thus the caregiver has the initial burden of recognizing incontinence and arranging for further evaluation of the patient. Urinary incontinence is an issue of quality of life that should be neither ignored nor denied.

RELUCTANCE TO ADMIT INCONTINENCE

In the early stages of Alzheimer's disease, when the patient still has insight into his condition, he may try to conceal his incontinence so as not to draw the attention of his cohabitants and social contacts. The patient knows he has a problem with his mental state, which he may find difficult to cope with and may try to hide from his immediate social contacts. Rather than admitting the additional problem of urinary incontinence and seeking medical advice, he often resorts to concealing it. He may hide soiled clothes or wear towels in his underwear. Often the patient feels ashamed of having lost control over his bodily functions and may be embarrassed to mention the problem. Finally, the patient may be afraid that he will be forced to accept institutional care and give up his possessions and independence. In fact, urinary incontinence often is the factor that convinces relatives and caregivers that institutionalization is necessary.

URINARY INCONTINENCE

Frequently, urinary incontinence seen in the early stages of Alzheimer's disease is not related to the disease itself but is caused by an unrelated condition that often can be easily treated. Unfortunately, the patient often feels that the urinary incontinence represents another step in his gradual and relentless deterioration and loss of control over his mind and body. This attitude usually leads to profound depression punctuated by bouts of irritability when the patient becomes angry with himself and fails to understand what is happening to him.

In late stages of Alzheimer's disease, urinary incontinence often is the result of the underlying condition and the global reduction in the number of cerebral cortical neurons (nerve cells). Because of this reduction in neurons, no inhibitory impulses are sent out from the micturition center in the brain to the urinary bladder. Alternatively, the patient may urinate in inappropriate places because he is unaware of his environment and disoriented. When the patient reaches that stage he may also become incontinent of feces.

DISCUSSING INCONTINENCE

The treating physician and other caregivers must be alert to the problem of urinary incontinence and need to be prepared to discuss it openly with the patient before its impact undermines the patient's self-confidence, worsens his general condition, and disrupts his precarious equilibrium with his environment. The caregivers must stress that urinary incontinence is not necessarily related to Alzheimer's disease and that it may be possible to correct it. Unfortunately, a conspiracy of silence often develops when the patient, the relatives, and the caregivers know that the patient is incontinent and yet pretend not to have noticed it.

It is remarkable how often the patient's relatives try to conceal the problem. When questioned, they may deny that their relative is incontinent until the situation becomes intolerable, in which case often little can be done apart from seeking institutional care. This situation is unfortunate because, even in late cases, a reversible cause for urinary incontinence sometimes can be found and treated.

COMMON TYPES OF URINARY INCONTINENCE

A number of classifications for urinary incontinence have been put forward. However, patients often have more than one type simultaneously. The various types are not mutually exclusive; in fact, one type often potentiates another.

Stress Incontinence

Stress incontinence characteristically occurs when a patient stands up, coughs, laughs, or sneezes. The patient usually is dry in between these episodes and at night. Stress incontinence is caused by weakness of the urinary sphincter and/or perineal muscles, which allows small quantities of urine to be passed when the intraabdominal pressure is suddenly increased, as occurs during sneezing, laughing, and coughing.

Stress incontinence also may result from anatomical changes that interfere with the urethrovesical angle (the angle between the urinary bladder and urethra). In women, the change may be a result of several pregnancies and childbirth or surgical interventions. In addition, estrogen deficiency in postmenopausal women often leads to urethral inflammation, which is associated with senile vaginitis that may further aggravate stress incontinence. In these instances the diagnosis can be suspected by the appearance of the vagina and can be confirmed by microscopic examination of a mucosal smear.

Stress incontinence often is aggravated by diseases that cause muscle weakness or interfere with the patient's mobility, such as Parkinson's disease, strokes, or osteoarthritis. In these circumstances the patient may need to strain or heave himself as he struggles to get up from his chair. Such straining increases the intraabdominal pressure, which is transmitted to the urinary bladder. If this pressure exceeds that of the urinary sphincters, urinary incontinence results. A similar situation may arise when a patient tries to get up from a very low chair. Stress incontinence is more common in women and usually responds well to pelvic floor and perineal muscle exercises (Kegel exercises).

Urge Incontinence

Urge incontinence, or detrusor instability, results when uninhibited contractions of the detrusor muscle (the muscle layer lining the urinary bladder) are strong enough to overcome the pressure of the internal urethral sphincter. This type of urinary incontinence, also known as unstable bladder, spastic bladder, or uninhibited bladder, is the most common kind occurring in old age. It is characterized by the almost continuous passage of small quantities of urine, with the pa-

tient being wet most of the time, day and night. The patient may fe
the desire to micturate but be unable to postpone the act.

In late stages of Alzheimer's disease, detrusor instability is cause
by decreased cortical inhibition because the number or the integri
of the neurons in the micturition center of the brain is affected, i
which case uninhibited contractions of the bladder occur before th
bladder reaches its full capacity. Stress incontinence often potentiate
detrusor instability.

Detrusor instability also may be caused by local or pelvic processe
including inflammation, infection, prostatic hypertrophy, neoplasms, f
cal impaction, uterine or bladder prolapse, and foreign bodies such a
calculi in the urinary bladder.

When urinary tract infections are responsible for this type of ur
nary incontinence, the incontinence usually is associated with a ce
tain amount of dysuria (pain or burning sensation while passin
urine). It must be emphasized, however, that although acute bladde
infection often is responsible for incontinence, chronic infection doe
not always lead to urinary incontinence.

Overflow Incontinence

As with other types of urinary incontinence, overflow incont
nence occurs when the pressure inside the bladder exceeds that of th
internal urinary sphincter. Unlike all other causes of urinary incont
nence, however, overflow incontinence is caused by an actual obstruc
tion to the flow of urine through the urethra. As a result of this ob
struction, urine is retained in the bladder, which progressivel
increases in size. The pressure in the bladder also increases until
exceeds the pressure obstructing the flow of urine, at which poir
urine is discharged from the bladder until the pressure in the bladde
falls below that of the obstructing lesion. Characteristically, patient
with overflow incontinence have grossly distended bladders that ca
be palpated clinically, and the urine flow rate is significantly reduce
often amounting to no more than a dribble.

One of the main problems associated with overflow incontinenc
is incomplete emptying of the bladder. A residual volume of urin
frequently is present, even at the end of a bout of incontinence (there
fore the bladder is palpable). This residual urine invites bladder ir
fections, which may spread to the kidneys via the ureters.

Many causes may be responsible for urinary obstruction an
overflow incontinence, including fecal impaction, pelvic tumors, ure
thral stricture, bladder neoplasms, and calculi. In men, one of th

most common causes of obstruction to the flow of urine is prostatic hypertrophy. In women, uterine or bladder prolapse may be responsible. The obstructing lesion may distort the urethra enough to cause an angulation that obstructs the flow of urine, thus interfering with micturition. Often when these patients try to micturate but cannot, they strain and increase the intraabdominal pressure, which is transmitted not only to the intravesical pressure but also to the base of the bladder and the structures surrounding the urethra. As a result of this increased pressure, the angulation of the urethra becomes more pronounced and further increases the obstruction and difficulty in initiating micturition.

Then another problem develops. As the intraabdominal pressure increases during straining, the venous return from the abdomen to the heart is reduced; this change causes pelvic congestion and may further increase the volume of the obstructing lesion or the already distended prostate and complicate the initiation of micturition. The solution to this problem is a simple exercise that consists of taking deep breaths to decrease the pressure in the thoracic cavity and to increase the flow of blood from the abdomen and pelvic cavity to the heart. This action reduces the intraabdominal and intrapelvic congestion (including that of the pelvic structures and urethra), thus lessening the obstruction to the flow of urine and allowing micturition to take place.

Drug-Induced Urinary Retention and Overflow Incontinence

Occasionally, urinary retention and overflow incontinence are precipitated by medications, which include over-the-counter or prescribed antihistamines, sedatives, and other psychoactive drugs with anticholinergic properties. Many hypotensive medications affect continence via smooth muscle relaxation. This relaxation causes a dysfunctional bladder that allows urinary overfill.

Certain drugs that cause constipation (narcotic, antidiarrheal, and antidepressant drugs) may lead to fecal impaction. In severe cases the fecal masses in the rectum may distort the urethra, alter the angle between the urethra and the urinary bladder, and cause urine retention and eventually overflow incontinence.

Functional Incontinence

Functional incontinence is caused by factors outside the urinary bladder and its nervous connections, which remain intact. The patient

is incontinent of urine because he is unable to postpone the act o
micturition until a suitable place for voiding is reached. In othe
words, the patient feels the desire to micturate, may start taking ap
propriate steps to go to the toilet, but does not have enough time t
reach the toilet before micturition takes place. Stress incontinenc
often potentiates this type of urinary incontinence.

Incontinence and Curtailed Patient Mobility

Functional incontinence commonly results when a patient be
comes less mobile. For instance, patients with severe osteoarthritis
Parkinson's disease, stroke, or any other condition that limits thei
physical capabilities may suffer from functional incontinence. I
these situations it is often useful to advise patients to anticipate whe
the urinary bladder is likely to be filled and to attempt to empty it a
regular intervals of 2 to 3 or 4 hours rather than waiting to feel th
urge to micturate.

Incontinence and Inability to Locate Toilet

Patients with Alzheimer's disease are prone to develop functiona
incontinence because they cannot find their way to the toilet. The
may become incontinent because the toilet is located too far from
their bedroom or sitting area. The maximum distance between toile
and room or sitting area should be approximately 100 feet.

Similarly, if the way to the toilet is not clearly illuminated, or i
there are many obstacles on the way to the toilet, the patient may no
be able to reach the toilet before his bladder empties. Since a patien
with Alzheimer's disease is likely to forget the way to the toilet, it i
important to make sure that the patient has easy access to the toilet
that he knows the way there, and that the way is well marked with
signs. Easy access is particularly important in institutions where a
patient may wake up at night wanting to void his bladder but i
confused and cannot recognize the way to the toilet. This situation i
especially likely to occur during the first few days after admission to
a nursing home or other similar institution.

If a patient with Alzheimer's disease cannot remember to empty
his bladder at regular intervals, the caregiver may need to remind
him. Alternatively, an alarm clock may be used to remind the patien
to go to the toilet at certain intervals. In residential institutions a
bladder-emptying schedule individualized for each patient may be
helpful.

Incontinence and Physical Restraints

Functional incontinence may result from the use of physical restraints, which frequently are applied to patients who tend to wander, fall repeatedly, or become aggressive, such as those who have Alzheimer's disease. Even though patients in restraints may feel the urge to micturate, they cannot free themselves to reach the toilet in time. The development of urinary incontinence in such patients often is a serious setback and may considerably increase their degree of frustration, irritability, and even violence. Such behaviors serve to reassure the caregivers that using restraints was justified, and thus a vicious cycle is begun. Often the rate of deterioration is dramatically increased when sedatives are also prescribed to "quiet" the patient. As a result, the patient's condition declines rapidly, and the complications of being bedridden quickly appear. Nurses who use restraints must make sure that the patients empty their bladders at regular intervals to avoid the problem of functional incontinence.

Incontinence and Inability to Communicate

Patients with anomia, aphasia, or other speech problems common to individuals with Alzheimer's disease may not be able to notify the nurse appropriately of their desire to micturate. For this reason nurses who care for such patients must develop a set of vocabulary signals or a ritual by which the patient notifies them of the desire to micturate. If such communication is not possible, regular toileting should be instituted. This subject is discussed in greater detail in Chapter 17.

Drug-Induced Functional Incontinence

Functional incontinence can also be precipitated by drugs. Loop diuretic drugs (e.g., furosemide, bumetanide, and ethacrynic acid), which suddenly increase the volume of urine several fold, may lead to functional incontinence, especially if the patient does not expect this result after taking the tablets. By suddenly increasing the volume of the bladder, loop diuretic drugs also may lead to pelvic congestion. In some instances, particularly in men with prostatic hypertrophy, this increased volume may lead to obstruction of the flow of urine and eventually to overflow incontinence.

Characteristically, incontinence induced by loop diuretic drugs develops shortly after these tablets have been taken. Therefore patients who take these drugs and their relatives or the nursing staff should be warned about the sudden increase in volume of urine that is likely to occur after this medication is taken. It should be emphasized that the patient must be taken to the toilet at regular intervals after taking the tablets. Also, patients taking loop diuretic drugs must be kept near a toilet, and they must know their way to the toilet. Similarly, these patients should not be encouraged to go on outings or for walks within a few hours of taking the diuretic drug without making sure that they have ready access to a toilet. It must be remembered that a bout of urinary incontinence, even an isolated one, can be so humiliating for the patient that it completely undermines his confidence and significantly accelerates his rate of decline.

Functional incontinence may occur during deep sleep and sometimes is induced by potent hypnotic drugs, when the patient's sleep is so deep that even though impulses are reaching the micturition center in the brain, they do not elicit any response from the other areas of the brain. Since no inhibitory impulses reach the sacral plexus, micturition takes place. In addition, alcohol use in the elderly should not be forgotten because of its potential for polyuria, urinary frequency, urinary urgency, sedation, delirium, and immobility.

INFORMATION FOR THE PHYSICIAN

Although the patient's physician must diagnose the cause of the urinary incontinence, this task can be eased considerably if the right information is provided. The caregiver therefore plays an active and important role in diagnosing and managing the patient who has urinary incontinence.

Even before referring the patient to a physician, the caregiver should attempt to determine whether the patient has genuine urinary incontinence or whether the leakage of urine was accidental, for example, having spilled from the urinal bottle or bedpan, as often happens with patients who are bedridden or confined to bed by either physical restraints or guard rails.

Characteristics of Incontinence

Once it has been established that the patient is genuinely incontinent of urine, the caregiver should determine whether the incontinence is of recent onset or has been a long-standing problem. Incontinence of recent onset has a better prognosis since it is usually the result of some reversible disease.

Attempts should be made to find out whether the patient is incontinent of urine all the time or whether the incontinence tends to occur at specific times of the day or is related to taking certain drugs. Urinary incontinence that is worse late in the morning could be caused by loop diuretic drugs taken earlier in the morning. On the other hand, incontinence that is worse at night could be related to hypnotic preparations, which may profoundly inhibit the higher cortical (brain) functions. This condition is particularly likely if the patient is taking large doses of hypnotic drugs.

Since there are other possibilities for drug-induced urinary incontinence, it is essential to know all the medications that the patient is taking and whether they were prescribed by a physician or bought over the counter. Certain over-the-counter drugs intended to assist in weight loss may contain diuretic preparations. Other drugs prescribed for allergies or the common cold induce sedation or produce anticholinergic side effects that may lead to urine retention and eventually to overflow incontinence.

It must be remembered that elderly patients and those with Alzheimer's disease may take or may be given medications that were prescribed for their friends, neighbors, or relatives. Therefore it is essential to inquire in detail about *all* medications that the patient is taking. The management of drug-induced urinary incontinence is fairly simple and consists of discontinuing the offending drug or substituting a less offensive one. Nevertheless, it is important to consult the patient's physician before discontinuing any prescribed medication, even if the drug is believed to be responsible for the urinary incontinence.

Next, the caregiver must determine whether the urinary incontinence is related to any of the patient's activities, such as standing up, coughing, laughing, or sneezing. If the patient tends to be incontinent while doing any of these activities, the diagnosis is probably stress incontinence. As noted earlier, this type of incontinence often responds to pelvic floor and perineal muscle exercise.

If the patient is not incontinent all the time, it is helpful to know how many times he needs to micturate, the amount of urine passed, and whether there is any associated urgency, dysuria (pain on urination), scalding, difficulty in starting micturition, or dribbling. Urgency, dysuria, or scalding suggests a lower urinary tract infection. Difficulty in initiating micturition or dribbling suggests prostatic hypertrophy. Finally, the patient should be asked whether he has any bladder sensation and whether he can voluntarily initiate and interrupt the act of micturition.

If the physician is given all this information before seeing the patient, the task of diagnosing the condition will be much easier and the diagnosis is more likely to be accurate. It is also important that the physician be told about the patient's mobility and physical capabilities. Patients with disorders that interfere with their mobility are more likely to have urinary incontinence (functional incontinence) than are fully mobile patients. Obesity may be a factor in aggravating urinary incontinence by weakening the pelvic floor muscles.

Clinical Examination

Although the clinical history is frequently enough to suggest the type of urinary incontinence and its underlying cause, a thorough physical examination is also necessary. The examination should include a rectal examination and, in women, a vaginal examination. In stress incontinence, urine leakage can be checked for when the bladder is full and by asking the patient to strain. Feeling a distended, enlarged bladder after the patient has voided suggests bladder outlet obstruction or a weak bladder muscle. Pelvic examination is done to identify inflammation of the urethra or vagina, pelvic muscle laxity, and pelvic masses. Rectal examination should also help to identify perianal fissure, anal sphincter muscle tone, prostate size, and nodules.

Laboratory Investigations

After the physical examination, laboratory studies may be indicated, including a urinalysis, urine culture, blood chemistry profile, prostate-specific antigen (as a screening test for prostate cancer in males), and x-ray imaging of the urinary tract. Fiberoptic cystoscopy with a direct view into the bladder is sometimes necessary to check for the anatomy of possible lower urinary tract obstruction and to note intrinsic bladder lesions, inflammation, or tumor. Urodynamic studies may also be indicated, especially if it is suspected that there is more than one cause for the incontinence.

FECAL INCONTINENCE

Fecal incontinence is the involuntary passage of stool. Established fecal incontinence is both socially isolating and a common cause of institutionalization of the demented patient. Like urinary incontinence, fecal incontinence is commonly denied by the patient and underreported by the caregivers. Both situations are unfortunate because the majority of affected patients can be helped.

MAINTENANCE OF FECAL CONTINENCE

Normal fecal continence relies on a properly functioning anal sphincter that transmits appropriate signals to allow the individual to discriminate between solid, liquid, and gas in the rectum. In addition, the sphincter must be able to defer fecal evacuation for a convenient time and place.

In anatomical terms, there are two anal sphincters. The internal anal sphincter is under the control of the autonomic nervous system. At rest, this sphincter remains in a tonically contracted state. When the anorectal region is distended by flatus or feces, the internal sphincter relaxes and the external sphincter, which is under volitional control, contracts unless the individual is ready to defecate.

COMMON CAUSES OF FECAL INCONTINENCE

Fecal Impaction

Fecal impaction is the most common cause of fecal incontinence in the elderly. It is often precipitated by the injudicious use of anti-diarrheal agents, which commonly are abused by elderly patients and their caregivers. Initially, these compounds may be taken because of a bout of diarrhea or loose stool. If the patient continues to take the agent after the diarrhea has been controlled, he may become constipated. In severe cases, fecal masses may become impacted in the rectum and later in the descending colon. Water is gradually absorbed from these fecal masses, which become hardened (fecaliths). In turn, these masses irritate the mucosal lining of the descending colon and rectum and increase the production of mucus. This occurrence may be interpreted by the patient as another bout of diarrhea, and he may take more constipating agents. As time goes by, the fecal masses may reach the proximal part of the descending colon, where the fecal matter is semisolid. At this stage the fecal material bypasses the fecaliths and may reach the rectum. The patient may not be able to control its evacuation and may think that he is having another bout of diarrhea. As a result, he may take more constipating agents, thus completing the vicious cycle and worsening his condition.

Management of fecal incontinence includes cleansing enemas used repeatedly. Such enemas are used to clear the lower rectal vault and allow distal passage of the more proximal stool. Oil retention enemas (olive oil) given over a 2-week period and followed by Fleet enemas may be helpful. For prevention of constipation and recurrence of impaction, daily phosphate enemas or bisacodyl suppositories may also be beneficial. Increased exercise, fluid intake, and dietary fiber are important adjuncts. Even bedridden patients may benefit from arm exercises.

Many elderly patients are highly conscious of their bowel habits and think that they should have a bowel movement daily. They report feeling terrible if they are not "regular." Therefore laxative use and abuse are rampant among the elderly. However, since daily use limits the effectiveness of the laxative as a cathartic, it allows constipation to persist.

Medications

Medications frequently taken by the elderly, either prescription or over-the-counter drugs, are always suspect in contributing to constipation. Iron supplements, for example, can cause intestinal irritation and have been reported to aggravate constipation. Diuretics, given for hypertension, congestive heart failure, or edematous states, by inducing urinary potassium loss and dehydration, may reduce stool hydration and adversely affect colon motility. Similarly, calcium channel blocking agents relax smooth muscle in the bowel wall, thus impairing gut propulsion. Sedatives prolong immobility and slow gut activity but may also affect sphincter control. Codeine and other narcotic analgesics can cause constipation and are occasionally used for severe diarrhea. Aluminum-containing antacids are also frequent offenders. Clonidine may cause constipation by affecting autonomic neuromuscular bowel control. This drug has been used successfully in controlling neuropathic diarrhea in patients with diabetes. Hypothyroidism that is severe enough to cause frequent symptomatic constipation can be easily screened through blood studies.

Neurogenic Factors

Fecal incontinence may be caused by neurological disorders such as strokes, spinal cord disease, and autonomic neuropathy resulting from diabetes mellitus. Patients with neurogenic fecal incontinence are not incontinent of stools all the time, as is the case with patients whose incontinence results from impaction. Instead, such patients tend to be incontinent once or twice daily, usually following the intake of food, when the gastrocolic reflex is stimulated, and the stools are usually well formed. This association between intake of food, gastrocolic reflex, and incontinence can be used successfully in the management of such incontinence. A rectal glycerine suppository may be given on wakening or prior to breakfast. A bedside commode chair is advisable for less mobile patients who are confined to bed. Velcro clothes fasteners are also helpful aids for patients who lack normal dexterity and cannot undress easily. Some patients with Alzheimer's disease may not appreciate the need to postpone the desire to defecate until reaching an appropriate setting. In addition, some patients may not be able to distinguish flatus from feces.

Gastrointestinal Conditions

Severe diarrhea of any cause may lead to incontinence, particularly if the patient's mobility is reduced. Diarrhea may result from a variety of conditions, ranging from acute infections of the bowel to neoplastic lesions. Acute infections may be the result of food poisoning, which is particularly likely to occur in patients who live alone and are provided with previously cooked food, whether through a senior citizens program or prepared by relatives. Instead of consuming such food promptly, they commonly store it, often unhygienically, and reheat it later to a temperature that is insufficient to kill possible pathogens. The introduction of the microwave oven, with its tendency to heat nonuniformly, may worsen the situation by promoting a false sense of security. Other gastrointestinal causes of fecal incontinence are the same as those in patients who do not have dementia and include irritable bowel syndrome, ulcerative colitis, diverticulitis, neoplastic tumors of the colon and rectum, and the pseudomembranous colitis that often complicates antibiotic therapy.

CLINICAL EVALUATION

Recently discovered or prolonged and sustained fecal incontinence mandates a search for reversible and treatable disorders. Nurses should be able to note the frequency and consistency of the stools and any associated symptoms, including abdominal or rectal pain, bleeding, abdominal cramps, or abdominal distention or bloating. Pertinent questions to be answered include the following:

1. Are there any new focal signs of weakness that suggest recent stroke?
2. Is the patient physically able to get to the toilet, or is he limited by arthritis or muscle weakness or poor eyesight?

3. What medication does the patient routinely take (both pre scribed and over-the-counter drugs)?
4. Is the patient's physical environment "user friendly"? In other words, is it free of obstacles in the patient's path? Does it afford good lighting and bed rails? Is clothing easy to unfasten?
5. Can the patient remember the way to the toilet?
6. Has the patient had noticeable or documented weight loss?

Having obtained this history, a complete physical examination should be done with the preceding questions used as an outline of focus.

A neurological evaluation is needed to determine the patient's mental status, mobility, and motor strength. The abdominal examination should focus on any abdominal distention, activity of bowel sounds, enlarged organs or masses, or tenderness in palpation. Digital rectal examination helps to define anal sphincter tone, masses, or impaction. A stool specimen should be obtained to check for occult blood. A "high" impaction may be present but not detectable on rectal examination. Therefore a plain film of the abdomen may be necessary to evaluate this possibility. Other investigations may be indicated to diagnose uncommon causes of incontinence.

SUMMARY

Urinary and fecal incontinence have profound implications on the quality of life of both patient and caregiver. It must be emphasized that neither type of incontinence is a diagnosis per se and that an appropriate evaluation is recommended. In many instances neither condition is directly related to Alzheimer's disease and may stem from causes that can be treated successfully. It is important to adopt a positive attitude toward the management of incontinence and to try to identify the underlying cause or precipitating factors. Even if the incontinence cannot be corrected, a number of aids can be used to make the management of incontinent patients easier and to lighten the burden on the caregivers. These aids are discussed in detail in Chapter 17.

BIBLIOGRAPHY

Barrett JA: Colorectal disorders in elderly people, *Br Med J* 305:764-766, 1992.

Diokno AC, Wells TJ, Brink CA: Urinary incontinence in elderly women: urodynamic evaluation, *J Am Geriatr Soc* 35:940-946, 1988.

Fantl JA and others: Efficacy of bladder training in older women with urinary incontinence, *JAMA* 265:609, 1991.

Hilton P: Urinary incontinence in women, *Br Med J* 295:426-432, 1987.

Leach GE, Yip CM: Urological and urodynamic evaluation of the elderly population, *Clin Geriatr Med* 2(4):731-755, 1986.

Orr WC: Fecal incontinence in the elderly, *Geriatr Med Today* 7:112, 1988.

Ouslander JG: Diagnostic evaluation of geriatric urinary incontinence, *Clin Geriatr Med* 2(4):715-730, 1986.

Parks AG: Fecal incontinence. In Mandelstam D, editor: Incontinence and its management, ed 2, Sydney, 1980, Croom Helm.

Parks AG, Swash M, Urich H: Sphincter denervation in anorectal incontinence and rectal prolapse, *Gut* 18:656, 1977.

Resnick NM: Urinary incontinence in older adults, *Hosp Pract* 27(10):139-184, 1992.

Resnick NM, Yalla SV: Management of urinary incontinence in the elderly, *N Engl J Med* 313(13):800-805, 1985.

Schnelle J: Treatment of urinary incontinence in nursing home patients by prompted voiding, *J Am Geriatr Soc* 38:356, 1990.

Smith RG: Fecal incontinence, *J Am Geriatr Soc* 31:694, 1983.

Straatsma BR and others: Aging-related cataract: laboratory investigation and clinical management, *Ann Intern Med* 102:82-92, 1985.

Teri L, Larson E, Reifler B: Behavioral disturbance in dementia of Alzheimer's type, *J Am Geriatr Soc* 36(1):1-6, 1988.

Thomas TM and others: Prevalence of urinary incontinence, *Br Med J* 281:1243-1245, 1980.

Urinary Incontinence Guideline Panel: Urinary incontinence in adults: clinical practice guidelines, AHCPR Pub No 92-0039, Rockville, Md, 1992, US Department of Health and Human Services.

US Department of Health and Human Services: Urinary incontinence in adults, *Consensus Development Conference Statement* 7(5):1-11, Rockville, Md, 1988, National Institutes of Health.

Wells TJ, Brink CA, Diokno AC: Urinary incontinence in elderly women: clinical findings, *J Am Geriatr Soc* 35:933-939, 1987.

Williams ME, Pannill FC: Urinary incontinence in the elderly, *Ann Intern Med* 97:895-907, 1982.

Winograd CH, Jarvik LF: Physician management of the demented patient, *J Am Geriatr Soc* 34:295-308, 1986.

Winogrond IR, Fisk AA: Alzheimer's disease: assessment of functional status, *J Am Geriatr Soc* 31(12):780-785, 1983.

Wold A: Biofeedback therapy for fecal incontinence, *Ann Intern Med* 95:146, 1981.

17

Management of urinary incontinence

Mary M. Lancaster

The treatment of urinary incontinence is receiving greater attention from health care personnel and the general public. In 1988 the National Institutes of Health issued a Consensus Development Conference Statement on "Urinary Incontinence in Adults." Recently, the Alliance for Aging Research and the National Institute on Aging issued a clinical bulletin entitled "Treating Patients with Urinary Incontinence." In the public arena, the topic of incontinence has been discussed on national news and talk shows.

Urinary incontinence is a disturbing and often distressing problem for both patients and caregivers. The onset of incontinence frequently results in the institutionalization of the affected person. Management of incontinence can be costly and time-consuming. With the increased costs of health care and the shortage of adequately prepared staff in long-term care facilities, the problem of urinary incontinence is compounded. When magnified by the decreased mental ability of patients with dementia, the management of incontinence can become a seemingly insurmountable task. However, several strategies exist that can help lessen the strain of incontinence on caregivers and patients.

GENERAL GUIDELINES

Finding the most appropriate form of management is the first step. Jeter and associates have provided guidelines for the selection of products for managing urinary incontinence. According to them, the ideal product should do the following:

1. Contain urine completely and prevent leakage onto clothing, bedding, and furniture.

2. Be comfortable to wear and protect vulnerable skin from maceration, chafing, and pressure sores.
3. Be easy to use.
4. Disguise or contain odor.
5. Be inconspicuous under clothing, without bulk or noise.
6. Be easy to dispose of or clean.
7. Be reasonably priced and readily available.

Additional criteria that nursing staff should keep in mind are the patient's physical and mental capabilities and quality of life issues. The easiest method of managing incontinence may not always be the safest, the best for the patient, or the most cost-effective. Products are designed only to manage incontinence, not to treat it. Therefore it is always recommended that any patient with a new onset of urinary incontinence receive a complete workup to rule out any reversible (treatable) cause.

SPECIAL CONSIDERATIONS WITH ALZHEIMER'S DISEASE

For management of urinary incontinence in the patient with Alzheimer's disease, nursing personnel must consider the nature of the disease. To successfully reverse or achieve complete independent management of urinary incontinence requires an intact central nervous system. Because the central nervous system of the patient with Alzheimer's disease is continually undergoing degenerative changes, the individual may no longer "feel" or "recognize" the need to void, may be immobile or restrained, may not be able to communicate the need to void, may not be able to control the urge to void, may not recognize the appropriate place to void, or may not be able to remember a toileting schedule. Therefore managing incontinence requires a caregiver, either a family member or health care personnel, to be readily available.

Mobility Factors

In many older adults, especially those afflicted with Alzheimer's disease, impaired mobility, slow gait, or the presence of restraints may cause incontinence. Simply being able to reach the bathroom in time becomes a real challenge. All too often health care personnel contribute to incontinence by restricting a patient's movement with restraints, geriatric chairs, or siderails. The best strategy for managing such problems is to make the toilet facilities easily accessible and available. A situation in which the person must climb stairs to reach an upstairs bathroom invites accidents when impaired mobility or urge incontinence is a factor. Also, the pathway to the bathroom needs to be uncluttered, well marked, and well lit. For patients who require restraints, nursing personnel must assess their need to void on a regular schedule. For patients who cannot remember where the bathroom is, signs and drawings can be used in hallways and on doors to help them find the correct place to void.

Manual Dexterity

Since manual dexterity may be impaired in the older person with Alzheimer's disease, such steps as unzipping pants or removing hosiery may interfere with the patient's ability to stay dry. There are many ways to be creative with clothing to make it easier to remove and thus keep cleaner and dryer. Velcro strips can be used to replace snaps, buttons, and zippers. Clothing with an elastic waistband can be quickly and easily removed. Undergarments are available with flap openings that eliminate the need to remove the undergarment. Wraparound skirts and dresses are convenient and inexpensive. Because not all "accidents" can be prevented, it is recommended that the patient's clothing be of a durable wash-and-wear material.

Access to Toileting Facilities

When getting to the bathroom constitutes a major problem, other methods may be more appropriate. If the patient is fairly mobile, portable commode chairs (potty chairs) can be used. Medical equipment suppliers usually have these chairs for rent. The chair can be placed in the area of the patient's environment where he spends most of the day. There are several different types of commode chairs, and selection should be based on the individual needs and capabilities of the patient and the caregiver. Some chairs have wheels that allow easy movement from place to place. Others have pans that slide underneath the seat and can be easily removed for cleaning. Many of these chairs can be rolled directly over the existing toilet, allowing the patient to use the bathroom facilities. Some commode chairs are upholstered and have lids and can double as regular cushioned chairs. Health care personnel and family caregivers should always check to make sure that any commode chair that has wheels also has wheel locks. These locks should be used whenever the patient is in the chair.

Flexibility

Since older adults have less flexible hip and knee joints, going to the bathroom can be difficult and uncomfortable. Simply sitting down on the toilet and getting up from it can be problematic. Elevated seats that increase the height of the toilet seat are available and may make going to the bathroom easier and less painful. In addition, handrails can be installed for added support and safety while sitting down and getting up. If the patient has trouble maintaining an upright position or has a tendency to fall to the side, chair arms that can be placed around the toilet to provide an additional degree of safety are also available. Nursing homes and other long-term care facilities are required by licensing agencies to have these types of supports and protective/assistive devices installed in their bathroom facilities.

Immobility

Urinals

For completely immobile patients or those who spend a great deal of time in wheelchairs, hand-held urinals for both men and women are available. Nursing personnel are usually familiar with the types of urinals designed for male patients but not with those for female patients. There are various types of female urinals, but they all have a funnel with a wide opening and a collection device. The collection device may be similar to a plastic jug, or it can be tubing connected to a drainage bag. In general, it is easiest for the female patient to use this type of device in a sitting position. If this type of equipment is not available, a plastic milk jug can be adapted as a male urinal and a plastic bowl can be used as a female urinal. Both male and female patients who use urinals should be checked regularly to make sure that spillage has not occurred.

Bedpans

The bedpan is probably the most well known device used for incontinent patients. Although generally used only for patients who are confined to bed, a bedpan can be placed on a chair to create a toilet type of arrangement. Problems associated with the bedpan include the difficulty of voiding in the lying position, the difficulty in cleaning the patient after the bedpan has been used, and the possibility of spillage in the bed. A bedpan is also awkward and uncomfortable if used for any length of time. Nursing staff must be attentive to helping patients remove themselves from the bedpan as soon as they are finished voiding. Patients must be cleansed well after using a bedpan. Such cleansing is usually best accomplished by turning the patient on his side.

Scheduled toileting

For the more mobile patient, particularly the patient who is in the earlier stages of the disease, bladder training or "scheduled toileting" can be successful in preventing accidents. True bladder training in which the patient achieves or regains control of voiding is rarely accomplished in the patient with Alzheimer's disease. The only time that bladder training may be successful is when the incontinence is brought about by an acute disease process such as an infection, surgery, or hospitalization that stresses the patient's abilities. Once the stress has been resolved, efforts can be made to retrain the patient. Scheduled toileting consists of reminding the person about or taking him to the bathroom at frequent regular intervals (every 2 to 3 hours). It is generally unrealistic to expect the patient to remember on his own to go to the bathroom this frequently. Scheduled toileting is advantageous because it helps to maintain the patient's dignity and self-esteem; it also keeps the patient mobile and using the bathroom facilities. This method is very cost-effective because no devices or special clothing are required. If accidents are prevented, clothing does not need to be cleaned.

Drainage and collection devices

If the patient's incontinence is not a result of any of the problems discussed here but caused by some medical or physical problem, there are drainage and collection devices and absorbent/protective devices that can make management much easier. Drainage and collection devices are closed systems by which the patient's urine passes into either an internal or external catheter and flows through the drainage tubing into a reservoir.

Internal drainage/collection systems are commonly called indwelling or Foley catheters. These systems consist of a rubber or silicone tube, or catheter, that is passed through the urethra into the bladder. The catheter remains in place by means of an inflatable balloon. The external end of the catheter is connected to a larger and longer piece of plastic tubing, which in turn drains into a bag. The urine is emptied directly and continuously from the bladder and flows to the collection device. Because this device is inside the bladder and continuously drains it, a catheter is generally used only when other management strategies have proven ineffective. Some problems associated with the use of indwelling catheters are infection, trauma to the urethra or bladder, and loss of bladder tone. Extreme care must be exercised when a catheter is being inserted so that trauma is avoided. Forcing a catheter during insertion should never be done. If resistance is met, the procedure should be abandoned and referral to an expert in catheterization should be made. The loss of bladder tone can be especially problematic if the catheter must be removed and the person retrained in voiding. If it is known that the patient's catheter is to be removed, time should be spent over several days clamping and unclamping the catheter to allow for increasing periods of urine collection in the bladder.

The external catheter provides a safer alternative to the indwelling catheter. For men, the condom catheter is the most frequently used drainage and collection device. This device is usually a thin latex condom that fits over the penis and connects to a drainage tube and bag. The condom should have some sort of firm molding at the connecting end to prevent the condom from coming twisted and closing off the drainage of urine. An external catheter is usually held in place by an elastic adhesive strip that fits either between the penile skin and the condom or directly over the top of the condom. Some companies make external catheters that have an adhesive inner surface that adheres to the penile skin. If an external catheter with an adhesive strip is being used, it must be wrapped snugly around the penis to hold the catheter in place. However, extreme care must be taken not to make the adhesive strip too tight because doing so can result in impaired blood circulation to the penis. If swelling or a change in skin color is noted, the adhesive strip is too tight and should be removed immediately. Care must also be taken to avoid taping the pubic hair with the adhesive because doing so can cause great discomfort when the catheter is removed.

External catheters should be removed daily. The skin should be washed with warm, soapy water, rinsed thoroughly, and dried well before a clean catheter is applied. Some patients may demonstrate an allergy to the latex condom; if a reaction occurs, another brand should be tried. In addition, some patients, regardless of proper hygiene, will develop skin irritation underneath the catheter. Such irritation can be healed quickly by discontinuing use of the external catheter for a few days and relying on another form of management.

A few external drainage and collection devices are available for female patients. However, the female anatomy poses difficulty in using these products successfully. The female incontinence system usually consists of a pliable, funnel-shaped device that fits snugly over the vulva and is held in place by pressure, straps, or adhesive. Some of these systems also use an undergarment that is worn to hold the funnel in place. Much more work must be done in designing an external collection system for women that is easily applied, comfortable, and effective. As with men, the female collection device should be removed and changed (or cleansed) daily and good perineal hygiene should be followed.

Urinary tract infection, the most common problem associated with the use of internal catheters, occurs frequently with the use of external collection devices. The risk of such infection increases dramatically the longer the catheter remains in place. Urinary tract infection can have serious consequences, ranging from increased length of hospital stay to death. In fact, septicemia that complicates urinary tract infection is one of the most common causes of death of patients with Alzheimer's disease. Every effort should be made to find a noninvasive method of managing incontinence. Because the catheter remains in the bladder, it provides a direct route for bacteria to enter the body. Therefore sterile technique must be used for insertion of an indwelling catheter. The drainage bag should always remain lower than the patient's bladder to prevent urine from flowing back into the bladder.

Indwelling catheters should be changed on a regular basis, and the area where the catheter enters the body should be cleansed at least daily with an antibacterial solution (e.g., Betadine). The patient's urine should also be monitored for signs of infection, including odor, cloudiness, and the presence of mucus or blood. Such monitoring is important because acute infection in the older adult often occurs atypically. Caregivers should be alert to evidence of pain, tenderness in the abdomen or back, fever, increasing restlessness, pulling at the catheter, increasing lethargy, or confusion. Any patient with an indwelling catheter should be encouraged to drink plenty of fluids. Fruit juices that are acidic are also recommended to help make the urine a less desirable medium of growth for bacteria. Cranberry juice is frequently the preferred choice.

Drainage bags or reservoirs for both indwelling and external catheters come in two basic forms, a leg bag and a chair/bed bag. The leg bag is a much smaller unit that holds less urine. The bag is strapped to the leg, which allows it to be concealed underneath clothing and enables the patient to engage in social activities without embarrassment or the need to carry around a larger bag. Leg bags are ideal for short trips, parties, or shopping. If the bag needs to be emptied while the patient is away from home, the urine can be easily drained into any toilet.

The larger bedside bag or chair bag is used mainly when the patient is at home, in the hospital, or away for longer periods of time. Because these bags hold larger amounts of urine, they require emptying less frequently and are ideal for nighttime urine collection. The larger bag usually is transparent (at least on one side), which allows the caregiver to monitor the characteristics of the patient's urine. The bag is marked in graduated increments, which is useful when monitoring the patient's total output. Because most bags do not have one-way valves but work by gravity, the collection bag and tubing should always be lower than the level of the patient's bladder.

Absorbent and protective products

Absorbent and protective products either directly contain the urine or serve as a barrier that protects clothing, bedding, and furniture. These products come in many styles and shapes, may be washable or disposable, and have various names. They have become extremely popular over the past few years and have been marketed extensively as "the answer" to adult incontinence problems.

Although many of the products work in essentially the same manner, serious considerations are involved in choosing the most appropriate product. The availability of laundry facilities, the cost of the various products, and the degree of absorbency should be considered. Disposable products have the advantages of being simpler and less time-consuming than nondisposable types. However, their cost may be greater in the long run. Also, the degree of absorbency and the ease of use may vary greatly. If the patient voids large quantities of urine, the volume of urine that the product will effectively contain should be of primary concern. On the other hand, if the patient's problem is occasional dribbling, a pad that is more comfortable and less bulky may be considered. Regardless of the type chosen, absorbent products have made life much easier and more dignified for many older adults. Because most of these products can be concealed under clothing, the individual can return to an active and social life.

One of the most readily recognized incontinence products on the market today is the adult diaper. Basically fashioned after diapers used for infants, adult diapers are good for people who are incontinent of both bowel and bladder. This product usually comes in sizes (S,M,L) and is fastened with adhesive strips or pins. Adult diapers have been improved greatly by incorporating comfort measures and "accident prevention." Most adult diapers now have elastic waistbands and legbands to help prevent leakage, and many have stay-dry liners. Adult diapers can be used with ambulatory and nonambulatory patients. Although one of the bulkiest types of absorbent products, adult diapers can be worn underneath loose outer clothing. They can also be easily applied to bedridden individuals.

Most adult diapers have absorbent inner layers covered by a waterproof outer layer. Frequently the layer closest to the perineal skin will pull the urine toward the outer layer, thereby preventing moisture from remaining in constant contact with the skin. Patients who use adult diapers must be checked regularly for changing.

Adult briefs or pants are similar to underwear, but they have a pocket into which a thick absorbent pad can be placed. When soiled, the pad is removed and replaced with a clean, dry one. This product also has a waterproof covering that prevents soiling of clothing. Adult briefs generally come in sizes according to waist measurements, thus offering a good fit. They can be pulled on with an elastic waistband or snapped closed. The product is slightly less bulky than the diaper and is more suitable for patients who are socially active.

Because the slip-in pad may not be as absorbent as the adult diaper, the brief works best with patients who void smaller amounts or have a dribbling problem. Newer adult briefs are made of a very light, stretchable material with a waterproof area surrounding the pad. These products also have the stay-dry lining next to the skin, reducing the incidence of perineal rashes and excoriation. In contrast to disposable diapers, many adult briefs can be washed and reused, with the pad being the only item that requires replacement.

Protective pads come in both reusable (washable) and disposable forms. The major purpose of this type of product is to protect linens and furniture from becoming soiled with urine or feces. Several different sizes are available, depending on the size of the area to be protected. When used to protect bed linen, the pad should cover an area that stretches from approximately midback to midthigh and extends to the sides of the bed. Such coverage will promote protection when the patient turns and moves around in bed. A much smaller area can be covered when the patient is sitting in a chair since less movement will take place.

At minimum, the protective pads should have a thin layer of absorbent material backed by a waterproof cover. Because an underpad is usually less absorbent than a diaper, it may need to be used in conjunction with one of the other incontinence products. Caution and care must be used with the protective pads because they tend to become rolled or wadded underneath the patient when he moves. This situation can result in undue pressure on certain areas of the body and, if the pressure is not relieved, can eventually lead to skin breakdown. The protective pad should be straightened and all wrinkles removed on a regular basis.

Regardless of the type of product chosen to aid in the management of incontinence, particular and regular attention must be paid to providing good hygiene and skin care. Urinary incontinence is one of the major factors underlying the development of skin irritation and breakdown. Skin breakdown can lead to increased length of stay, increased costs of care, potential for infection, and extreme discomfort for the patient.

The pad, pants, and diaper should be changed whenever they become saturated, and the patient's skin should be cleansed with warm and soapy water, rinsed well, and thoroughly dried. The patient should be checked regularly (every 2 hours) to see if care is needed. The perineal area needs to be assessed frequently for signs of rash or irritation. Many skin care products used to prevent and treat diaper rash in children are suitable for use with adults. If a rash or irritation occurs, the incontinence product should be removed for several days to allow for healing. Often simply exposing the irritated area to air can help the skin to heal. If the rash or irritation persists, the physician should be notified. Occasionally, patients are sensitive or allergic to materials used in the products. If an allergic reaction occurs, another brand or a hypoallergic product can be tried.

SUMMARY

Many of the products discussed in this chapter are not covered by health insurance policies, Medicare, or Medicaid. Insurance policies should be checked carefully to determine whether or not incontinence management is a covered service. Because incontinence products can be expensive, an adequate workup for ruling out reversible causes of the incontinence is suggested.

Urinary incontinence is a treatable and manageable problem faced by millions of people. It need not control the life of the patient or the caregiver. When the physician, family, and nursing personnel work together, a successful and amenable management plan can be developed. This approach leads to fewer worries, eases the burden of caring, and allows a more normal and enjoyable life for patient, family, and staff.

BIBLIOGRAPHY

Brink C, Wells T: Environmental support for geriatric incontinence, *Clin Geriatr Med* 2:829-840, 1986.

Jeter KF: The use of incontinence products. In Jeter KF, Faller N, Norton C, editors: *Nursing for continence*, Philadelphia, 1990, WB Saunders.

Lincoln R, Roberts R: Continence issues in acute care, *Nurs Clin North Am* 24:741-749 1989.

Long ML: Managing urinary incontinence. In Chenitz WC, Stone JT, Salisbury SA editors: *Clinical gerontological nursing: a guide to advanced practice*, Philadelphia 1991, WB Saunders.

Mulholland G: Urinary tract infection, *Clin Geriatr Med* 6:43-51, 1990.

National Institute on Aging and Alliance for Aging Research: *Controlling urinary incontinence: information for health care providers*, Clinical Bulletin, Winter 1991 Washington, DC, The Institute.

Palmer M: Incontinence: magnitude of the problem, *Nurs Clin North Am* 23:139-155 1988.

Rousseau P: Urinary collection devices in geriatric incontinence, *J Enterostom Therapy* 18(1):26-31, 1991.

Smith D: Continence restoration in the homebound patient, *Nurs Clin North Am* 23:207-217, 1988.

Thomas A, Morse J: Managing urinary incontinence with self-care practices, *J Gerontol Nurs* 17(6):9-14, 1991.

Wanich C, Reilly N: Incontinence care products: non-surgical management of urinar incontinence, *Ostomy Wound Management* 34(3):45-51, 1991.

Warkentin R: Implementation of a urinary continence program, *J Gerontol Nurs* 18(1):31-36, 1992.

18

Safety and accident prevention

Mary M. Lancaster and Warren Clark

Patients who have Alzheimer's disease are prone to a number of accidents. The type of accident and its prevention depend greatly on the classification of the patient's condition according to the three stages of the disease.

STAGE 1 (EARLY STAGE)
Driving a Car

Traffic accidents often are one of the earliest signs that alert an individual's relatives to the fact that something is wrong with the person's mental functioning. Common driving problems include becoming lost and failing to stop at traffic lights, stop signs, or yield signs.

As discussed in Chapter 8, a patient who is in stage 1 of Alzheimer's disease may appear normal or just "eccentric" (at least to people who do not know him), although he has definite impairment of memory and other cognitive functions. Because of this apparent normalcy, the decision about whether to stop the person from driving is always a difficult one, especially since driving may represent the individual's only means of independence. It is surprising that many persons with Alzheimer's disease are able to drive themselves to the local shopping center or to the home of a relative or friend. They do so almost automatically. Nevertheless, because these individuals have definite mental impairment and their reaction time is slower than normal, they are a hazard to other drivers, to pedestrians, and to themselves.

Persons with Alzheimer's disease may forget the meaning of road signs, may confuse the meaning of red and green traffic lights, may incorrectly gauge the distance between vehicles, or simply may forget which way to go. Any one of these mistakes can cause a serious accident.

Individuals who are in the early stage of Alzheimer's disease also find it difficult to integrate and understand the meaning of several stimuli received simultaneously. As a result, they are easily distracted which is often a cause of traffic accidents. For instance, the person may be distracted by road construction and may not notice that a traffic light has changed to red, that they are about to crash into a nearby car, or that they may run off the road.

Persuading a person with Alzheimer's disease that he should not drive a car can be difficult. When explaining to the individual that he is no longer capable of driving, simply providing specific details may not work. It may be necessary to hide the person's car keys. Also, having a physician tell the patient that he can no longer drive may be effective. As a last resort, the car can be sold or the engine can be altered so that it will not start (e.g., by disconnecting the distributor).

Becoming Lost

Persons with Alzheimer's disease frequently lose their way. Since they cannot integrate various stimuli and orient themselves, they are often unable to retrace their steps. In many instances individuals with Alzheimer's disease have taken a bus, a car, or the train and later have been found wandering miles from home. Patients in the early stage of Alzheimer's disease generally have a specific purpose or destination in mind when they leave home (e.g., shopping or visiting). However, once away from the familiar surroundings of their home, they no longer recognize the way to the store or their friend's home and they are lost. Because of this tendency to become lost, such persons run the risk of being mugged, becoming victims of other forms of violence, or being exposed to extreme weather.

The problem of becoming lost that occurs in the early stage of Alzheimer's disease differs from that of wandering, seen in the next stage of the disease. Persons with Alzheimer's disease appear to have a deep rooted need to keep moving, a phenomenon that seems even more pronounced in the second stage of the disease. This problem raises the issue of how to constrain the person. Yet deciding whether to prevent him from leaving the house presents another difficult matter, since this measure often increases his agitation and irritability.

Poor Judgment and Gullibility

In the first stage of Alzheimer's disease, affected persons may not be fully aware of the risks they take or the consequences of their actions. Their ability to weigh risks and benefits or to accurately determine the steps and "equipment" necessary to complete a task is impaired. For example, a person may not remember to make sure that traffic is clear before crossing the street and consequently can be hit by a car. Similarly, at home a person may use a poorly balanced ladder to try to reach an object on a high shelf.

Because many persons in stage 1 of the disease are still relatively independent and able to communicate, it is not unusual for unscrupulous people to take advantage of their impaired mental functioning. The affected person may be approached by someone who persuades him to part with his money or property, and complex legal problems may ensue. Therefore, if the person's judgment is considered to be poor, power of attorney probably should be granted to a more capable person. It is also important to remember that individuals with Alzheimer's disease may invite strangers into the home and that these strangers may abuse them.

STAGE 2 (MIDDLE STAGE)

In stage 2, persons with Alzheimer's disease are easily recognized as having some mental abnormality since their mental functions are grossly impaired. The main concern for the individual's safety in this stage focuses on falls and other personal injuries.

Falls

Falls commonly occur in older persons, but particularly in those with Alzheimer's disease. On average, approximately half of the falls among older persons are secondary to an intrinsic problem such as orthostatic hypotension, arrhythmias, Parkinson's disease, neuropathies, and epilepsy. The other half are caused by environmental factors such as poor lighting, loose carpeting, or cluttered surroundings. Persons who have trouble perceiving their surroundings because of diminished vision or hearing also are more likely to fall.

In addition, persons with Alzheimer's disease often take unnecessary risks. For example, the person may place a chair atop a table and attempt to climb on both to reach an item on a high shelf, and the results are often disastrous. Similarly, the person may decide to paint a room, repair a window, or clean out the gutters and in doing so may take risks that increase his chances of falling.

The person with Alzheimer's disease reacts more slowly than normal, which makes it difficult for him to regain his balance if he starts to fall. This slow reaction time is one reason that it is so important to ensure that the person's surroundings are free of any potential hazards that might cause falls. Such hazards include poorly placed electrical wires, uneven floors, and throw rugs. Friends and family members who visit the affected person should be reminded not to rearrange his furniture or place things on the floor. They need to understand that the person cannot easily adapt to changes in his environment and that he performs best in familiar surroundings. When furniture or household items are moved, the person may bump into them and fall.

Throw rugs are very dangerous to elderly people, especially persons with Alzheimer's disease. Loose rugs are hazardous because the person may catch his foot underneath the edge, trip, and fall, possibly suffering a broken hip. All rugs should be made slip-proof for everyone's safety, but particularly for the elderly person with Alzheimer's disease. Certain throw rugs or decorative rugs may have been in place for many years and therefore may have great sentimental value to the family. In addition, they may help with the person's orientation by keeping the surroundings familiar. Such rugs should be given nonslip backing, or the edges should be secured to the floor with nails or double-sided adhesive tape. Bulky rugs should be replaced by thinner ones that are not so high off the floor.

Removing obstacles from the common path of traffic throughout the house is important. If large pieces of furniture must remain where they are, any sharp edges or corners should be padded to prevent serious injury. All traffic areas, pathways, and rooms commonly used should be well lit. Bedrooms, bathrooms, hallways, and stairwells also require good lighting. Highly polished floors and direct sunlight in rooms should be avoided since both produce glare, which presents a difficulty for older people. Glare can be reduced by using low-luster polishes on floors and by placing sheer curtains over windows.

Persons with Alzheimer's disease may not be able to gauge the height of steps, curbs, and door thresholds accurately, a situation that often leads to falls. The edges of steps can be highlighted in a bright color to help draw attention to the steps. As an alternative, barriers can be used to block stairways; however, the barriers should be high enough that the person will not try to walk over them. Doors leading to basements should be kept locked.

As the dementia of Alzheimer's disease progresses, the person may develop an ataxic gait and may be at even greater risk of falling, even in the safety-conscious environment of an institution. Although little can be done to affect the processes underlying these changes, there are many other factors that increase the risk of falls for patients with Alzheimer's disease in a residential care setting. Controlling those risk factors provides a major opportunity for reducing the injuries associated with falling in this category of residents. One of the major activities of nursing staff should be assessment of the effect of medications on the risk that a resident will fall. Since antipsychotics, antidepressants, sedatives/hypnotics, vasodilators, and diuretics are particularly associated with increased risk of falls, they should be used in the smallest doses that will achieve the desired effects. The administration of drugs at bedtime can be done to allow some of the sedating effects to wear off during the resident's sleep.

The nurse should consistently assess the resident's stability during standing, ability to change positions safely, and balance and coordination. All these skills may deteriorate in the resident with advancing dementia. Sometimes assistive devices such as walkers or wheelchairs can be used by the resident to provide support during ambulation. However, because of the resident's poor memory and impaired learning, he cannot be relied on to use these devices each time he is walking or to use them correctly. Offering general activities to maintain strength, ensuring that sensory deficits are corrected with eyeglasses and hearing aids, and constantly assessing for environmental risks may be all that can be done practically to prevent falls.

In the past, physical restraints were often used to prevent falls in these residents. However, it is becoming increasingly obvious that the negative effects of this practice, such as increased agitation and deterioration in overall physical and mental condition, make this an option of last resort in the management of residents at risk of falling.

Fire and Electrical Hazards

Persons with stage 2 Alzheimer's disease are at high risk for personal injuries and for causing injuries to others through improper or inappropriate use of household equipment and devices. The person's poor memory, curiosity, and poor coordination and judgment are responsible for most of these injuries. For example, after deciding to cook a meal, the person may turn on the gas but forget to light it, or he may forget about the food he has put on the stove to cook.

Persons with Alzheimer's disease inadvertently pose frequent fire hazards because they often do not appreciate the significance of many of their actions, and they can be easily distracted. Electrical appliances,

stoves, heaters, and matches pose particular dangers. Frequently th
person may turn on one of these appliances and leave it unattended
Changing or removing control knobs from stoves and heaters can help t
prevent accidents. Gas stoves are especially hazardous because if the ga
is turned on but not lit, gas poisoning or an explosion can result. Also
electrical outlets should be covered when they are not in use. Fuse boxe
and circuit boards should be secured to prevent the person from tam
pering with the power supply.

Bathing

Often, persons with Alzheimer's disease are easily distracte
while preparing to bathe. As a result, the faucet may be left on and th
person may not realize that the water is overflowing the tub. Person
may scald themselves with bath water that is too hot or expose them
selves to hypothermia with water that is too cold.

Similarly, affected persons may forget to (or be unable to) turn o
the heat. They may not realize that although the heat is on, the hous
will not become warm if the windows are open. They also may b
unable to appreciate the need to dress appropriately. These person
tend to go outside inappropriately dressed and are likely to suffe
from the effects of inclement weather. Because of their impaired mem
ory and poor judgment, hypothermia appears to be a significant ris
for persons with Alzheimer's disease.

Poisoning and Pica

Accidents with common household cleaners, caustic agents, an
poisons are more likely to happen to persons who have Alzheimer'
disease in comparison to unaffected individuals. The affected person'
inability to read or recognize labels, forgetfulness, and inquisitiv
nature are responsible for many of the accidental poisonings and in
gestions that occur. Many substances are ingested because the perso
no longer recognizes or understands the appropriate use of the sub
stance. Therefore all potentially hazardous materials and substance
should be kept secured.

In cases of food poisoning, the person's diminished senses of smel
and taste may prevent him from noticing a strong smell or "off" tast
in spoiled food. Thus he may not be able to recognize food that ha
gone "bad." Similarly, the person may forget to return food to th
refrigerator.

Pica, that is, the craving for or eating of unusual foods or substances, is a trait that is not uncommon among persons with Alzheimer's disease. The person with Alzheimer's disease can have a very curious nature, and, just like a child, he may use his mouth to investigate both liquids and solids. Therefore all cleaning products, medications, and other poisonous substances must be kept safely locked in a cabinet. The person may no longer recognize which things are appropriate to eat and may pick up items such as soap, cigarette butts, and flowers and put them in his mouth. Products such as mouthwash, toothpaste, and liquid detergent also should be kept out of sight; although not actually poisonous, they can make a person very ill if taken in large amounts.

Medications

Persons with Alzheimer's disease are likely to take the wrong medicine, the correct medicine at the wrong time, or too much of any medication. One patient known to us who was in stage 2 of Alzheimer's disease took his sleeping medication first thing in the morning and his diuretic the last thing before going to bed. Consequently, he tended to be lethargic and sleepy most of the day and incontinent and fully awake at night. It was generally assumed that these two conditions were the result of his Alzheimer's disease, but, in fact, the problems were caused by the inappropriately taken medication.

An individual with Alzheimer's disease must not have uncontrolled access to medications. He may take a sleeping tablet, then forget that he took it, and a few minutes later take another one. This sequence may be repeated several times until the patient has taken an overdose of hypnotic medication. A number of devices can be used to prevent the person from taking more medication than is required. For instance, all the day's medication can be placed in a small compartment of a special container while the main compartment, which contains the rest of the medication, remains inaccessible. A note can be left in the container saying that, since no tablets are left, the medication for the day has been taken and the person should not try to take any more. This reminder may prevent the patient from becoming agitated at not being able to take additional medication.

The same risk of overdose applies to a person who is in pain, who has analgesic preparations at hand, and who tries to relieve the pain. Because the person's memory is poor, he may forget having taken an analgesic tablet and therefore may take too much of this medication.

Overdosage of many preparations, such as hypotensive medications and medications that act on the heart, may be associated with serious side effects. Therefore no medication should be left lying around. As much as possible, the person should be given his medication on a day-to-day basis.

It is wise to have the caregiver take charge of all the person's medication and administer it as prescribed. The caregiver must be instructed about how and when to give the medication and should know the common side effects. In this way the caregiver will be prepared and able to consult with the physician if any side effects should occur.

Wandering

Wandering is a problem many caregivers must face with persons who have Alzheimer's disease. Nursing homes with special units for these individuals have an advantage because they usually have an area that is locked for safety yet allows the person to move about freely. Although the person should be granted as much independence as possible, the prevention of accidents caused by wandering outside the house must be considered when it is no longer safe for the person to be out alone.

Doors leading to the outside should be kept locked. Often, simply changing to a new type of lock that the person is not familiar with can solve the problem. If this step does not work, deadbolt locks requiring keys should be installed. Regular door handles can be replaced with child-proof models that require a combination of actions to turn the handle. The person with Alzheimer's disease probably will not be able to figure out the sequence necessary to open the door. Doors may be concealed with drapes, pull-down shades, or portable decorative screens. However, one of the dangers of this approach is fire. In each town the local fire marshall often will have specific suggestions to deal with this problem.

Alarm systems on doors also can be helpful. These systems allow the door to be opened but signal that the person is going outside. Sometimes the alarm itself is enough to scare the person so that he will close the door and stay inside. Many types of door alarms are available, and they vary in sophistication and cost. It is wise to shop around to find the system best suited to the living arrangement and the budget. Many nursing homes use alarm systems on the outside doors of buildings.

If the person in stage 2 can go outside, fencing around the yard can serve as added protection. This arrangement allows the person to get some fresh air and to exercise in an enclosed safe area. The yard should be kept clear of branches or other objects that might cause harm. In addition, the person should have adequate identification on his body, such as a bracelet or locket with his name and the name and phone number of the individual to be contacted if the person becomes lost. The family also should have a recent photograph of the person that can be given to the neighbors or the police if a search should become necessary. Neighbors and friends should be told of the person's condition so that they can notify the caregiver if they see the person wandering outside. The phone numbers of the police department and the neighbors should be kept readily accessible. Caregivers should be encouraged to contact the local chapter of the Alzheimer's Association in their area to see if the chapter offers a "wanderer's program." Such a program registers the person with Alzheimer's disease with the local chapter, local police, and 911. Then, in the event that the person wanders away from home, one phone call will activate search procedures.

Some persons will not go outside unless they are wearing their favorite jacket or shoes or carrying their purse or wallet. This practice is probably a lifelong habit that the person with Alzheimer's disease has maintained. Putting these articles out of sight until they are needed can help prevent the person from wandering.

In the institutional setting wandering becomes a safety issue when the resident is able to wander into a section of the facility that is unsafe for him or to leave the facility altogether. Many institutions now have mechanisms to alert staff when a resident wanders beyond safe limits. Such devices allow a staff member to locate the resident, accompany him briefly, and then redirect him to a safe area. Wandering behavior often can be contained by having cues that anchor the resident to a safe area, such as the presence of familiar or pleasing items.

In some instances, residents must be placed in special care areas where wandering can be restricted. Such restriction can be achieved through the use of extensive monitoring systems or by locking doors to prevent exit. These units should be designed to maximize the resident's freedom to move about and should include access to indoor and outdoor recreational activities.

Some wandering residents can be contained by manipulating the environment to make it seem more restrictive than it actually is. Complicated opening mechanisms on exit doors are often enough to frustrate the resident with cognitive impairments. This illusion of containment also can be fostered by including noxious stimuli, such as rough walls or disorienting designs near exits.

In spite of the institution's efforts to deal with the wanderer, occasionally a resident will wander away from a facility. The facility should have a clearly defined procedure for searching for missing residents and for notifying appropriate authorities and family members. The use of identification bracelets and the presence of a current photograph can be lifesaving in such situations.

STAGE 3 (LATE STAGE)

In stage 3, the person with Alzheimer's disease has several physical disabilities in addition to mental impairment. Because of his failing physical status, the person with late-stage Alzheimer's disease is much more likely to be confined to a chair or bed. In some ways this confinement reduces the risk for many of the accidents previously described; however, different concerns for overall safety arise. This person is at greater risk for falling (if still ambulatory), for becoming incontinent of urine, for developing decubitus ulcers, and for becoming dehydrated (see Chapters 8 and 16).

In addition to failing physical status, the person's mental abilities decline. As the patient's degree of confusion increases, he may wander more or may become agitated or combative toward caregivers or others in his environment. This combination of mental and physical decline frequently results in placement of the person in a hospital or nursing home. Safety in these institutions is complicated by the presence of a number of residents with similar behaviors and by the necessity for staff to closely monitor the idiosyncrasies of individual residents.

Safety is the paramount concern in institutional settings. Institutions generally have policies and procedures aimed at ensuring the safety of their residents. Issues addressed in these policies include environmental safety, mealtime safety, fire safety, use of restraints, wandering, and risk of falling.

Environmental Safety

Environmental safety in an institutional setting encompasses a program for the evaluation of all aspects of the environment in regard to the safety of residents and staff. One of the major safety risks posed by the person with severe dementia is the tendency to place objects in his mouth. This tendency may be caused by confusion over whether or not the item is food, or it may represent a need for oral stimulation. Whatever the reason for this action, any item that could be swallowed or aspirated must be placed out of the resident's reach. Staff must be particularly careful to alert family and other visitors to this risk and must inspect all personal items left with the resident. Institutions should have policies concerning the identification and storage of unsafe items and the supervision of residents during potentially risky activities. This safety measure includes monitoring the use of medical devices and appliances and even monitoring routine activities of daily living such as bathing or shaving.

Mealtime Safety

Related to the tendency to place foreign objects in the mouth is the high risk for choking and aspiration during mealtimes. The resident with advanced dementia may eat rapidly without paying attention to the consistency of the food he is eating. He also may stuff his mouth with food without swallowing between bites. Choking often can be prevented by attention from staff during mealtimes, by reminders to eat slowly, and by avoiding the tendency to rush residents through meals. It may be advisable to limit the amount of food available to the resident at any one time. In some instances it may be necessary to prescribe soft or pureed foods when the choking risk is determined to be very high. If residents are identified as being at risk for choking, their families should be instructed about the necessary precautions and the methods for identifying respiratory distress and for immediately notifying staff of such occurrences.

All staff caring for residents with Alzheimer's disease should be trained in the use of the Heimlich maneuver for relieving airway obstruction. It is also wise to encourage family members to learn this procedure. Portable oxygen and suction equipment also should be available in areas where residents are eating.

Fire Safety

Another major component of institutional safety concerns fire hazards. All the precautions regarding fire hazards cited already also should be considered in a fire safety program in an institutional setting. When the institution houses residents with Alzheimer's disease, particular attention should be paid to the need for an evacuation plan that can be followed with as little assistance by residents as possible. Advanced de mentia makes smoking a very high risk behavior that should be allowed only under close supervision. The severe confusion and curious nature of many patients with Alzheimer's disease may lead to resident-initiated false fire alarms. This problem usually can be addressed by having two-step process for initiating fire alarms, one that is too complicated to be mastered by a resident with dementia.

Use of Restraints

Physical restraints or restraint achieved by means of drugs can be used to ensure the resident's safety. The objective in using restraints is to protect the person from falls and self-injury. Because the use of restraints conflicts with the overall treatment goal of maintaining independence, all alternative measures for safety should be exhausted before restraints are prescribed. Restraints never should be seen as the first or the definitive solution to a safety problem. They also should not be used solely for the convenience of the caregiver or staff. In an institutional setting it must be remembered that a physician must order any restraint and the order must be time-limited. In addition, the need for restraint must be clearly documented in the medical record. Whenever a restraint is used, the goal is to eliminate it as soon as possible. Success in achieving this goal is measured by how quickly this elimination can be accomplished. It must be remembered that restraints restrict the person's movement and deny him independence and a sense of freedom.

A common unwanted side effect of restraints, especially when used with persons with Alzheimer's disease, is aggressive and agitated behavior. Often the person does not comprehend the reason for the restraint and begins to fight it. He may think that he is being tied down or punished. Conversely, some individuals may exhibit regressive behavior and retreat further into isolation by not interacting. In either situation the person's confusion, isolation, and dependence will probably increase. If this situation occurs, engaging the person in some activity and using therapeutic touch can help to decrease the person's agitation by distracting his attention from the restraints.

Many types of restraints are available: vests, waist and ankle restraints, bar restraints, and belts. Each type has advantages and disadvantages, which should be considered when selecting the one most appropriate for the person's needs.

Vest restraints are used frequently because they allow free movement of the arms and legs while supporting the upper body. This type of restraint is particularly useful for persons who tend to lean forward and are at risk of falling out of a wheelchair. Vest restraints also can be effective for persons who try to climb out of bed. A disadvantage of the vest restraint is that the person can slide down and wiggle out of the vest. This situation can be dangerous if the restraint becomes caught underneath his chin and lodges around his neck because the person is, in effect, hanging himself. Vest restraints always must be applied properly and according to the manufacturer's specifications to help prevent respiratory distress or strangulation.

Many persons can get out of a restraint even if it has been correctly applied. By no means should the restraint be considered a sure safeguard against falls and accidents. The person in restraint should be checked frequently to ensure that the restraint remains in place and that circulation and respiration are not restricted. The person's needs for toileting, food, fluid, and activity also must be assessed and met by releasing the restraints every 2 or 3 hours. All checks on the restrained person should be recorded in the nursing notes or on a flowsheet. In addition, there must be documentation in the nurse's notes regarding the person's response to the restraint and the assessment performed for continued justification for the restraint.

A restraint always must be secured to a stable object. Restraints used for persons confined to bed should be secured to the bed frame, not to the siderail. The person should be able to roll from side to side in a vest restraint. Restraints for a person in a wheelchair should never be fastened to a movable part of the chair. Belt restraints can be securely fastened underneath the seat of the wheelchair. This type of restraint is best used with cooperative persons who need reminding only to call for assistance when they want to get up.

Siderails are a form of restraint that helps to remind the individual to stay in bed. When rails are used, the bed should always be in the low position. If the person should decide to climb over the siderails and the bed is in the high position, the added distance that the person will fall can significantly increase injury. It is probably wise to use a vest restraint in conjunction with siderails for persons with Alzheimer's disease. Because their judgment and reasoning are impaired, they frequently do not understand the need for siderails and will try to climb over them. Most individuals who climb over siderails or fall from bed report that they were trying to get to the bathroom. Therefore it is vitally important for staff and caregivers to attend to the person's elimination needs frequently.

Arm, leg, or wrist restraints are used less frequently than other methods. They should be used only when the person's agitation is severe and this method is the only way to keep the person from harming himself or others. This type of restraint should be used only for short periods because it completely restricts movement of the extremity. Sedatives are frequently used in combination with arm, leg, or wrist restraints. If the person requires this type of combination restraint, he must be assessed at regular intervals, and this assessment must be documented. Because arm or leg restraints severely restrict movement, ethical and legal issues must be considered. Hand mittens, which allow free movement, can be used instead of wrist restraints for persons who try to remove their intravenous lines or feeding tubes. The ankle or wrist restraint must be removed frequently, and the extremity must be massaged and placed through range-of-motion exercises. The area where the restraint is applied must be assessed for tissue injury.

The use of restraints is a controversial issue. Each state and local institution must have a policy outlining the requirements and procedures for using physical restraints. In addition, each situation must be analyzed individually. New regulations and guidelines are being enforced that mandate that restraints, in any form, be used only when absolutely necessary and then only under a physician's order and for a limited period of time. Health care workers must be aware that the use of restraints adversely affects behavior and outcomes. The person's safety and well-being must be weighed against the risks and side effects of restraints, and the goal of using restraints for the least amount of time possible must always be kept in mind.

Families are becoming more involved in decisions related to restraints. Family conferences are the ideal setting for discussing the pros and cons of restraint, explaining why temporary restraint may be needed, and assessing the family's beliefs and attitudes about the use of restraints. If a family is opposed to the use of restraint for maintaining the person's safety, this decision should be entered in the record during the family conference and all in attendance should sign the note (including family members).

SUMMARY

Safety and accident prevention for persons with Alzheimer's disease pose many difficulties for staff and caregivers. Being aware of potential hazards and realizing that the affected person can no longer be responsible for his own safety is the first step in preventing accidents. Providing a safe environment, either at home or in the institution, can help lessen the strain on caregivers. Considerable patience and creativity are required to make an environment safe yet stimulating for persons with Alzheimer's disease.

BIBLIOGRAPHY

Chenitz WC, Kussman H, Stone J: Preventing falls. In Chenitz WC, Stone JT, Salisbury SA, editors: *Clinical gerontological nursing: a guide to advanced practice*, Philadelphia, 1991, WB Saunders.

Counseling to prevent household and environmental injuries, *Am Fam Physician* 42: 135-138, 1990.

Eigsti D, Vrooman N: Releasing restraints in the nursing home, *J Gerontol Nurs* 18(1): 21-23, 1992.

Gross Y and others: Why do they fall? Monitoring risk factors in nursing homes, *J Gerontol Nurs* 16(6): 20-25, 1990.

Hall GR: This hospital patient has Alzheimer's, *Am J Nurs* 91(10):44-50, 1991.

Josephson K, Fabacher D, Rubenstein L: Home safety and fall prevention, *Clin Geriatr Med* 7:707-731, 1991.

Kaszniak AW, Keyl PM, Albert MS: Dementia and the older driver, *Hum Factors* 33: 527-537, 1991.

Namazi KH, Rosner TT, Calkins MP: Visual barriers to prevent ambulatory Alzheimer's patients from exiting through emergency doors, *Gerontologist* 29:699-702, 1989.

Strumpf NE, Evans LK, Schwartz D: Physical restraint of the elderly. In Chenitz WC, Stone JT, Salisbury SA, editors: *Clinical gerontological nursing: a guide to advanced practice*, Philadelphia, 1991, WB Saunders.

19

Daily care and management

Mary M. Lancaster

During the early stages of Alzheimer's disease, the patient will begin to demonstrate a lack of attention to personal hygiene and grooming. This development may be caused by changes in memory that interfere with the patient's ability to perform tasks that require sequential steps or by his simply ignoring the need for personal hygiene. Whatever the cause may be, patients with Alzheimer's disease soon forget to bathe, change clothes, or use the bathroom. To caregivers, these tasks seem quite simple, but to someone whose memory is impaired, the tasks of daily living can be frustrating and overwhelming.

Activities of daily living are actually quite complicated when broken down into steps. Forgetting any one of the steps can block the patient's ability to perform the task. For example, brushing teeth requires the patient to recognize all the equipment used (toothbrush, toothpaste, sink) and to remember how to use each piece of equipment. In addition, the patient needs to remember to find the equipment, put the toothpaste on the toothbrush, brush his teeth, and rinse his mouth. Early in the disease, providing assistance with the one step that is forgotten may be all that is needed for the patient to finish the task. Eventually, the entire activity will need to be performed for the patient.

Task breakdown is a very useful tool in keeping the patient with Alzheimer's disease functioning on his own. The caregiver needs to be present to coach the patient through the task verbally. However, if the patient is allowed to actually perform the activity, he will retain the ability longer. Completing tasks for the patient is not always the best approach. Providing cues such as labeling, breaking tasks down into very simple steps, giving verbal reminders and prompts, placing equipment and clothes out in view, and offering demonstrations are all useful in keeping the patient functioning. Maintaining set routines for the activities of daily living will also help to keep the patient functioning independently. It is most important to remember that, for the patient with Alzheimer's disease, once a skill has been lost, it is virtually impossible to regain.

Family caregivers and health care providers need to continually assess the patient's skill in performing activities of daily living since this skill level can change on a daily basis. Expecting the patient to perform an activity that he cannot do will lead to frustration for the caregiver and the patient. Catastrophic reactions occur frequently when the patient becomes overwhelmed and frustrated by expectations. Therefore caregivers must be attuned to the patient's general hygienic needs and to the specific areas of impairment in order to promote good personal hygiene, independent functioning, and strong self-esteem.

ORAL CARE AND HYGIENE

Care of the mouth is one area of daily hygiene that is most often neglected when patients no longer perform the task independently. However, it is vitally important that oral care be provided, even if the patient wears dentures. Improper or inadequate oral care can result in serious problems with both teeth and gums and can lead to systemic infection. When neglected, the gums can quickly become irritated and inflamed, resulting in pain, bleeding, and exposure of the root of the tooth, and provide an excellent site for infection. In addition, a mouth that is not properly cleansed causes bad breath and an associated decrease in self-esteem.

If the patient has his natural teeth, attention must be given to proper brushing at least once a day. All surfaces must be brushed to remove food particles and plaque. The gum line needs to be brushed to stimulate circulation and remove imbedded food. If the patient is performing the activity himself, caregivers may need to provide assistance. It is very important for the caregiver to check the patient's mouth to make sure he is adequately cleansing his teeth, gums, and tongue. The mouth should be inspected frequently for signs of gum inflammation, swelling, or tenderness. Adaptive equipment, such as long toothbrushes, suction toothbrushes, and toothbrushes with large handles, is available to make oral care easier. Ingestible toothpaste can be used for the patient who tends to swallow after brushing instead of spitting. If the patient cannot brush his own teeth, the caregiver must assume this task. Props designed to keep the patient's mouth open are available from medical equipment suppliers, or they can be made from tongue blades padded with gauze.

The patient who no longer has any natural teeth still requires daily oral care. It is a myth that patients who are edentulous do not require oral care. All the soft tissues of the mouth should be cleansed at least once a day. A soft toothbrush, sponge, or washcloth wrapped around a finger can be used to clean the edentulous patient's mouth. If the patient wears dentures, particular attention must be given to oral care. The dentures should be removed at least once a day and scrubbed with a soft brush and cleanser. This practice helps to remove the food particles that adhere to the dentures. The top and bottom of each denture should also be cleansed to remove any trapped food, mucus, and adhesive. Ideally, the patient's dentures should be removed each evening, cleansed, and stored in a denture cup filled with water until the next morning. Just before the dentures are to be placed in the patient's mouth, they should be rinsed.

Dentures can improve the patient's chewing ability, looks, and speech. The patient should be assisted in inserting his dentures each morning. Certain problems unique to denture wearers need to be noted. If the patient has lost a significant amount of weight, which is not uncommon in Alzheimer's disease, the dentures may become very loose and actually inhibit chewing and speech. If the dentures do not stay in place, a dentist should be consulted. "Wobbly" dentures and ones that are left in place for long periods can be sources of soft tissue irritation. Large ulcerations can develop and interfere with eating and speaking. They can also cause significant pain. The accompanying box illustrates the impact of inadequate denture care on health and functioning.

Periodic examinations by a dentist or hygienist should be continued as long as possible. Some dentists will make trips to the home or the nursing home if the patient is unable to come to the office. It is recommended that edentulous patients have a yearly oral examination and those patients with natural teeth be checked twice a year. In addition, all patients who are entering a long-term care facility should have a comprehensive oral assessment by a dentist to provide a baseline for treatment and management.

INADEQUATE DENTURE CARE

Mrs. W. is a 72-year-old woman who has been residing in a nursing home for the last 4 years. She was diagnosed as having Alzheimer's disease 3 years ago. Her daughter comes to visit every day at supper time to encourage her to eat. For the past several weeks Mrs. W. has become more agitated and irritable and has been losing weight. She has also been noted rubbing her face. Because of this agitation, Mrs. W. has been given increasing doses of a tranquilizer. She now sits slumped over in her chair, and her speech is slurred. Mrs. W.'s daughter is quite concerned about her mother's rapid deterioration and her grimacing during eating. As a last resort, she consults her own dentist and asks him to see her mother.

The dentist arrives and finds Mrs. W. in her usual position slumped in her chair. He inspects Mrs. W.'s mouth and sees that she has all her natural lower teeth but has an upper denture. The lower teeth are in good repair, except that they need brushing. The dentist asks Mrs. W. if she is having any problems. Mrs. W. pulls at her upper denture and shakes her head. After removing the upper denture, the dentist finds a large ulcer on the hard palate covered with a thick layer of mucus and food. After cleansing the area, the dentist is relieved to note that the ulcer is superficial. He recommends that the denture be left out for 1 week, after which it is to be used only when eating. He also leaves instructions for cleansing of the denture and Mrs. W.'s mouth (hard palate in particular) after each meal.

Two weeks later, the dentist comes to see how Mrs. W. is progressing. He is amazed to find a woman who is sitting up, communicating, and eating very well. The staff report that the dose of the tranquilizer has been greatly reduced and that Mrs. W. has gained 3 pounds.

BATHING

As Alzheimer's disease progresses, the patient experiences increasing difficulty in locating the bathroom and may even begin to resist bathing. There are numerous possible causes for this resistance toward bathing. Some causes are fear, lack of privacy, the overwhelming aspect of the mechanics of bathing, changes in hot/cold sensations, embarrassment, and depression. The patient may associate a shower with being out in the rain, he may fear what will happen if he undresses, he may no longer recognize the person who is helping him, or he may have forgotten how to turn the water on. It is very important for caregivers to investigate the possible cause of the patient's reluctance so that appropriate corrective action can be taken.

To begin, the caregiver needs to evaluate the best time of day for bathing. This decision should take into consideration the patient's past routine. Some persons bathe in the morning, whereas others bathe before bedtime. In any case adequate time is needed to avoid making the patient feel rushed. Once a bath time has been established, it should be followed consistently on a daily basis. The bathroom needs to provide privacy and warmth. A shower chair may prove useful for the older individual. Placing out all the needed supplies, such as soap, washcloth, and towel, will provide cues that the patient can use. In the early stages of the disease, simply reminding the patient of the bath and drawing the water may be all that are necessary to begin the routine. The patient must be assessed for his ability to distinguish between hot and cold and to regulate water temperature so that injuries can be avoided. If the patient has mobility or balance problems, a bath is generally safer than a shower. A bath also can be very therapeutic.

Consideration also needs to be given to making the bathroom a safe environment for the patient. Temperatures on water heaters should be adjusted so that the water is not dangerously hot, locks on doors should be removed, and all containers used should be plastic instead of glass. The addition of handrails in the bathtub and on the walls, the use of nonslip bathmats, and care taken to wipe up any puddles of water can help to prevent falls and broken bones. All electrical appliances such as razors and hairdryers need to be out of the patient's reach. Finally, a hand-held spray attachment can be useful in rinsing the patient and makes hair washing much easier.

An elderly patient usually does not need a complete bath every day; three times a week is normally sufficient. However, the patient does require daily cleansing of the face, hands, axillae, and perineal areas. Age changes in the skin result in reduced elasticity, moisture, and oil secretion. Daily bathing with soap can compound the problems of dry skin, itching, and fragile skin. Mild soaps and emollient lotions should be used to help decrease skin dryness. Bath oil or lotion should be applied after the patient has gotten out of the bathtub to avoid the possibility of slipping. Special attention must be given to thoroughly drying skin creases and folds. Unscented powders and cornstarch can be used to keep these areas dry; however, care needs to be taken not to allow these powders to accumulate.

Assisting the patient with his bath is an opportune time to assess joint mobility, skin condition, and lesions or moles. It also offers the chance to obtain an overall picture of the patient's condition. If the patient should become extremely agitated and combative, it is generally best to stop the bath, remove the patient from the area, and try again later, when the patient has calmed down. If the patient is bedridden, adequate care can be provided with the patient in bed. Adaptive equipment for washing hair is available, for example. While giving a bed bath, the caregiver should pay particular attention to the condition of the skin at bony areas. Regardless of the type of bath, bathing is a very personal and private activity. The loss of independence in this area can be extremely difficult for the patient. Caregivers must recognize that the person with Alzheimer's disease may be experiencing strong feelings about this loss and that such feelings may be contributing to his resistance to bathing.

DRESSING

Inappropriate dressing may be one of the problems faced by persons caring for patients with Alzheimer's disease. The patient may no longer be able to coordinate colors, may put on a shirt backward, or may fasten buttons in the wrong order. Affected patients often put on many layers of clothes, or they may want to remove clothing at inappropriate times. The act of dressing is as complex as any of the other activities of daily living.

In the early stages of the disease, simply organizing the patient's clothes in outfits and colors can be very useful. Labeling the closet and dresser drawers with large letters (e.g., SOCKS, UNDERWEAR) can help the patient locate certain clothing. Placing an outfit out on the bed for the patient can help avoid catastrophic reactions that may occur when the patient becomes frustrated by trying to coordinate colors or choose clothing. Eliminating clutter and distractions while the patient is dressing will help keep his attention focused on the task.

As Alzheimer's disease progresses, the patient loses fine motor skills. A noticeable stiffening of the muscles also may occur. Both of these physical changes make the act of dressing much more difficult than it would normally be. The patient may not be able to manipulate small buttons, hooks, or zippers. Clothing that has been adapted with large zippers or Velcro closures makes dressing easier for the patient. Pull-on skirts and pants are also easier for the patient to use. Clothing that is pulled on over the head may prove problematic because of poor joint mobility but also because the patient may feel threatened if his head is temporarily covered. Clothing should also be made of easy-care fabric to lessen the burden on the caregiver since patients with Alzheimer's disease can easily go through several pieces of clothing a day.

Putting away rarely worn or out-of-season clothing can help to simplify choosing what to wear. Accessories such as belts and ties should be hung with the appropriate outfit to make dressing easier. All the articles of clothing needed for an outfit can be placed in sequential order on the patient's bed to enable him to dress himself. The pattern of the fabric should be relatively simple, since wild, busy prints can be distracting to the patient. Shoes should be slip-on type or have Velcro closures instead of strings or ties. If the patient wants to wear the same clothes day after day, this issue should not become a point of argument. It is generally easier to buy several sets of the same outfit to accommodate the patient.

Some patients tend to undress frequently, which can be both embarrassing and inconvenient for caregivers. It is important to investigate the cause of this action. The patient may be too hot, the material may be scratchy, the patient may be bored, or he may need to go to the bathroom. In any case, caregivers must remember that the patient with Alzheimer's disease no longer understands what is appropriate and usually is not undressing himself to be provocative. On the other hand, some patients develop a habit of putting on many layers of clothes, regardless of the weather. Again, this practice can be embarrassing to the caregiver. It also can be potentially dangerous if the environment is very warm. First, a determination needs to be made about whether the patient is cold. Then, the possibility of danger associated with the layers of clothes should be considered. If no danger is involved, the practice can be allowed. If the patient needs to have several sweaters or coats removed, more appropriate clothing can be substituted when the original clothing is removed. Removal of the layered items should be done with patience and the understanding that the very same thing will need to be done again later.

TOILETING

As Alzheimer's disease progresses, the patient will begin to experience problems related to emptying the bladder and/or bowel. Initially, the problem may be related to the fact that the patient no longer recognizes the body signals of a full bowel or bladder. At this point a patient with Alzheimer's disease may need to be reminded to go to the bathroom frequently to empty his bladder. With many patients, setting up a regular schedule for toileting has proven effective in avoiding accidents. The patient may also forget where the bathroom is located, or he may not recognize the toilet as the appropriate place to urinate. Such a patient will need to be taken by the hand, led to the bathroom, and seated on the toilet. Sometimes labeling the bathroom door will be helpful to the patient. Regardless of the cause, the onset of toileting problems and incontinence is distressing to both family and health care personnel. The causes, treatment, and management of urinary incontinence are discussed in greater detail in Chapters 16 and 17.

Maintaining normal bowel function in the patient with Alzheimer's disease takes creativity on the part of the caregiver in addition to advice from health professionals. Generally, problems with bowel function do not arise until later in the disease; however, constipation can develop at any time. Changes in the digestive system that occur with aging tend to make the older person more prone to constipation. Constipation and fecal impaction can cause a high degree of discomfort and distress in the patient, which can lead to unwanted behavioral problems. Therefore it is extremely important for caregivers to continually assess and monitor the patient's bowel function.

In initiating a bowel maintenance program, it is necessary to know the patient's usual pattern of bowel movement. This pattern includes frequency and time of day. Once this pattern has been established for the patient, all efforts should be geared toward maintaining it. Patients should not be permitted to go longer than 3 days without a bowel movement because of the high risk for fecal impaction. Taking the patient to the bathroom at the same time every day and having him sit on the toilet will help to "train" the bowel to empty at this particular time. The next step is to use the natural methods of stimulating bowel function. Diet, activity, and fluids are the mainstays of preventing constipation and preserving normal bowel function. Particular attention must be given to diet in the patient with Alzheimer's disease since chewing and swallowing problems are often encountered. Increasing the amount of whole fiber in the patient's diet is very important because fiber acts to pull water into the bowel to soften the fecal mass. Whole-grain breads, pastas, cereals, vegetables, and fruits are good sources of fiber.

The patient needs to be kept as active as possible because physical activity helps to facilitate bowel motion. Taking the patient for a walk twice a day, involving him in an exercise class (if possible), or simply moving him from one chair to another throughout the day can help add to the patient's activity level. For the bed-bound patient, turning him every 2 hours and helping the patient to sit up in a chair several times during the day can aid in increasing bowel motility. Finally, increasing the amount of fluids that the patient consumes will assist in preventing constipation. Older individuals sometimes drink less fluid to reduce urinary frequency and incontinence. Others will simply forget to drink unless the caregiver is attuned to this need. Water is definitely needed throughout the day. Some fruit juices are also good and offer nutritional value. Coffee and tea should not be used as substitutes for water because these liquids tend to act as diuretics and thus decrease body fluid. Sometimes a cup of hot liquid, such as coffee or prune juice, taken a few minutes before toileting can help to stimulate bowel action. If activity, fluids, and fiber are given a 2- to 4-week trial and fail to regulate bowel function, laxatives may be needed. This decision should always be discussed with the patient's physician because drug interactions may occur with some laxative preparations.

Before the use of laxatives is initiated, valid indication for the laxative should always be determined. Laxatives can lead to serious complications, such as fecal incontinence, intestinal obstruction, mental disturbances, and urinary retention. Therefore appropriate use must be followed, and continuing assessment of the patient's need for the laxative must be done. Laxatives are generally grouped into five categories: bulk-forming, osmotic (saline), surfactant (wetting agents), contact (stimulant/irritant), and lubricant (emollient). The action of each varies, and the laxative chosen should be based on the patient's needs.

Bulk-forming laxatives are basically fiber-containing mixtures (bran, methylcellulose, psyllium hydrophilic mucilloid). These agents act by retaining water in the intestine so that the fecal mass remains large and soft. This type of laxative is traditionally tried first because it tends to restore bowel function in the most natural manner. The effects of bulk-forming agents can be realized within 24 hours or may take as long as 3 days. One important factor is the need for additional fluids with these agents to prevent dehydration and obstruction. Each dose should be administered with at least 8 ounces of water. The side effects of bulk-forming laxatives include gaseousness and abdominal fullness and discomfort. Patients with diabetes must be aware that some of these preparations contain large amounts of dextrose.

Osmotic laxatives act by attracting water into the intestine to soften the fecal mass. These agents work faster than bulk-forming agents, taking only 2 to 6 hours, but they have more serious side effects. Since these agents are often salts of magnesium, sulfate, or phosphorus, patients with impaired kidney function may not be able to clear the body of the extra salt load. Also, the serum levels of magnesium and phosphate ions may rise. Lactulose is an osmotic agent that has been used a great deal. However, because it contains digestible sugars, lactulose must be used with caution in patients with diabetes. Lactulose can also cause cramping, diarrhea, and electrolyte imbalance if taken at higher than recommended dosages. As with bulk-forming agents, additional water needs to be provided to the patient to prevent possible dehydration.

Surfactant or wetting agents are recommended for patients who have normal bowel tone but hard, dry stools. These agents react with the fecal mass, allowing it to be penetrated by water and fat. Dioctyl sulfosuccinates make up this category of laxatives. These agents have a relatively quick action, within 6 to 8 hours, and are recommended for temporary use. When used on a long-term basis, they do not appear to have much effect on preventing constipation. Therefore, after the immediate problem of hard, dry stool has been corrected, the patient should be given bulk-forming agents for long-term management.

Contact, or stimulant, laxatives are recommended only for temporary relief of constipation or for bowel cleansing before a procedure. These agents act directly on the intestinal mucosa to increase activity and motility, thereby stimulating the propulsion of the fecal mass. Severe cramping and diarrhea can result, and some agents remain in the system for several days, causing continued action. Chronic use of this type of laxative can lead to serious problems, such as intestinal mucosal damage, fluid and electrolyte disturbances, and malabsorption. The tablet form of these laxatives should not be crushed or chewed because this practice causes irritation of the stomach mucosa.

Lubricants or emollients, such as mineral oil, act by coating the fecal mass to prevent loss of water and facilitate passage of the mass through the colon. Mineral oil can interfere with the absorption of vitamins A, D, K, and E. In patients with swallowing difficulty, aspiration of mineral oil can lead to lipid pneumonia, a very serious complication. Large doses of mineral oil may leak through the anal sphincter and cause soiling of the patient's clothes and bed linens. Enemas should be used for only the most difficult cases of constipation, and they should be provided only by persons educated in proper administration. Fluid and electrolyte imbalance and perforation of the colon have been associated with the incorrect administration of enemas.

In the debilitated, bed-bound patient, a bowel movement can sometimes be produced by lightly massaging the lower abdomen. If this method is unsuccessful, a glycerine suppository can be used to stimulate a bowel movement. Sometimes just digitally stimulating the anal sphincter can produce a bowel movement. This type of patient does not need to have a bowel movement every day, but, as mentioned previously, should not go longer than 3 days without bowel evacuation. If a patient begins to have small, diarrhetic stools, leakage of small amounts of feces, or abdominal cramping and pain, he should be checked for a fecal impaction, which often produces these symptoms. A laxative or an enema will help to remove the impaction. With any patient, the frequency of bowel movements should be monitored to avoid impaction, and the quantity and characteristics of the stool should be noted.

OTHER HYGIENIC TASKS

Eventually the patient will need help with other tasks related to overall hygiene. Fingernails and toenails should be trimmed and filed on a regular basis. They should be kept short to prevent accidental scratching. Toenails should be trimmed straight across, whereas fingernails should be rounded at the ends. An opportune time to perform nail care is after the bath since the nails are generally softer and easier to manicure at that time. The nails should be cleaned regularly to remove dirt, feces, oils, and dead skin, which accumulate under the nail. In the patient whose fingers are severely contracted, the nails must be kept short to prevent them from cutting into the palm of the hand. Also, the patient must have his hands thoroughly washed and dried in the palm and between the fingers to remove dirt and dead skin. If this step is not performed, the area under the contracted fingers will quickly become macerated and possibly infected.

The patient's ears should not be neglected. The outside part of the ear can be cleansed easily with a washcloth wrapped over a finger. Cotton swabs can be used, but the tip should always be visible (i.e., the ear canal should not be entered). Improper use of swabs serves only to push wax farther into the ear. The ears should be inspected periodically to detect the buildup of hard packed wax. Such buildup occurs commonly in the older person and can lead to a substantial hearing loss. This problem can be easily corrected by having the ear canal irrigated by a health professional to remove the impacted wax.

Shaving is another task that requires safety and supervision. Once the patient's coordination and judgment have become impaired, an electric razor can be used to keep the patient independent and safe while performing this activity. If an electric razor is used, shaving should be supervised to ensure that electrical safety practices are followed (e.g., not shaving with water in the sink and correct plugging/unplugging of the cord). Rechargeable battery–operated razors can be used to avoid such hazards. Beards and mustaches should never be shaved by a health care professional unless the family has been consulted first. Most of the time, a beard or mustache can be left, but it needs to be kept short, neat, and regularly cleaned. Because food particles often become embedded in a beard or mustache, the area should be thoroughly cleansed after each meal. Applying a small amount of after-shave lotion can help the patient feel good about himself.

For female patients, cream depilatories can be used on legs and underarms. However, a skin patch test should be performed before the product is used to note any sensitivity to it. Female patients who have previously worn makeup should be encouraged to continue the practice because doing so helps their self-esteem. The patient should be supervised when applying makeup so that it may be done appropriately. The makeup should be thoroughly removed each night to avoid skin problems. Finally, many women in this age group have had a lifelong habit of having their hair professionally cut and styled. All efforts should be made to continue this practice as long as possible since this routine will make the patient feel better about herself. Once the patient can no longer visit the hair salon, arrangements can be made to have someone come to the nursing home once a week to style the patient's hair. Health care personnel should strive to style the patient's hair each day in the patient's usual fashion.

Hygienic practices may seem simple and well ingrained in everyone. Yet each task requires decision-making, judgment, memory, and coordination. Since each of these abilities is impaired in the patient with Alzheimer's disease, the caregiver must continually assess the patient's abilities and provide guidance and assistance as needed. Helping the patient to complete each task with the least amount of assistance helps to improve his self-esteem and body image and to keep him functioning longer.

TERMINAL CARE

As the patient progresses through the stages of Alzheimer's disease, he becomes more and more incapacitated and eventually requires total care, since he is unable to perform any task for himself. Difficulty with swallowing and loss of speech and movement compound the problems already discussed and set the stage for serious complications such as pneumonia and pressure sores. It is at this stage that institutionalization often occurs. Although patients in the last stage of Alzheimer's disease can be cared for at home (as many are), the physical and emotional needs of the patient are often greater than the family alone can meet. Helping the family to find assistance in their caregiving activities is one option. Placing the patient in a nursing home is another, but this decision can be particularly difficult for the family. Feelings of helplessness and guilt accompany the decision to institutionalize the patient, but many families also recognize the need for assistance and relief from caregiving. The family must weigh the toll of 24-hour caregiving against its own physical and emotional well-being. Whatever the decision and wherever terminal care is provided, the care must be based on the particular needs and problems of the patient. Astute observation and assessment are required because the patient can no longer verbally communicate his needs. The terminal stage of Alzheimer's disease must be confronted and the reality of death must be faced so that the patient can be assisted toward a peaceful and dignified death.

A patient in the terminal stage of Alzheimer's disease is usually bedridden and has developed a rigid body posture. Therefore moving him presents a problem. Although the patient's needs related to daily hygienic care remain much the same, the method of meeting these needs changes. The caregivers must perform all tasks for the patient. Because the patient has usually lost his ability to communicate, it becomes important to anticipate his needs and recognize any subtle changes in body language. Caregivers must continue to talk with the patient, and this dialogue must be supplemented with the comfort of touch. The patient should be approached in a calm manner, and explanations of care should be provided to avoid the possibility of frightening him. In addition, some special concerns must be addressed, including skin care, mobility, nutrition, and resuscitative and supportive measures.

SKIN CARE

The patient in the end stage of Alzheimer's disease has specific skin care needs. Because he is usually bedridden, movement is very limited and relief of pressure becomes problematic. Because of aging and impaired nutrition, the patient's skin is very thin and fragile. Loss of subcutaneous fat tissue places bony prominences such as the heels, elbows, sacrum, and hips at risk for breakdown. Therefore special attention must be given to protecting the skin from breakdown. Prevention is the key because once breakdown has occurred, it is extremely difficult and costly to heal.

The immobile, bedridden patient must be turned regularly, at least every 2 hours. Turning relieves pressure on bony areas and allows the return of circulation to the tissues. Side-lying, prone, and dorsal recumbent positions all can be used if the patient tolerates them. The body should always be kept in good alignment, and the dependent areas should be supported with pillows or props.

In the side-lying position, the legs should be bent at the hips and knees and pulled forward to keep the patient from rolling over. A pillow can be placed behind the patient's back to provide additional support. The ankles and knees should have pillows or padding placed between them to prevent them from pressing against each other. When the patient is placed on his back, a small pillow or towel roll should be placed under the lower legs to elevate the heels from the mattress. In the prone position, a small pillow should be placed at the lower abdomen to relieve pressure on the back and the chest wall. With each position, the patient needs to be assessed in regard to the effects of the position on respiration. When the patient is turned, care must be taken to avoid dragging the patient across the bed. Shearing forces can easily damage the skin and lead to tissue breakdown.

The skin, especially the skin surfaces that are against the bed, must be kept clean and dry. Any effects of incontinence should be taken care of as soon as possible, and clean, dry sheets should be placed on the bed. Lotions can be applied to the skin to help prevent moisture loss. Heavier ointments can be used for the perineal area to protect the skin from the irritation of urine and feces. Linens need to be kept free of wrinkles and crumbs of food and other objects. If the patient has a catheter, care must be taken to avoid having the patient lie on the tubing. Pressure-relief devices such as foam mattresses, water mattresses, and sheepskin pads are also recommended for the bedridden patient. These devices help to distribute the patient's weight over a greater area. Adequate nutrition and fluid intake are also needed to keep the skin in good condition.

The skin should be assessed daily, and all bony prominences should be examined at each turning. If the redness over a bony area persists longer than 1 hour after relief of the pressure, the patient should not be placed back on that area until the redness has disappeared. Particular attention should be given to monitoring less conspicuous areas, such as the ears, the back of the head, and the shoulders. Finally, it may be advisable to pad the bedrails to prevent blunt injury to the patient during turning or seizure activity.

MOBILITY

As Alzheimer's disease progresses, the patient tends to experience increasing muscular rigidity. This rigidity produces stiffening of extremities and sometimes joint contractures. If left untreated, the patient could become completely immobile, which would compound the problems of daily care. Range of motion exercises are an extremely important part of daily care of the patient. Each joint and extremity should be put through its normal motions to keep it flexible. Bathing activities are an ideal time to perform range of motion. These exercises, if performed twice a day, can help combat progressive rigidity and stiffening.

With the aging process and the decreasing activity level of advanced Alzheimer's disease, the bones tend to become more fragile and are much more likely to break. Care must be taken to prevent the patient from falling out of bed. When turning the patient, it is important to have adequate help to avoid pulling on an extremity or roughly handling the patient.

The musculature of the chest wall also becomes stiffer, making breathing more difficult. Elevating the head of the bed 30 to 45 degrees will help the patient to expand the chest wall and lower the diaphragm, thus allowing fuller ventilation. If the patient does not have a hospital bed, he can be propped up with pillows or wedges. Because of inactivity and shallower respirations, secretions will begin to pool in the bases of the lungs. Turning the patient becomes vitally important to keep the secretions mobile. The patient should be encouraged to breathe deeply and to cough several times each day. If the patient has lost the ability to cough effectively, suctioning equipment may be needed to help keep the airways clear. This equipment can be purchased or rented from medical equipment suppliers.

NUTRITION

Maintaining adequate nutritional intake in the patient with end-stage Alzheimer's disease is a challenging task. Despite the best efforts of caregivers, most patients lose weight in the terminal stage. There are several reasons for the eating difficulties that these patients experience. The profound memory loss interferes with the recognition of food, the need to eat, and the mechanics of eating. Changes in level of arousal may interfere with the patient's responding to the signals of hunger. The patient may experience a return of reflex actions (e.g., sucking, biting, and tonic neck reflexes) that interfere with eating. Some patients may also resist attempts at being fed by the caregiver. As damage to the brain continues, chewing and swallowing become impaired, leading to a high risk for aspiration. In this stage of the disease, the patient becomes totally dependent on his caregivers for nutrition.

Choosing foods of the highest nutritional value that supply many calories becomes very important because the quantity of food and fluid that the patient consumes is usually reduced. Many nutritional supplements are available to increase the patient's intake. These supplements, when mixed with ice cream, make a palatable and nutritious snack. Providing foods that can be chewed and swallowed easily is also important. Caregivers can prepare meals that include ground meats and soft foods, or the food can be placed in a blender and pureed. Baby food can also be used, but it tends to be less palatable and is more costly.

Often patients will experience choking on thin liquids such as water and juices. However, both are still needed to maintain the patient's hydration. Many of the patient's favorite liquids (e.g., coffee, water, milk, juice) can be thickened with cornstarch or unflavored gelatin to add enough substance to the fluid to make it easier to swallow. Gelatin dessert and ice pops also can be given to provide the needed amounts of water.

In this stage of the disease, a tremendous amount of time is needed to feed a patient. It may take 1 to 2 hours just to get the patient to complete one meal. This situation is problematic in nursing homes where a caregiver may have four or five patients to feed. Plenty of time for chewing and swallowing each mouthful of food is required.

Verbal cues from the caregiver may also be needed. Sometime patients will hold the food in their mouths and not swallow. Swa] lowing can sometimes be stimulated by instructing the patient t swallow or by gently stroking his throat. Care must also be taken nc to place too much food in the patient's mouth at one time. Famil members provide valuable and much needed assistance to the nur: ing home staff when they come in to feed their loved one.

As swallowing becomes affected by the disease, correct positior ing for eating is extremely important. The patient needs to be place in an upright, sitting position. The head of the bed should be elevate to the highest position tolerated by the patient. Pillows and prop can be used to help the patient maintain this position. The patien should remain sitting upright for approximately 30 minutes after th meal has been completed, and the mouth should be checked an cleansed of any remaining food. Because of the danger of aspiratio during eating, all caregivers, both family and health professional: need to know how to perform the Heimlich maneuver. Equipment fo suctioning the mouth and upper airway should also be available a the patient's bedside.

If the patient has a feeding tube, especially a nasogastric tube, it i imperative to keep the head of the bed elevated at least 30 degree: Patients with a feeding tube receive the feeding by either bolus o continuous drip. If the patient receives bolus feedings, the head of th bed should remain elevated for 30 minutes to 1 hour after the feeding However, if the patient is receiving continuous feeding, the head of th bed should remain elevated at all times since the stomach is neve empty. Placement of the tube must also be checked periodically. Fo bolus feedings, the tube can be checked just before each feeding. Fo continuous drip feedings, tube placement should be checked every hours; the amount of residual feeding in the stomach also should b noted at this time. Patients receiving either type of feeding requir additional water to maintain adequate hydration. A 150 ml bolus c water can be given four to six times in a 24-hour period. The wate should not be added to the feeding in continuous drip feedings becaus the amount of calories the patient receives would then be reducec Rather, the feeding should be momentarily interrupted, and the wate should be given as a bolus.

RESUSCITATIVE AND SUPPORTIVE MEASURES

As the patient enters the end stage of the disease, family member are confronted with very difficult decisions. Among these are th placement of feeding tubes to maintain nutrition, resuscitation in the event of cardiopulmonary arrest, and the aggressive treatment of infections. These issues need to be discussed before the onset of any crisis situation. Family members should be encouraged to openly discuss their desires and wishes among themselves. On admission to any health care facility that accepts Medicare/Medicaid, health care personnel are now required by law to inquire about the existence of advanced directives that the patient may have signed. This requirement has opened the door for questions, discussion, and decisions on these issues. Nursing personnel, in particular, prefer to have a decision on these issues as soon as possible in the event that it is needed in the middle of the night, when neither the physician or a family member is present. Whatever decisions the family makes, health care professionals need to be supportive of their decisions. If a health care professional feels at odds with the family's decision, the professional needs to find someone else who can work with the patient and the family in her place.

Supportive nursing measures for the patient include attending to all his daily needs. In addition, the patient may require comfort measures such as oxygen and pain medications. When the patient receives oxygen, particular attention must be given to providing good oral hygiene since the oxygen has a drying effect on the oral tissues. Even if the patient is not receiving oxygen, good oral hygiene is needed if the patient is breathing through his mouth. The oral cavity should be swabbed every few hours with water or another moisturizer. The caregiver needs to inspect the face and ears of the patient on a daily basis to make sure that the nasal cannula, oxygen mask, or elastic straps are not irritating the skin or causing pressure breakdown. The oral cavity and upper airway will most likely require suctioning whenever there is a buildup of secretions since most patients no longer can swallow.

The patient needs to be assessed frequently for any signs of discomfort or pain. Such assessment takes astute observation and an understanding of how the patient has manifested pain in the past. Correct positioning of the patient may be all that is necessary to provide comfort. If pain medication has been prescribed for the patient, the caregiver must evaluate how well the medication relieves the pain. If it does not appear to comfort the patient, the caregiver should discuss the situation with the physician.

The family will also need the support of health care personnel during this final stage. Allowing the family to visit the patient and to participate in the patient's care can help them to feel a part of the patient's life. Encouraging the family members to talk with the patient and relive precious times will help the family and the patient through this difficult time. Referrals to chaplains, psychologists, or social work counselors may also aid the family in resolving any problems. Many emotions—anger, guilt, and despair—must be dealt with as the patient's death nears. The professional caregiver must be sensitive to the patient's needs and the family's wishes while helping the patient to have a dignified death and the family to accept the passing of their loved one.

BIBLIOGRAPHY

Beverley L, Travis I: Constipation: proposed natural laxative mixtures, *J Gerontol Nurs* 18(10):5-12, 1992.

Burd C and others: Skin problems: epidemiology of pressure ulcers in a skilled nursing facility, *J Gerontol Nurs* 18(9):29-39, 1992.

Burgener S, Barton D: Nursing care of cognitively impaired, institutionalized elderly, *J Gerontol Nurs* 17(4):37-43, 1991.

Donahue P: When it's hard to swallow: feeding techniques for dysphagia management, *J Gerontol Nurs* 16(4):6-9, 1990.

Heacock P and others: Caring for the cognitively impaired: reconceptualizing disability and rehabilitation, *J Gerontol Nurs* 17(3):22-26, 1991.

Kelley LS, Mobily PR: Impaired skin integrity, *J Gerontol Nurs* 17(9):24-29, 1991.

Lee VK: Language changes and Alzheimer's disease: a literature review, *J Gerontol Nurs* 17(1):16-20, 1991.

Marzinski LR: The tragedy of dementia: clinically assessing pain in the confused, nonverbal elderly, *J Gerontol Nurs* 17(6):25-27, 1991.

Monicken D: Immobility and functional mobility in the elderly. In Chenitz WC, Stone JT, Salisbury SA, editors: *Clinical gerontological nursing: a guide to advanced practice*, Philadelphia, 1991, WB Saunders.

Norberg A, Athlin E: Eating problems in severely demented patients, *Nurs Clin North Am* 24(3):781-787, 1989.

Norman L: Terminal care of patients with Alzheimer's disease. In Hamdy RC and others, editors: *Alzheimer's disease: a handbook for caregivers*, St Louis, 1990, Mosby–Year Book.

Robinson A, Spencer B, White L: *Understanding difficult behaviors*, Ann Arbor, Mich, 1989, Geriatric Education Center of Michigan.

Sand BJ, Yeaworth RC, McCabe BW: Alzheimer's disease: special care units in long-term care facilities, *J Gerontol Nurs* 18(3):28-34, 1992.

Stone JT: Managing bowel function. In Chenitz WC, Stone JT, Salisbury SA, editors: *Clinical gerontological nursing: a guide to advanced practice*, Philadelphia, 1991, WB Saunders.

Tanner F, Shaw S, editors: *Caring: a family guide to managing the Alzheimer's patient at home*, New York, 1985, New York City Alzheimer's Resource Center.

Yakabowich M: Prescribe with care: the role of laxatives in the treatment of constipation, *J Gerontol Nurs* 16(7):4-11, 1990.

20
Programming for activity

James M. Turnbull and Elizabeth A. Turnbull

Day care programs for patients with Alzheimer's disease offer much more than respite for the caregivers, as valuable as that service may be. A well-structured program provides a mechanism for the design and coordination of plans between health care providers and caregivers. Most important, it offers an opportunity for patients to maintain a sense of community and self-worth in the face of increasing isolation and an inevitable decline in abilities.

Creating day care programs for patients diagnosed with Alzheimer's disease is a simple, though multifaceted, task. Most conventional day care centers for the elderly lack important elements that are essential for patients with this disease. The characteristics of these patients impose requirements for staffing and facilities that are beyond the level that most day care centers routinely offer. The unexpected and often disruptive behavior of patients, the inability to complete tasks without step-by-step instruction, and the tendency to wander all must be accommodated.

An effective program is based on a careful evaluation of each individual patient's strengths and needs. The lack of familiarity that accompanies memory loss can lead to constant insecurity and social impotence. The strengths that patients retain are their only links with productive life. Through careful planning and guidance, these strengths may be called on, returning meaning and productivity to a life of seeming chaos.

PATIENT NEEDS

Alzheimer's disease often leaves a patient in a state of conflict, wanting to be active and involved while limited in the ability to function. The patient may react with irritability and restlessness, demonstrated in

265

social withdrawal, a resistance to anything new, and a disinterest in ongoing activities. An effective program attempts to establish alternate modes of functioning that minimize this conflict.

The hierarchy of needs developed by Abraham Maslow provides a useful framework for analyzing patient needs. The basic needs include the physiological ones, such as thirst, hunger, shelter, and warmth. Security becomes the focus when these basic needs have been met. When the need for security has been satisfied, psychosocial needs, such as self esteem, autonomy, identity, control, and meaningful communication with others, emerge. Meeting the security and psychosocial needs is of paramount importance in effective program planning for patients with Alzheimer's disease.

A sense of security or safety is essential. The symptoms of Alzheimer's disease make the patient's world frighteningly unpredictable. A predictable, calm, and nonthreatening environment can relieve the insecurities that memory loss and perceptual impairments create, enabling the patient to make full use of the abilities that he has retained.

Nowhere is the devastation of Alzheimer's disease more profound than on a patient's identity. The deficits caused by the symptoms of Alzheimer's disease can be reversed by using the patient's remaining abilities. Tasks that the patient can still accomplish, such as drying dishes or folding clothes, can help to reinforce his feelings of control and autonomy. Being included as a member of a group can deter the effects of Alzheimer's disease that often lead to social isolation and low self-esteem. These needs must be recognized in program planning. Light chores, grooming, and group activities are simple activities that can contribute to meeting both psychosocial and security needs.

PATIENT STRENGTHS

Although the disabilities of patients with Alzheimer's disease must be considered, programs should capitalize on their functional abilities, that is, their strengths and retained abilities, particularly emotional awareness, remote memory, primary sensory and motor functions, perseveration, and retention of well-learned or habitual tasks.

Pleasant emotions can be promoted through activities such as interaction with animals or babies, group sharing sessions, and reminiscence sessions. Remote memory, or recollection of one's distant past, can provide pleasure by creating a link with more stable times, reaffirming the patient's self-esteem. Such life-review activities can help to create a balance between the patient's current abilities and past accomplishments. Music and fragrance activities are particularly effective in helping the patient recall sensory memories when abstract memory has been lost. Negative emotions such as frustration and anger can be used in vigorous physical activities. When a patient with Alzheimer's disease displays inappropriate emotional reactions, staff often tend to discount that person's feelings and emotions. Instead, these emotions should be acknowledged, validated, and used in the patient's behalf.

Since most primary motor and sensory functions are left intact in Alzheimer's disease, these functions can be used productively within an effective program. If perceptual problems are taken into consideration, retained strengths such as muscular control, dexterity, and strength can enable the patient to accomplish tasks and successfully engage the day care environment. Rhythm also appears to be a very effective mode of sensory stimulation. Use of these strengths is an effective antidote to inactivity and isolation.

Perseveration, the tendency to repeat a motion repeatedly until interrupted, can be an asset in performing certain tasks. The ability to repeat one simple step often eliminates the frustration of forgetting the next step. Activities that require repetitive motions, such as raking leaves or vacuuming, are well suited to this disturbance.

Habitual and well-learned activities, those that have been learned and practiced repeatedly throughout a person's life, are often retained, at least in part. Activities that incorporate these routines can be especially reinforcing because of the familiarity of the behavior and the self-confidence that performing without constant instruction imparts. Problems may occur when an inappropriate routine is evoked or when a distraction interrupts the flow of activity during performance.

PROGRAM DESIGN

The physical environment, staffing, and selection of program activities, scheduling, and pacing of program activities should contribute to making the patient feel as productive, autonomous, and secure as possible.

Physical Environment

The perceptual difficulties experienced by patients with Alzheim er's disease require an effort to make the environment predictable and consistent in order to avoid confusion. For example, floors and wall should be perceptually distinct from each other (e.g., different colors and should be clear of any markings that may be perceived as obsta cles. Furniture should be distinct, have clear edges, and be placed outside high traffic areas, where it might become an obstacle. The space should be divided into specific permanent activity areas (e.g one for meetings and another for crafts). The permanent arrangemen helps the patient feel more secure and capable of getting around Restrooms should be clearly marked as "Men" and "Women" to avoid confusion. Well-marked exits are very important so that patients de not have a sense of being trapped, but the exit should be monitored so that a patient cannot wander off unattended. Gardens and walking areas can be used by patients to safely work off their restlessness Orientation to time and place can be effectively achieved by using clocks, calendars, and decorations appropriate to current season and holidays.

The location of the program in a nonmedical building tends to lessen feelings of anxiety on the part of patients. A large room located within a community facility, with an adjoining restroom and coat room, and having activity areas clearly segregated by furniture group ings is an ideal setting for a day care program.

Staffing

Zgola has recommended that two professional staff member (e.g., nurse, physical therapist, or occupational therapist and/or rec reation therapist) and four volunteers be provided for every seven to eight patients. Although the number may vary from activity to activ ity, this amount suffices for most activities. The initiation period of an activity demands a one-to-one ratio that can be slowly altered to ac commodate the patient's reactions and abilities. Highly structured activities such as group discussion and meal preparation may require fewer staff (two or three staff to eight patients). Having too many staff members for activities in which some staff are uninvolved tends to overwhelm patients and reduce independent activity. It is best for the uninvolved staff to withdraw but remain available in case assistance is needed.

ACTIVITIES

Patients with Alzheimer's disease are capable of performing a variety of activities that fulfill their need to be active. These activities include exercise and other gross motor activities, grooming, socializing, meal preparation, housework, crafts, light work, and special events (see box on pp. 270 and 271).

Exercise helps to maintain muscular strength, joint dexterity, and body awareness. It also provides a gentle cardiopulmonary workout and can be utilized to avoid the restlessness or agitation that a surplus of physical energy can cause. Simple games such as beanbag toss, shuffleboard, and bowling, which have an obvious objective and are generally considered adult games, are most acceptable. More complex games such as croquet can be used by simplifying the goal (e.g., hitting the ball the farthest).

Grooming activities help to build self-esteem. Initiation and assistance are often required. Staff members who assist can identify helpful techniques that can be shared with caregivers for use at home. Staff may also be aware of a physical problem that the patient "forgets" to mention but may lead to further complications if left untreated.

Socialization can be promoted in many activities. During the orientation held at the beginning of the day, patients should be encouraged to contribute to discussions and to planning the day's activities. Coffee and tea breaks offer the opportunity for self-directed interactions that help maintain good social skills. A scheduled "wind-down" at the end of the day helps the patient to recall his accomplishments during the day's events. Communication is difficult for many patients with Alzheimer's disease and should be facilitated by program staff. Patients need to feel safe and accepted regardless of their communication skills. Since memory loss can inhibit the recollection of material, direct questions targeted at specific information should be avoided unless it is certain that the patient can answer them. The interactions that develop among the patients within the program are probably the single most valuable benefit of participation in a day care program.

Tasks at which the patient was once proficient offer special opportunities for participation. Washing and drying dishes, dusting, sweeping, chopping vegetables, or mixing prepared ingredients can give a patient the opportunity to be useful and to accept gratitude. Activities involving many steps need to be broken into several simple steps so that the patient can accomplish the task and proceed to the

SAMPLE ACTIVITIES

Orientation

Welcome, introduce new members
Discuss/plan daily activities

Household Chores

Dust, sweep, polish, mop
Sort, fold, hang laundry
Wash and dry dishes
Water and pot plants
Rake leaves, vacuum
Organize drawers and closets

Grooming and Hygiene

Dress
Brush teeth/dentures
Comb hair, wash face, apply makeup
Polish shoes

Meal Preparation

Chop, peel, clean vegetables and fruits
Cut or shape cookies
Stir, knead, mix
Grate cheese or vegetables
Set table

Crafts

Knitting, crocheting, embroidery, making pompom animals
Dried flower cards, nature plaques, refrigerator magnets
Woodworking, carving, wreaths
Stenciled notes, Christmas decorations, bookmarks

Work-Oriented Activities

Staple papers, fold newsletters
Stuff/stamp envelopes
Punch holes

Special Events

Birthday and holiday parties
Outings to parks, picnics, museums
Bus trip, river cruise
Demonstrations of fashion, makeup, decorating

Gross Motor Activities

Exercise, walking, dancing
Floor games: beanbag toss, ring toss, shuffleboard, bowling

Sample Activities—cont'd

Social Activities

  Coffee or tea break
  Table games, bingo, checkers, dominoes
  Sing-along, storytelling
  Guided reminiscence

Sensory Activities

  Perfumes, makeup
  Music, art, picture books
  Animals, children, touching objects (fur, fabric scraps, stones)
  Rocking chair
  Massage
  Food tasting (hors d'oeuvres, finger foods)

Modified from Zgola JM: *Doing things: a guide to programming activities for persons with Alzheimer's disease and related disorders,* Baltimore, 1987, Johns Hopkins University Press.

next step with confidence. Meal preparation is most successful when recipes have assembly-line organization and do not require precise proportions of ingredients.

Crafts can be satisfying if they are modified to accommodate the limited abilities of patients with Alzheimer's disease. Work-oriented activities, such as stapling papers, stuffing envelopes, or folding newsletters, are preferred by those who are not interested in housekeeping or crafts.

Special activities associated with the holidays offer the opportunity to celebrate and to enjoy decorating, food preparation, and sing-alongs. These celebrations should be brief in order to avoid overstimulation and overtiring. Field trips to local points of interest are enjoyable if large crowds and bad weather are avoided. Films are not recommended because the perceptual changes that characterize Alzheimer's disease make films difficult to follow.

Selection of Activities

The plan for the individual patient should be based on a comprehensive evaluation that includes information from a variety of sources, including physical and neurological examinations, neuropsychological testing, and psychiatric consultation. A social history that includes an evaluation of the patient's home environment and support systems helps staff and caregivers to translate program gains to the home setting. The individual plan must be grounded in an accurat assessment of the individual's needs, abilities, and limitations.

Functional Evaluation

Functional evaluation assesses the patient's level of functionin in terms of basic senses and functions, cognitive and behavioral skill interpersonal relations, self-care skills, and mobility. A useful fram work for functional evaluation, developed by Zgola, includes th seven w's:

What can the patient do?

What does the patient do?

In what way does the patient do it?

Which part of the task is the patient unable to do?

Why is the patient unable to do it?

Where does the patient perform best?

When does the patient perform best?

Ongoing evaluation is essential. Staff and caregivers can assis each other by sharing perceived problems and highlighting an changes that need to be considered. A notebook containing the day plan and notes on accomplishments (Table 20-1) is sent to and fror the day care program and home and serves as a means of commun cation between family members and staff on matters of importanc ensuring that the therapeutic program can be updated as the patient needs dictate.

Appropriate activities are selected, graded according to difficult and analyzed in regard to each individual's capabilities and needs. A activity should be a voluntary effort. It is essential that the patier understand the activity's purpose and perceive the activity as mear ingful and achievable. In addition, it is necessary for the intellectua physical, and perceptual demands of an activity to be achievabl given the abilities of the patient.

Grading an activity permits variation of the degree of involve ment of each patient, allowing a decrease or increase of the activity demands to match each individual's abilities. If the activity is bakin cookies, for example, one patient might be able to mix the ingredient (a fairly high grade) and another patient could successfully partici pate at a lower grade by holding the cookie sheet while the cookies ar portioned for baking. The second patient is able to participate suc cessfully even though the grade of activity is lower. Activities wit several steps are preferable since individuals can work together, a various levels, to complete an activity.

Table 20-1 Sample schedule/communication sheet*

Time	Type of Activity	Options
10:00 AM	Orientation	Make coffee and discuss plans for day
10:30 AM	Housekeeping	Dust, vacuum, or fold clothes
		Note: Needs help getting started, but great at vacuuming
11:00 AM	Prepare lunch	Soup, sandwiches, or cake
11:45 AM	Lunch	*Note:* Ate well but refused soup
12:15 PM	Cleanup	Clear table, wash or dry dishes
12:45 PM	Craft	Bookmark or wreath

Modified from Zgola JM: *Doing things: a guide to programming activities for persons with Alzheimer's disease and related disorders*, Baltimore, 1987, Johns Hopkins University Press.
*By jotting notes in the margin, staff can communicate with the patient's caregivers. Sharing this record helps keep them in touch and communicates the most effective activities, difficulties encountered, and suggestions or concerns.

Analyzing activities in terms of their task demands also aids in matching abilities to the individual's functional levels. Analysis can be accomplished by asking the following questions:
1. What physical abilities (dexterity, strength, flexibility, coordination) are necessary to complete this activity successfully?
2. What sensory abilities (sight, smell, hearing, feeling, balance) are required?
3. What perceptual processes (spatial relations, eye-hand coordination, visual activity) are required?
4. What cognitive functions (memory, organization, problem-solving, communication, and attention) are required?

By also analyzing an activity in terms of its potential to contribute to the patient's psychosocial needs (e.g., identity, autonomy, inclusion), the program design can ensure both productivity and social interaction in even patients with the greatest disability.

Highly repetitive activities are often very successful. They create a sense of continuity and competence through the absence of worry about the "next step." Activities that have a wide range of successful outcomes are effective in avoiding failures. The best are those that give the patient a sense of accomplishment and social interaction.

Scheduling

Scheduling of activities should take into account the patient's fluctuating energy levels and their effects on the patient's predictability and behavior. The patient's comfort and security are often acutely affected by these changes. Since energy levels tend to be highest at the beginning of the day, it is most effective to schedule the most demanding activities in the morning.

The duration of an activity is also important. Simple, nondemanding activities, such as grooming, games, singing, or simple crafts, are enjoyed for longer periods since repetitive patterns can be established after the sometimes difficult initiation phase has been overcome. Unstructured activities, such as free-flowing group discussions and free times, are usually tolerated for 30 minutes or less.

Provision of Guidance

Without the skillful guidance of the staff, patients would face numerous obstacles in attempting activities. The following aspects of supervision aid in avoiding or overcoming the problems that arrest activity in patients with Alzheimer's disease: (1) organization and presentation of the activity, (2) assistance in initiating the activity, and (3) guidance during task performance.

Organization of activities helps to overcome the ambiguities that can confuse patients. Staff and volunteers need to be aware of the activity's objectives, that is, the intended benefit for the patient. The goal might involve evoking a positive emotional reaction, for example, by making a heart magnet for a grandchild or by discussing memories recalled after regarding a family photograph. The actual completion of the task is only one objective.

Next, the activity must be broken down into logical, simple steps. This approach includes checking to be sure that the proper materials are at hand, reviewing the instructions, and eliminating possible sources of interference. Staff should have already completed portions of the task that the patient is no longer able to accomplish. Last, interference can destroy a patient's focus on an activity, and therefore a distraction-free area that is already set up for the activity is needed.

An orderly, careful initiation to the activity is necessary to combat the paralyzing fears and doubts that lead to inactivity in many patients with Alzheimer's disease. A simple, concise statement ("Let's go to the restroom") with a visual or concrete tactile clue (pointing toward the restroom) is more effective than an abstract statement ("Would you like to go to the bathroom?"), which may be unclear to the patient with Alzheimer's disease. Simple instructions that help in beginning the task, such as "Hold this" or "Sit down," can be used to overcome inertia. Fortunately, patients often experience the pattern of action taking over once the activity has been initiated.

For craft activities, a brief explanation of what will be made, its uses, and a chance to see a sample will help in overcoming patients' fear of the unknown.

Making the purpose of the activity known (e.g., a snack for the group) helps to motivate the patient. Each step needs to be explained, and a demonstration of how it is accomplished should be given. The patient should not be expected to remember every step, and it should be made clear that the instructions will be repeated as often as needed. This reassurance eases some of the anxiety that keeps patients from attempting new activities. Observing the staff performing an activity is often effective as a first step toward further participation, such as holding or passing something. The grading of the activity serves as a good marker for the patient's ability and his potential level of involvement. If the patient resists an activity completely, it is best to stop and move on to another activity while noting problems that the patient might be experiencing, such as fatigue, or allowing a short break.

The successful outcome of an activity largely depends on the quality of guidance after initiation has been achieved. *Only as much guidance as is needed should be given.* Standing back yet being prepared to help if necessary allows patients to fully utilize their own initiative and ability.

The prior evaluation of the patient's abilities indicates whether verbal, visual, or manual guidance is preferable for a patient. Simple cues aid in reinforcing learning and establishing a pattern. Verbal cues should be concise and simple, and repetition using the same wording should be done to avoid confusion. Cues that involve touching the patient should occur within the patient's visual range since unexpected contact can be frightening to patients with Alzheimer's disease. It may be helpful to prepare the patient for contact by saying, "Let me show you how to hold your fingers." Force should never be used to push or pull the patient because this approach tends to elicit either total passivity or resistance. Gentle touching or firm pressure will comfort the patient and provide guidance. All guidance should be slowly withdrawn when it is no longer needed.

Coping with problems and failures in any task is an important aspect of guidance. Staff should be able to perceive problems and effectively help the patient to overcome them. A patient with Alzheimer's disease, for example, might be asked to bring the sugar to the mixing table and find that she cannot recognize the sugar. The inactivity that results might be easily overcome if the staff member restates the directions as, "Bring the white jar with the red lid." If a task seems to require too much guidance and too little patient participation, it is best to stop and evaluate the appropriateness of the activity or the level of participation. The activity may be attempted again with additional preparation or with the staff providing more assistance. Reducing the negative impact of failure is a critical aspect of guidance.

Effective reinforcement preserves dignity and capitalizes on the innate sense of accomplishment associated with the task. A simple nod or smile will let the patient with Alzheimer's disease know that he is doing well. The patient should not be distracted with too much praise. A simple "thank you" is preferable to overpraise since the sense of accomplishment is the most important reward.

Assistance with Mobility

An effective program offers accommodation for a patient's impairments in mobility. Seemingly simple actions, such as walking, sitting, or arising from a sitting position, become major challenges for the patient. Selecting a route that is free of obstacles or initiating movement may not be possible without assistance. Close observation can offer clues to the cause of difficulty and reveal effective ways to assist the patient.

The following suggestions are given for those assisting patients with difficulty in walking:
1. Lead the patient with your arm rather than by pushing or pulling.
2. Break long excursions into smaller segments.
3. Clearly state the destination.
4. Warn the patient of obstacles or irregularities in the surface.
5. Create a walking rhythm with your body while holding the patient's arm to help normalize his gait.
6. Rhythmic, single-word directions such as "step, cane; step, cane" help to coordinate movement when walkers or canes are used.

The following step-by-step procedure is effective in helping patients to rise from a seated position:
1. Have the patient move forward in the seat.

2. Position the patient's feet just under the rim of the chair or toilet, with heels raised slightly.
3. Instruct the patient to lean forward, put his weight over the feet, and push off with hands on the knees.
4. Offer an arm to the patient to help him balance, but do not pull; let the patient be in control.
5. If a walker is used, place the walker in front of the patient and guide it gently while he pulls up on it.

Sitting down can also be difficult, but the following techniques are helpful:

1. Clearly direct the patient to the chair or toilet.
2. Approach the chair or toilet from the front. Help or direct the patient to bend slightly and grasp the handrail or chair arm on the opposite side. A toilet chair with rails placed over the toilet is helpful for severely impaired patients.
3. Help the patient to retain grasp of the chair and direct him to take small, turning steps until the chair is directly behind him. Applying firm pressure to the patient's hip and nudging him in the right direction can be helpful.
4. Direct the patient to reach back for the other arm of the chair and lower himself.
5. A little downward pressure on the nape of the neck may help a patient who has trouble flexing the hips become seated.

Many maneuvers, such as getting in or out of an automobile, become even more difficult if the patient is given too much time to think about what to do. A casual distracting conversation with the patient while opening the door and gently positioning him to enter or exit can be very helpful. Established patterns tend to take over at this point. Only as much assistance as the patient needs should be given since too much assistance is as confusing as too little.

PATIENT REACTIONS

Alzheimer's disease leaves many patients with a constant feeling of insecurity and fear. These problems can persist for a long time since memory loss, perceptual difficulties, conceptual difficulties, and temporal distortions severely hamper a patient's ability to cope with change. Support for both patient and caregivers is essential during stressful periods, particularly the early stages of participation in the day care program.

Ideally, the introduction to the program is made in the patient's home by a staff member who will be a consistent contact for the patient and family. The home visit allows the staff member to effectively assess the patient's ability to benefit from the program. To be effective, the program must fit the needs of both the patient and the caretakers. The patient's anxieties and fears must be acknowledged, but the staff member should point out the positive and beneficial aspects of the program and invite the patient and caretakers for an observational visit. The patient may politely agree to attend and then voice negative feelings to the family. The family should be prepared for this reaction. They should be advised to keep a positive attitude, avoid confrontations while acknowledging negative feelings, and stress the benefits that the program offers to the patient.

Leaving home to go to the program for the first time is often a highly stressful event, even if the patient is enthusiastic about participating. Patients often become ambivalent and even resistant when the actual time to leave arrives. If possible, it is helpful for the staff member who made the initial contact to accompany the patient to the program. Having family members accompany the patient during the initial visit may also help to ease the insecurity and doubt that are caused by the novelty of the situation. The staff member, sensitive to the patient's needs and anxieties, may use an approach that varies from calm reassurance to firm direction, depending on the patient's reactions. Breaking the processes down into smaller steps is often helpful. For example, if the staff member escorts the patient on a walk during the initial home visit, leaving for the program on a later day is less unfamiliar and anxiety-provoking. Consistency in attendance is essential because the program is generally held only 1 day per week. If the routine of preparing for and attending the program is rigidly structured, the patient adjusts to the routine more easily.

Some patients may continue to experience episodes of distress and anxiety. Memory loss may cause the patient to forget that he will be picked up by a loved one at the end of the day. Frequent reassurances and distracting the agitated patient by involving him in a task can decrease this distress. Caregivers of such patients are encouraged to seek psychiatric consultation; day care programs may not be well suited for these patients' needs.

Sometimes an individual will routinely become distressed at a certain time of day. These episodes of agitation can often be identified as being related to the loss of an activity always scheduled at that time in the past (e.g., early afternoon episodes may be associated with the time when the children used to get picked up from school). An engaging activity similar to the former task may be effective in combating these episodes. Sometimes a 5-minute break, to allow a little respite, will help the patient return to the activity more calmly.

If paranoid delusions or hallucinations frighten the patient, creating a desperate wish to leave the program, staff should be alert to recognize the episode's beginning and to distract or reassure the patient before it turns into a crisis. Staff should confirm the patient's feelings of anxiety and distress and give support. Physical restraint and arguments tend to increase the patient's agitation and anxiety. Unobtrusive supervision while the patient walks outside or goes to another time-out area is usually most effective. Often two staff members, one playing the role of friend and the other being directive, can stage a "rescue" without being perceived as threatening. A patient who demonstrates such persistent behaviors should be referred for psychiatric intervention and should be assured that staff will not react negatively. To prevent disruption of the program, it is essential that episodes of anxiety and distress be dealt with promptly.

Occasionally, a patient is identified who does not react positively to any activities offered and for whom the program may not be suitable. Individuals who were previously independent, demanding, and somewhat asocial may, for example, find it difficult to function in group settings that foster dependence and enjoyment of leisure activities.

CAREGIVER REACTIONS

Caregivers often need assistance in adjusting to the day care program. Rather than enjoying the respite, they may experience feelings of guilt for subjecting their loved one to the stress of a new environment and may worry that he is suffering. Patients may anxiously relate negative messages that do not pinpoint a specific cause of distress but encompass the whole experience. Caregivers must be advised that these complaints are common and should not be a reason for early withdrawal from the program. Regular meetings between staff and caregivers can provide opportunities for caregivers to feel involved. It is essential that both staff and caregivers be secure in the knowledge that the patient is receiving benefits from the program.

Caregivers are essential in providing an accurate case history since the patient's own ability to retain information and make rational judgments may be limited. Caregivers and staff must make decisions that are based on accurate evaluations of the patient's ability and emotional state and the origins of negative emotions that are expressed. A case history should include the history of the manifestations of the symptoms, the reactions of the patient to these changes and to the diagnosis of Alzheimer's disease, an evaluation of the patient's progress in the program and at home, and a record of emotional reactions to various situations. This information aids the staff and caregivers in designing a program that benefits the patient both at home and at the program.

SUMMARY

The loss of familiar roles and tasks and the sense of self-worth that accompanies them is an inherent part of the decline facing the patient with Alzheimer's disease. Activity programs designed to accommodate both the needs and the strengths of the patient can replace the activities that have been lost, provide achievable roles, enhance self-esteem, and improve the quality of the life that remains.

In addition, a well-designed program is an effective antidote to the prevalent notion that, barring the discovery of a cure, there is little of value that can be done for the patient with Alzheimer's disease. This fatalistic attitude, an important source of burnout in staff and caregivers, cannot be maintained in the face of evidence that supporting the simple activities of daily living and social interaction is a powerful therapeutic tool.

BIBLIOGRAPHY

Cox KG: Milieu therapy, *Geriatr Nurs* 6(3):152-154, 1985.

Eisdorfer C, Cohen D: Management of the patient and family coping with dementing illness, *J Fam Pract* 12(5):831-837, 1981.

Haight BK, Burnside I: Reminiscence and life review: conducting the processes, *J Gerontol Nurs* 18(2):39-42, 1992.

Keyes B, Szpak G: Day care, *Postgrad Med* 73(4):245-250, 1983.

Tariot P and others: How memory fails: a theoretical model, *Geriatr Nurs* 6(3):144-147, 1985.

Zgola JM: *Doing things: a guide to programming activities for persons with Alzheimer's disease and related disorders*, Baltimore, 1987, Johns Hopkins University Press.

UNIT FOUR

SPECIAL ISSUES

21

Ethical issues

Sharon Turnbull

DECISIONS OF LIFE OR DEATH

Matthew J. is 62 years old and has a wife and three grown children. Two years ago he was diagnosed as having stage 1 Alzheimer's disease and was informed of this diagnosis. He has just recovered from a mild heart attack, and his cardiologist has told him that he requires cardiac bypass surgery if he is to live. He has refused the surgery, stating, "There is no point in living." The consulting psychiatrist confirms that Mr. J. is clinically depressed in addition to having Alzheimer's disease, and the psychiatrist believes that Mr. J. cannot make a rational decision.

ADMINISTRATION OF DRUGS

Shirley W. is a 74-year-old patient with Alzheimer's disease who lives in a nursing home. Over the past few months she has become increasingly difficult to spoon-feed because she spits, pushes the spoon away, and refuses to eat. When admitted to the home, while coherent and clear-minded, Mrs. W. had asserted that she did not want her life prolonged by artificial means. The physician orders feeding by a nasogastric tube, which Mrs. W. frequently pulls out. In response to complaints from the nursing staff, the physician prescribes tranquilizers for Mrs. W. to make her "more manageable."

CONFIDENTIALITY

Dave S. is taken to his family doctor by his wife and grown daughter to find out why he has become so irritable. He admits to angry outbursts for no apparent reason. He also says that he has trouble remembering and is finding it increasingly difficult to add and subtract. After extensive testing, the diagnosis is confirmed: Mr. S. has Alzheimer's disease. The doctor tells him about the diagnosis and gives him a broad outline of what he can expect. Mr. S. takes the news calmly, then states that under no circumstances does he want his wife or daughter informed.

PATIENT'S WISHES VS. SOCIETAL NORMS

Martha J.'s children have complained to the nursing home administrator that on their last three weekly visits, they have found Martha in her room, dressed only in her slip. The children have protested that "the nurses aren't even bothering to tidy her up." Actually, Martha recently had become combative each time a staff member had tried to make her dress for social activities. The nursing staff, with feelings of ambivalence, had decided to honor Martha's apparent wish not to dress as long as she was in her room.

Caregivers charged with responsibility for a patient with Alzheimer's disease continually wrestle with ethical issues. Simple day-to-day care demands a repeated confrontation with these dilemmas. Dealing with the complex problem of the elderly person with dementia arouses intense discomfort in the caretaker, especially when an ethical issue underlying the care emerges. Yet there are no simple answers and no agreed-upon formulas that will ensure that the rights of the elderly person with dementia are maintained and that the conscience of the caretaker will remain clear. Ultimately, all caregivers have a professional obligation to analyze carefully the ethical principles that must guide care, to explore their own moral boundaries, and to be aware of the need for respectful consideration of the impact of ethical issues on the quality of staff interaction and relationships.

ETHICAL PRINCIPLES GOVERNING CARE

Moral standards and the nature of moral decision-making are the concerns of ethics, and ethical reflection is an obligation of the caregiver. Moral obligations sometimes are thought of as rules and indeed may be codified into law, but ethical practice goes far beyond what can be reduced to rules.

Certain values are basic to any ethical system. These are moral obligations in the sense that, without them, no community or cooperative activity could exist. These central values include truthfulness, fairness, and respect for life. Besides these values, there are many others, such as not inflicting harm or suffering. Caregivers often must make decisions in the face of conflicting values; for example, telling the truth about the diagnosis of Alzheimer's disease in itself may cause suffering. Rules alone are not enough. Caregivers must thoughtfully consider whether actions and policies are consistent with moral principles and rules. Care of the patient with Alzheimer's disease presents many complex challenges to these moral principles, and the "good" choice is seldom obvious. However, caregivers are obligated to consider these issues carefully and to use them to frame moral choices to guide their behavior.

Three ethical principles are commonly applied to the dilemmas that arise in patient care:

1. Beneficence—that caregivers ought to produce good, preserve life, and prevent harm and suffering
2. Respect for persons—that the autonomy and dignity of individuals should be preserved and promoted
3. Equity—that the benefits and burdens of care be fairly and equitably distributed among individuals

PSYCHOLOGICAL REACTIONS OF CAREGIVER

The elderly patient with dementia, who is seemingly bereft of relationships and cognition, is often described by family and friends as "no longer here." In this sense caregivers in the institution may have an advantage because, not having known the "former self," they may find it easier than family or friends to see the patient as a full person, albeit one who is difficult, unpredictable, and complex. The family, on the other hand, grieves for the loss of the person they once knew and loved.

Caregivers themselves often experience powerful emotional reactions that profoundly influence their ethical decisions. Besides confronting their own mortality, they may see the frailties of patients with dementia as intimations of their own future losses, mental as well as physical. If the patient does not demonstrate a strong sense of individuality, a sense that depends largely on his ability to relate, the caregiver may project certain attributes onto him—often those of the caregiver's own parents—and respond to the patient accordingly. Many of the ethical dilemmas that caregivers face place them in a double bind situation in which any action taken evokes guilt. For example, on the issue of forced feeding, caregivers experience conflicting demands—to preserve life (by techniques such as nasogastric tubes that may inflict additional suffering on the patient) and to respect the patient's wishes (although refusal of food will shorten life). This double bind may increase the caregivers' sense of guilt or helplessness and impede ethical choices.

Little is known about the psychological mechanisms that caregivers use to manage their own feelings in these difficult situations. Undoubtedly many flee, choosing instead work that is less emotionally demanding.

Other caregivers distance themselves emotionally from the patient, becoming less sensitive to the patient's feelings and needs and eventually reducing their perception of the person to that of "a thing . . . handled routinely and mechanically, not nursed with tenderness and understanding" (Norberg and others, 1980).

Several hospitals, recognizing the impact of the psychological reactions of their staff, have created interdisciplinary bioethics committees that facilitate discussion of dilemmas being faced and foster a sense of shared responsibility for consideration of choices and decision-making. In addition, they support separate nursing ethics groups, which provide a vehicle by which all staff members have the opportunity to discuss their concerns.

OBLIGATION TO PRESERVE LIFE AND PREVENT SUFFERING

The rigid stereotyping of professional roles, such as those of the physician and the nurse, may decrease the possibilities for successful management. Although current therapeutic measures cannot cure Alzheimer's disease, they can improve the patient's functioning and quality of life. Team efforts to resolve problems such as urinary incontinence and nocturnal agitation, for example, are often successful. Optimum care requires the involvement and collaboration of family members, friends, and caregivers alike. The question of what type and degree of life support should be given is a troublesome one since loss of intellect often is equated with loss of humanness. Undoubtedly, the minimum ethical requirement is that the extent and irreversibility of the loss of cognitive function be established and that the patient be kept clean, adequately hydrated and nourished, and as free of pain and discomfort as possible.

The ethical code embodied in criminal law prohibits positive euthanasia, the performance of a lethal act, even if that act is motivated by a compassionate desire to prevent suffering. On the other hand, negative euthanasia, the decision to withhold treatment and let nature take its course, is more generally accepted. Since criteria for decision-making are not well defined, this situation creates ethical dilemmas for conscientious caregivers. The patient's wishes, if known and expressed while he was still competent, should be considered. Ethical caregivers must

walk a tightrope between resisting premature requests from weary relatives or staff to stop all life-prolonging efforts up to the last. . . . Situations in which health professionals are uncertain about what is best should be resolved in favor of extending life where possible. This should apply when friends or relatives strongly urge it. They will have to live with these decisions, in a way that health professionals do not, after the death of their loved ones. [Dyck, 1984]

At the same time, patients have the right to refuse life-extending treatment, and incompetence does not diminish that right. When a patient, family, and caregiver cannot agree on these serious matters, the decisions must be left to the courts.

OBLIGATION TO RESPECT PATIENT

Institutionalization inevitably involves a paternalistic attitude toward the patient. In a setting where most or all aspects of the patient's life are regulated by the staff, the patient's individuality is sacrificed to some extent. No longer able to select what to eat, what to wear, or when to sleep, patients often respond with either belligerence or psychological withdrawal and a steadily increasing dependence. However, research indicates that the degree of dementia improves, or at least progresses less rapidly, when patients stay active and are allowed some role in decision-making, even if only about minor aspects of their environment. The issue of competence to decide is obviously a matter of degree. Some patients are competent to make all decisions; some, most decisions; some, only a few; and others, virtually none. Individualized assessments that are repeated periodically can limit the overzealous application of paternalism. However, such assessments require considerable effort and reduce bureaucratic efficiency.

In general, individuals are presumed to be capable of discerning their own best interest and pursuing it. Seen as autonomous and competent, a normal person has the legal and moral right to choose and to refuse. However, it is this right to make reasonable choices that is the major issue in progressive Alzheimer's disease. What degree of autonomy can be left to the patient? Who is to decide, if not the patient? By its very nature, paternalism (limitation of a patient's freedom and authority by the "wise and loving father") exists to do good—to protect the patient from the dangers of his own freedom, such as the freedom to starve to death. Since much of the health care function is inherently paternalistic, this attitude probably cannot be totally avoided. However, an effort should be made to keep this element within proper bounds.

The right to decide is most controversial when it involves the refusal of treatment, particularly treatment that would extend life. Recent ethical debates and court decisions have done much to clarify the patient's rights and the caregiver's obligations in decisions involving patients who are still competent. It is clear that the patient should not be forced to undergo treatment that is against his wishes, even if the treatment is for his own good. Although caregivers have an ethical duty not to force treatment against a patient's wishes, they have the additional obligations of helping to educate the patient and helping him to work through the reasons for refusal. Two criteria have been identified as morally justified for refusing treatment: (1) if the treatment is useless, or (2) if it involves a grave burden for the patient or another.

Who should decide for the incompetent patient, and what criteria should be used? These questions are surrounded by great controversy. The concept of substituted judgment is increasingly being recognized by some states and validated by the courts in cases in which patients had expressed their wishes concerning care while they were still competent so that those wishes could be carried out even if they lapsed into incompetence, perhaps with the appointment of a guardian to ensure that their wishes were expressed. If the patient, while competent, does not express an intent (or if a patient has never been competent), other issues arise. In general, when the care of an incompetent patient without a guardian is debated, the courts must decide in favor of what they deem to be the best interest of the patient. However, the extent to which family members rather that the courts should have the right to decide among the reasonable courses of action available is unclear. Veatch and other authors have argued for a "limited familial autonomy" in which the family is given responsibility for carrying the patient's or the family's beliefs and values into the decision, with the caregiver seeking court intervention if the family is considered to be unreasonable and exploitative.

Advance Directives

Advance directives are designed to give patients an opportunity to direct their own care and to reduce the ambiguity that occurs when patients cannot communicate their wishes. There are two types of advance directives in current use: a living will and a durable power of attorney for health care. Ideally, a patient should have both types.

A living will is generally limited to decisions about withdrawing or withholding life-sustaining procedures for patients who are terminally ill or facing imminent death. A durable power of attorney for health care is designed for situations in which the patient is incapacitated, not necessarily terminally ill. Thus the durable power of attorney covers patients who are unconscious or mentally incompetent, including those with Alzheimer's disease. It is an instrument that allows patients, while still competent, to make and express decisions regarding treatment choices and to appoint representatives who can make health care decisions for them if they should become incompetent or incapacitated.

Nurses must be aware of the laws governing advance directives in their own states. The specific form, process, and procedures for valid advance directives are established by state laws, which vary considerably. In many states, for example, the durable power of attorney for health care requires the notarized signatures of two witnesses who are unrelated to the patient. In some states health professionals are prohibited from serving as those witnesses. Likewise, in some states specific procedures, such as the withholding of hydration or nutrition, are not included in the definition of "life-sustaining treatments" and must be mentioned specifically. Some states do not permit the withdrawal of artificial nutrition even if the patient desires such withdrawal. State-approved advance directive forms, including living wills, can be obtained from the Choice in Dying (formerly Concern for Dying/Society for the Right to Die),* as well as from other organizations. A medical directive form that allows the patient to specify his wishes regarding medical procedures, such as invasive tests, and provides space to note additional desires can be obtained from Harvard Medical School.† It is important that procedures not desired be specified because court involvement is often necessary when the patient's wishes are ambigu-

---

*Choice in Dying, 200 Varick St. New York, NY 10014-4810, (212) 366-5540.
†Harvard Medical School, Health Publications Group, Department MD, P.O. Box 380, Boston, MA, 02117.

ous. States also have varying rules regarding the longevity of an advance directive. To be kept current under the most restrictive statutes, advance directives should be revalidated every 5 years.

The Patient Self-Determination Act, which became effective in 1991, requires that all Medicare- and Medicaid-reimbursed agencies provide written information to patients at the time of admission concerning their rights to an advance directive for health care under their state law. In addition, the agency must document whether the patient has an advance directive and must comply with all state statutes regarding these directives. The agency is not compelled to adhere to provisions contained in a directive that is in conflict with the agency's policy. However, the agency must develop policies and provide information concerning these policies to the patient on admission. These policies should be detailed enough to communicate the philosophy of the institution regarding the discontinuation of life-sustaining treatment and indicate any specific limitations the agency might place on the implementation of advance directives.

OBLIGATION TO GIVE EQUITABLE TREATMENT

The principle of equitable treatment provides for impartiality and prevents discrimination. It ensures that the patient's rights to adequate treatment for the preservation of life or prevention of suffering are in no way diminished simply because the patient has certain characteristics, such as being elderly or having dementia. Too often the right to impartial treatment is overlooked or ignored in patients with Alzheimer's disease. When cognitive decline prevents conventional types of interaction between the caregiver and the patient, the patient often is viewed as an undesirable type. Yet being "undesirable" does not represent valid ethical grounds for disenfranchising a patient from the normal standard of care. Three of the numerous ways in which differential treatment can be seen involve disclosure of the diagnosis, different management of medical problems, and use of restraints.

Disclosure of Diagnosis

In the early stages of Alzheimer's disease, the patient can understand the diagnosis and prognosis. Should he be apprised of these facts at this time? Informing a patient of a diagnosis of Alzheimer's disease presents vexing issues. Under the principle of autonomy, the patient is seen as having a moral right to know. Adherence to the principle of beneficence, on the other hand, may lead to a decision to withhold this information if it is thought that it would be detrimental to the particular patient at that time. Although no studies have yet assessed the actual impact of being told the diagnosis, a study by Erde and associates suggests that an overwhelming majority of individuals (92%) indicated that they would want to be informed of the diagnosis. Reasons commonly given included being able to plan for financial and personal care (94%), wanting to seek a second opinion (62%), and wanting to settle family matters (36%).

Those persons who want to know the diagnosis were even more likely to want their spouse told (89%) if for some reason the information was withheld from them, and they also were more likely to state that not being told would make them angry (71%). The ethical caregiver balances the burden of being the bearer of bad tidings with a sensitivity to the patient's and family's needs—for timely presentation of small "parcels" of information, for support and information at times when they request it and are able to accept and process it, and for help in coping with the signs and symptoms of the disease and in preparing for its progression.

Management of Medical Problems

The first duty of patient care, and the least controversial, clearly is to provide care. Yet studies repeatedly have found that institutionalized persons and elderly patients with dementia seldom receive the aggressive medical care provided to patients who are more independent. Obviously, there is an ethical obligation to apply considerable effort, knowledge, and skills in reaching a diagnosis of Alzheimer's disease, particularly in searching for other possibly reversible causes of dementia. Likewise, the obligation to evaluate and treat fevers and physical illness is not diminished by the patient's age or mental state.

PHYSICIAN-ASSISTED SUICIDE AND ACTIVE EUTHANASIA

A national debate about the morality of euthanasia has been fueled by ballot initiatives in two states (both narrowly defeated) that would allow the terminally ill to choose physician-assisted suicide. The widely publicized case in which Dr. Jack Kevorkian, a retired pathologist, helped a woman diagnosed with Alzheimer-type dementia to self-administer a lethal injection stimulated a growing interest in the issues surrounding the right to die. Furthermore, the book *Final*

Exit by Derek Humphrey, which describes ways in which those seeking relief from terminal or debilitating illness can commit suicide became a bestseller in 1991.

Public opinion polls consistently reveal support for the general desire for "death with dignity" and for the notion that physicians should be allowed to comply with a terminally ill patient's request for help in dying. Surveys of physicians, however, reveal support for the patient's right to die but a reluctance to involve the medical profession in the process. Only 30% of primary care physicians and 26% of geriatricians favored easing restrictions on physician-assisted suicide. Numerous organizations, including the American Medical Association, the American Cancer Society, and the American Geriatrics Society, have stated positions opposing physician-assisted suicide.

Are acts of withholding treatment that allow a patient to die morally different from active euthanasia—the administration of a fatal injection, overdose, or deadly gas? This issue is the central question under debate. Those who favor voluntary active euthanasia argue that it is an individual right, the right to choose a painless and peaceful death. Opponents contend that the legalization of active euthanasia devalues life, abolishing misery from the human experience and diminishing the natural value that is bound to the preservation and protection of life.

If we as a society decide to honor patient requests for assistance with suicide, whose job should it be? Many in the health professions are reluctant to assume the obligation of this expanded role, which they think conflicts with their traditional roles, which are conceptualized as "life sustaining and death defying." Will a new profession be needed to carry out this role?

What safeguards are necessary to prevent abuse? Although withdrawal of treatment is a recognition of the limitations of medicine, active euthanasia raises the specter of medical omnipotence and omniscience. What controls will be needed to ensure that the physician, for example, acts (1) with the appropriate consent of the patient, and (2) only in situations in which the diagnosis is correct, life is intolerable or there is no hope of recovery, or death is ensured?

The experience in Holland, where active euthanasia and physician-assisted suicide have been allowed for two decades under guidelines developed by the courts, underscores the importance of adequate safeguards. The Dutch rules generally permit physicians to perform euthanasia for patients who are experiencing intolerable suffering and have no prospect for improvement, but only after consultation with an independent physician who is experienced with the disease. A court-sponsored study of the Dutch experience indicated that fewer than 3% of all deaths in Holland in 1990 involved active euthanasia and assisted suicide and that only one third of patient requests for euthanasia were honored. These figures suggest that euthanasia is not being used as an alternative to good terminal care. Most of these acts of euthanasia were conducted in the patient's home with the patient's family and physician in attendance.

However, critics point to disturbing findings amid the statistics in the study. Guidelines require that a patient's request be "well-considered, durable and persistent," yet in one third of the cases this standard was not met. A separate study of deaths resulting from euthanasia indicated that the time that elapsed between the patient's request and the euthanasia was less than 24 hours in 59% of the cases.

Most worrisome was the finding that 92% of the cases in which medical decisions were made to hasten the death of the patient (38% of all deaths during the same period) did not qualify for classification as euthanasia. These requirements include that there be explicit and repeated requests by the patient that leave no reason for doubt concerning his desire to die; that the decision be well informed, free, and enduring; that the mental or physical suffering be severe with no prospect of relief; that all other options for care have been exhausted or refused by the patient; and that a second physician be consulted. Only 2.9% of all deaths were recorded as euthanasia under these guidelines. However, 17.5% of all deaths resulted from the administration of opioids for the alleviation of pain and suffering at such dosages that death was either expected or intended, and an additional 17.5% of all deaths involved "passive euthanasia," or the withdrawal or withholding of treatment designed to prolong life. The finding that the physician had not discussed the medical decision with the patient in 60% of the opioid overdose cases and in 63% of the nontreatment decisions is particularly disturbing, although in many cases the patient had previously indicated a desire for euthanasia if his suffering became unbearable, even though these requests were not sufficiently documented. Patients whose lives were terminated without documented consent tended to be those who were comatose, demented, or otherwise thought to be mentally incompetent. In these cases physicians cited the following reasons for proceeding without consent: unbearable pain/suffering (30%), low quality of life (31%), no prospect of improvement (60%), and protection of the patient's family (32%).

Increasing public pressure for a system that ensures a patient' "right to die well" will undoubtedly bring change to the America health care system. If the legalization of euthanasia is to be adoptec it is clear that it should be preceded by vigorous, systematic deliber ation and debate and accompanied by a credible supervisory systen Alternatively, the health professions must acknowledge the wide spread public dissatisfaction with many factors related to dying an increase their efforts to assist the patient in dying well—to reliev pain; provide strength, comfort, and support; avoid burdensom treatments that are likely to prove futile; and communicate with pa tients and families, helping them to find meaning in their suffering

Restraint

The unpredictable behavior of patients with Alzheimer's diseas is often disturbing to caregivers. Disruptive behavior, "unprovoked assaults, and combativeness are not uncommon. If such behavior i bothersome rather than likely to injure the patient or others, restrain is viewed as unethical. Allowing the patient to stay in his robe rathe than get dressed, for example, may eliminate his resistance and pre vent an assault. Unfortunately, however, physical or chemical re straints often are used to manage bothersome behavior, resulting i. increased health risks from immobility, overmedication, and drug re actions and interactions. What are the patient's rights in such a situ ation? An ethical decision would demand the use of the least restrain possible to ensure safety, not staff convenience.

BROAD ETHICAL ISSUES

Numerous ethical issues surround the difficult dilemmas c Alzheimer's disease. For example, what special protections are needer in research on Alzheimer's disease? This disease requires experimen tation on humans since no animal models have been identified. Wha is the ethical responsibility of the health care professional for ensur ing that research into the cause and amelioration of this disease re ceive high priority? What are the implications for public policy? Wha choices should be made about the allocation of limited health car resources for this special group?

Underlying all these considerations, and central to the resolutioi of the ethical dilemmas presented by this disease, is a need for a unifying goal to serve as a guide in the care of the patient with Alzhei mer's disease. Faced with a patient's inevitable disintegration into a disabling dependent state that is devoid of meaningful relationships, the caregiver must ask, "What must be my goals?" The answer I would suggest is (1) to assist the family and friends in celebrating the individual personhood that once was the patient's and in grieving its passing and (2) to help make each moment for the patient "as gentle, as content, and as kindly as it can be" (Howell, 1984).

BIBLIOGRAPHY

Badzek LA: What you need to know about advance directives, *Nursing* 42(6):58-59, 1992.

Campion EW: Ethical issues in the care of the patient involved in Alzheimer's disease research. In Melnick VL, Dubler ND, editors: *Alzheimer's dementia: dilemmas in clinical research*, Clifton, NJ, 1985, Humana Press.

Cassell CK, Jameton AL: Dementia in the elderly: an analysis of medical responsibility, *Ann Intern Med* 94:802-807, 1981.

Dyck AJ: Ethical aspects of care for the dying incompetent, *J Am Geriatr Soc* 32:661-664, 1984.

Erde EL, Nadal EC, Scholl TO: On truth telling and the diagnosis of Alzheimer's disease, *J Fam Pract* 26:401-406, 1988.

Flarey DL: Advance directives: in search of self-determination, *J Nurs Admin* 21(11):16-22, 1991.

Goldman R: Ethical confrontations in the incapacitated aged, *J Am Geriatr Soc* 29:241-245, 1981.

Greco PJ and others: The Patient Self-Determination Act and the future of advance directives, *Ann Intern Med* 115:639-643, 1991.

Hermann HT: Ethical dilemmas intrinsic to the care of the elderly demented patient, *J Am Geriatr Soc* 32:655-656, 1984.

Hersh AR, Outerbridge DE: *Easing the passage*, New York, 1991, Harper Collins.

Howell M: Caretaker's views on responsibility for the care of the demented elderly, *J Am Geriatr Soc* 32:657-660, 1984.

Jacobs P: Initiative fuels debate over morality of euthanasia, *Los Angeles Times*, p. A20, October 31, 1992.

Norberg A, Norberg B, Bexell G: Ethical problems in feeding patients with advanced dementia, *Br Med J* 281:847-848, 1980.

Rouse F: Legal and ethical guidelines for physicians in geriatric terminal care, *Geriatrics* 43(8):69-75, 1988.

Van der Maas PJ and others: Euthanasia and other medical decisions concerning the end of life, *Lancet* 669-674, 1991. (see also comments in *Lancet* 338:952, 953, 1010-1, 1150, 1991).

Veatch RM: An ethical framework for terminal care decisions: a new classification of patients, *J Am Geriatr Soc* 32:665-669, 1984.

Watts DT, Howell T, Priefer BA: Geriatricians' attitudes toward assisting suicide of dementia patients, *J Am Geriatr Soc* 40:878-884, 1992.

22

Legal issues for caregivers

Marguerite Mettetal

At some point almost every family of a person with Alzheimer's disease must address legal issues. Therefore, a basic understanding of the provisions of guardianship and conservatorship laws is helpful to the family and to health care professionals. Familiarity with the law of durable power of attorney and the law on living wills is also beneficial since the use of these laws is appropriate for patients in the very early stages of Alzheimer's disease. Although specific laws vary from state to state, much of the following information has general application. Any person who is considering guardianship, conservatorship, or power of attorney should consult an attorney who practices in the state in which the patient lives.

A few states have enacted public guardianship laws. The training that public guardians receive in legal issues and the experience they gain with their clients enables them to present an overall view of matters of concern to persons with Alzheimer's disease and their families.

Financial problems often develop for patients in the early stages of Alzheimer's disease. It is at this time that family members are advised to gather all the financial information they can find while the patient is still able to help them. In particular, they should ascertain details about real estate holdings, income amounts and sources, bank accounts, and insurance policies. This information should be taken to an attorney in order to discuss steps that should be taken immediately to protect the patient's assets.

Many people are reluctant to contact an attorney because of expected high costs. However, most attorneys have an established hourly fee that they charge for office consultations. This fee is a small price to pay for competent advice about protecting a victim's assets or physical well-being. Anyone whose relative is suspected of having Alzheimer's disease is encouraged to seek the advice of an attorney.

REGULAR VERSUS DURABLE POWER OF ATTORNEY

In an article about the legal problems of persons with Alzheimer's disease and their families, the director of legal care projects for the Tennessee Commission on Aging stated that "in all cases in which the patient is capable of executing a contract, efforts should be made to obtain a Durable Power of Attorney." This instrument can eliminate the need for having a guardianship petition filed with the court. The durable power of attorney is a very important document that should always be discussed with and drawn up by an attorney.

The regular power of attorney, familiar to most people, becomes invalid when the person who granted that power of attorney (i.e., the patient with Alzheimer's disease) becomes incapable or incompetent. In other words, it ceases to be effective when the need for it is the greatest. In contrast, the durable power of attorney is specifically designed to remain effective regardless of the eventual mental or physical disability of the person who executed it. The person appointed in either form of power of attorney is called an attorney-in-fact, although this person does not need to be an attorney at law. The attorney-in-fact should be a trusted friend or relative. The specific powers granted to the attorney-in-fact should be clearly set out and may include the handling of any matters from a wide variety of business and legal affairs.

The durable power of attorney gives a tremendous amount of power to one person. The activities of an attorney-in-fact are not supervised by the court the way that guardianships and conservatorships are. As with any relationship based on trust, room for abuse exists. For this reason very careful study and seeking of advice are recommended before using the durable power of attorney. The person to serve as attorney-in-fact must be carefully chosen.

DURABLE POWER OF ATTORNEY FOR HEALTH CARE

A durable power of attorney for health care is a written document that allows one person ("principal") to give another person ("attorney-in-fact" or "agent") the power to make health care decisions for him if he is unable to speak for himself.

The agent can be any friend or relative, but the individual cannot be someone who is providing health care services to the patient. The principal must be mentally competent and must know exactly what responsibilities he is giving to the agent when he signs the document.

The durable power of attorney for health care gives the agent authority to consent, to refuse to consent, or to withdraw consent to any care, treatment, service, or procedure to maintain, diagnose, or treat a physical or mental condition. This power is subject to any limitations that the principal includes in the durable power of attorney. The principal may state in the document any type of treatment that he does not desire. The agent must act consistently with the desires the principal expresses in the durable power of attorney.

When the principal is unable to make his own decisions, the agent designated in the durable power of attorney has priority over any other person to act for the principal in all matters of health care decisions. The designated agent has the right to review the principal's medical records and to consent to their disclosure unless that right is specifically limited in the durable power of attorney. Unless otherwise specified in the durable power of attorney, the agent has the power to authorize an autopsy and to direct the disposition of the body.

The durable power of attorney for health care does not take away the patient's right to make decisions as long as the patient is able to understand the treatment being considered. In addition, no treatment may be given to the patient over the patient's objection. Health care that is necessary to keep the patient alive may not be stopped or withheld if the patient objects at the time.

The durable power of attorney for health care can be revoked by the principal at any time by notifying the agent, treating physician, hospital, or other health care providers orally or in writing.

Any health care provider must arrange for the prompt and orderly transfer of a patient to the care of others when, as a matter of conscience, the health care provider cannot implement the health care decisions made by the attorney-in-fact as provided in a durable power of attorney for health care.

Most states are very specific about the requirements that must be satisfied in appointing an attorney-in-fact for health care decisions. Usually, this durable power of attorney must be signed in front of a notary and two witnesses. Most states list certain groups of people who cannot sign as a witness, such as relatives or health care providers. The advice of an attorney should be obtained to ensure compliance with the law of the state in which the document is signed.

LIVING WILL

A written declaration called a living will allows a competent person to state in advance his wishes regarding the use of life-prolonging medical care if he becomes terminally ill and unable to communicate. A competent person is defined as an individual who is able to understand and appreciate the nature and consequences of a decision to accept or refuse treatment. Individuals in the early stage of Alzheimer's disease probably meet these criteria and should be given an opportunity to make this decision.

Most states have a law that allows an individual to sign a living will. This directs that anytime a person has a terminal condition that the attending physician determines is irreversible and will result in death, medical care can be withdrawn or withheld. The person may be permitted to die naturally with only the administration of medication necessary to provide comfortable care or to alleviate pain.

Recently, the law has been expanded in several states to permit a declaration directing the withholding or withdrawal of artificial nutrition or hydration when the preceding circumstances exist. Competent patients with Alzheimer's disease should be asked specifically if they want to be kept alive with food or water given through a tube. They should be asked if they want to be kept alive through the use of life-support machines if they are in a coma. If they do not want to be kept alive in that manner, they should sign a living will, which has such statements in it. If they want every effort made to prolong their life, they should not sign a living will.

Most states have a statute with a suggested form for a living will (Fig. 21-1). Legal Services or the Area Agency on Aging may provide a preprinted living will that meets the requirements in a specific state.

To be legal, a living will must be signed in the presence of a notary public. In most states it must be witnessed by two people, neither of whom can be a relative or a health care provider (e.g., physician or nurse or anyone who works for them). A witness cannot be anyone who operates or works for a health care institution such as a hospital or a nursing home. Finally, a witness cannot be anyone who will inherit or otherwise receive the person's money or property when he dies.

To My Family, My Physician, My Lawyer
And All Others Whom It May Concern

Death is as much a reality as birth, growth, and aging—it is the one certainty of life. In anticipation of decisions that may have to be made about my own dying and as an expression of my right to refuse treatment, I, _____, being of sound mind, make this statement of my wishes and instructions concerning treatment. _____ (print name)

By means of this document, which I intend to be legally binding, I direct my physician and other care providers, my family, and any surrogate designated by me or appointed by a court, to carry out my wishes. If I become unable, by reason of physical or mental incapacity, to make decisions about my medical care, let this document provide the guidance and authority needed to make any and all such decisions.

If I am permanently unconscious or there is no reasonable expectation of my recovery from a seriously incapacitating or lethal illness or condition, I do not wish to be kept alive by artificial means. I request that I be given all care necessary to keep me comfortable and free of pain, even if pain-relieving medications may hasten my death, and I direct that no life-sustaining treatment be provided except as I or my surrogate specifically authorize.

This request may appear to place a heavy responsibility upon you, but by making this decision according to my strong convictions, I intend to ease that burden. I am acting after careful consideration and with understanding of the consequences of your carrying out my wishes. *List optional specific provisions in the space below. (See other side.)*

Durable Power of Attorney for Health Care Decisions (Cross out if you do not wish to use this section)

To effect my wishes, I designate _____, residing at _____ _____, (phone #) _____, (or if he or she shall for any reason fail to act, _____, residing at _____ _____, (phone #) _____) as my health care surrogate—that is, my attorney-in-fact regarding any and all health care decisions to be made for me, including the decision to refuse life-sustaining treatment—if I am unable to make such decisions myself. This power shall remain effective during and not be affected by my subsequent illness, disability or incapacity. My surrogate shall have authority to interpret my Living Will, and shall make decisions about my health care as specified in my instructions or, when my wishes are not clear, as the surrogate believes to be in my best interests. I release and agree to hold harmless my health care surrogate from any and all claims whatsoever arising from decisions made in good faith in the exercise of this power.

I sign this document knowingly, voluntarily, and after careful deliberation, this _____ day of _____, 19_____.

_____
(signature)

Address _____
_____

I do hereby certify that the within document was executed and acknowledged before me by the principal this _____ day of _____, 19_____.

_____
Notary Public

Witness _____
Printed Name _____
Address _____
_____

Witness _____
Printed Name _____
Address _____
_____

Copies of this document have been given to:

This Living Will expresses my personal treatment preferences. The fact that I may have also executed a declaration in the form recommended by state law should not be construed to limit or contradict this Living Will, which is an expression of my common-law and constitutional rights.

(Optional) my Living Will is registered with Concern for Dying (Registry No. _____)

Distributed by Concern for Dying, 250 West 57th Street, New York, NY 10107 (212) 246-6962

Fig. 21-1. Living will and health care proxy. (From Choice in Dying [formerly Concern for Dying/Society for the Right to Die], 200 Varick Street, New York, NY 10014-4810, [212] 366-5540.)

A properly executed living will is effective from the date of its execution until it is revoked. If more than one document has been executed, the latest declaration known to the attending physician takes precedence. A declaration can be revoked at any time by the declarant, without regard to his mental state or competency. It can be revoked in writing or by simply telling the attending physician or other health care provider of the revocation.

Copies of an individual's living will should be widely distributed. In addition to the attending physician and the local hospital, copies should be given to close relatives.

No matter what the course of the disease, at some point the patient with Alzheimer's disease will no longer be able to sign legal documents or make appropriate decisions. Yet bills must be paid and assets need to be conserved. If no durable power of attorney is in place, legal action through the court will be necessary before anyone can act on behalf of the patient. There are basically two legal approaches available to assist and protect the patient: a full guardianship/conservatorship or a limited guardianship/conservatorship.

FULL OR LIMITED GUARDIANSHIP AND CONSERVATORSHIP

The differences between full and limited guardianship and conservatorship are defined by state laws. In general, the conservator handles the property, including real estate, personal property, and finances. The court also may appoint a guardian or a conservator to have charge and custody of the patient. Full control of both the patient and his property may not be necessary in all cases. Under such circumstances a limited guardian or conservator may be appointed and given only the responsibilities specifically enumerated by the court.

The actions of all guardians and conservators are supervised by the courts. For example, if real estate or other assets are to be managed, the guardian or conservator must file a sworn inventory containing a list of the property of the disabled person and a list of the source, amount, and frequency of each item of income, benefit, or other revenue. Specific approval must be obtained before any real estate or significant personal property can be sold. Court approval may be required for major purchases. Once a year an accounting is made to the court. This accounting requires a listing of all income and all expenditures. Bank statements and canceled checks are presented to the court. The overall rule is that the conservator must manage the financial affairs of the disabled person in the manner of a prudent person at all times.

In addition to handling financial assets, if the conservator or guardian has charge of the person, that person has other responsibilities. These responsibilities may include ensuring that the patient is adequately housed, fed, and clothed and receives appropriate medical care. A statement concerning the physical or mental condition of the disabled person is made to the court in the annual accounting. This statement must demonstrate to the court the need, or lack of need, for the continuation of services.

Another duty often placed on a conservator or guardian is to give informed consent for the care and medical treatment of the disabled person. It is important to note that the person who signs the forms as the responsible party when the patient is admitted to the hospital or nursing home does not automatically have the legal authority to make decisions or authorize treatment for a patient. The responsible party is only responsible for paying the bill. Only the guardian or conservator of the person who has the specific authority over health care decisions can authorize treatment. The conservator or guardian makes the health care decisions for the disabled person, decisions that would normally be made by a competent patient.

In some states it is not necessary to prove that the patient is legally incompetent before the court appoints a conservator or guardian. The laws of some states require only that the person be mentally and/or physically disabled or incapacitated and not able to handle his own affairs. Proper notice, medical evidence, and a hearing in court are definitely required. The decision as to whether the appointment is needed and appropriate is made by the court. The appointed guardian or conservator must be someone the court finds to be both willing and capable of serving in that capacity.

Often a willing relative may be too frail and disabled to handle the job. In other cases relatives simply do not want to take the responsibility. If there is no money to hire an attorney or a trust department at a bank, a public guardian may be appointed in states having such a program.

Procedures used to establish a full or limited conservatorship or guardianship are fairly similar. For a patient with Alzheimer's disease, the petition will most likely be for a full guardianship or conservatorship since the patient eventually may be unable to handle any of his affairs. The first step in the process requires a petition to be drawn up by an attorney and then filed with the chancery court. The petition can be signed by a family member or any other concerned person. Sometimes the state's department of human services signs the petition to the court. Social workers at hospitals or nursing homes also may sign the petition when they realize the need for such an appointment. Once the petition has been filed, a date is set for the hearing. Most states specify the number of days' notice that must be given to the person for whom a guardian or conservator is to be appointed. Notice also is given to the spouse, children, or next of kin, unless the person files the petition himself. The notice is sent by registered mail or served by a sheriff's deputy.

Before the court hearing (which can be delayed for 60 days or longer), the court usually appoints a guardian ad litem to serve for this one action only. The role of the guardian ad litem is to protect the interests of the person being considered for a guardianship or conservatorship. The guardian ad litem completes a thorough study of the patient's situation and reports his findings to the court. At the hearing he represents the best interests of the person by questioning the witnesses and the potential guardian or conservator.

The court may subpoena witnesses, such as nurses who have cared for the patient, neighbors, or anyone who has been involved in the case. The laws of most states require the testimony of at least two physicians; their testimony may be submitted in a written document, by deposition, or in person. The judge decides at the hearing if a guardian or conservator is needed. If such a finding is made, the judge then appoints the conservator or guardian.

After the appointment has been made, the court approves all fees, which are usually paid from the disabled person's funds. This includes the petitioning attorney's fee, the fee of the guardian ad litem, and the court costs. The procedure is not inexpensive. If the court decides that the appointment of a guardian or conservator is not appropriate, the person who filed the petition must pay the fees and costs.

A number of difficult choices face the conservator, guardian, or attorney-in-fact. As the patient's assets decline, he may become eligible for Supplemental Security Income and/or Medicaid. Therefore the laws and regulations governing these benefits need to be considered. If application for Medicaid is even a remote possibility, a consultation with someone well schooled in the requirements of this program is suggested.

SUMMARY

Immediate financial and legal planning is necessary as soon as Alzheimer's disease is diagnosed or even strongly suspected. The

plans should be developed under the guidance of an attorney. Appro
priate steps taken during the early stages of the disease will enable the
caregiver, family member, or appointed guardian or conservator to
make medical decisions consistent with the disabled person's wishes
and to ensure that the best use is made of all assets during the re
maining life of the person with Alzheimer's disease.

BIBLIOGRAPHY

Hirsh HL: Legal and ethical considerations in dealing with Alzheimer's disease, *Leg Med*, 1990, pp. 261-326.

Levine J, Lawlor BA: Family counseling and legal issues in Alzheimer's disease, *Psy chiatr Clin North Am* 14:385-396, 1991.

Overman W Jr, Stoudemire A: Guidelines for legal and financial counseling of Alz heimer's disease patients and their families, *Am J Psychiatry* 145:1496-1500, 1988

Silver HM: Alzheimer's disease: ethical and legal decisions, *Med Law* 6:537-551, 1987

23

Lawsuits related to Alzheimer's disease

J. Howard Frederick

CAREGIVER PROBLEMS

Many families of a person with Alzheimer's disease refuse to accept the fact that the individual is going through a steady downhill course. Some either give the person credit for more functional capabilities than he or she possesses or refuse to accept the significance of this progressive encephalopathy. An affected person who is improperly supervised, even for a very short period, may walk in front of a passing motor vehicle and become injured. As a result, the family may sue the driver. Innocent people in the environment may suffer property damages or physical harm caused by the affected individual. A person with Alzheimer's disease who is permitted to drive becomes a deadly menace to everyone on the highway, including himself. He may enter the exit ramp of an expressway and travel in the wrong direction, or he may drive on the wrong side of the road. Many suits have been generated by accidents caused by such drivers.

Family caregivers are often unable to accept the correlation between progress of the disease and its effect on the patient's recovery from surgery such as total knee replacement or hip fracture pinning. The condition of the patient with Alzheimer's disease may worsen as a result of the administration of anesthetic drugs. The patient may show little or no progress in physical therapy after surgery because of

Modified from Clinical Concepts, Southern Medical Association, 5(6):15-17, 1992.

his inability to remember to follow instructions for self-improvemen
As a result, the family may be angry with the physician and the car
facility because the family expects progress to occur when it is rea
sonable to anticipate little or no improvement. A lawsuit may ensue

By the time the patient can no longer be cared for at home an
has been moved to a nursing home, he may not recognize the family
Therefore the relatives may not visit him often. In one celebrated cas
in Houston, Texas, the family failed to keep the nursing home ir
formed of their whereabouts after a move. When the family could nc
be located to approve a hospitalization, the nursing home had th
court appoint a guardian. When the patient died and the family sti
could not be located, the guardian made arrangements for burial, nc
realizing that a burial fund had been a part of the patient's estate. On
month later the family arrived at the nursing home, after 6 month;
absence, to see the patient. They were very upset that the patient ha
died and had been buried without their knowledge. The nursing hom
was sued by the family. Although the insurance company's settlemen
for this case was a five-digit figure, the majority of the blame for thi
incident was clearly that of the patient's family.

Families often need to make a traumatic adjustment when thei
beloved relative must go to a nursing home. The guilt of the famil
may be manifested by long visits and a judgmental attitude towar
the caregiving nursing aides. This guilt is compounded if in the pas
the family promised the patient that a nursing home would never b
a part of his care. No family should ever make such a promise!]
creates too large a burden of guilt, which then affects the nursin
home and the physician, despite their best efforts.

In a case well known to me, a family paid extra personne
(usually off-duty nursing home employees) to stay with their belove
mother during certain hours of each day, even though there was n
legitimate need for this. One morning the patient was found to hav
large ecchymoses (bruises) around the knee. X-ray examination re
vealed a supracondylar fracture of the right femur. The family sue
the nursing home, citing negligence. There was no evidence t
support any trauma, although this condition was being presumed b
the patient's family. In the case analysis it was discovered that th
patient had a seizure disorder for which she had received no medica
tion for the preceding 4 years. It is medically accepted that a seizur
in a patient with knee contractures, as exemplified by the case here
may result in a fracture. This case was settled out of court.

PHYSICIAN PROBLEMS

Many physicians feel uncomfortable dealing with elderly people in general and patients with dementia in particular. Many of them were not taught geriatrics in medical school. Their lack of knowledge about how to give first-class care may lead to an aversion toward taking care of patients who cannot improve and are on an inexorable downhill course. As a result, physicians may tend to prescribe mild tranquilizers and other sedating drugs routinely for patients with dementia. Such medication may lead to confusion, agitation, disturbed sleep, a decrease in spontaneous muscle movements, and possible decubitus ulcers for these patients.

NURSING HOME PROBLEMS

Many patients with Alzheimer's disease eventually are placed in nursing homes. Many of these facilities rely heavily on reimbursement by the Medicaid program, and this compensation is notoriously low in many states. Because of the poor funding, most nursing home care is performed by nurse's aides, who are paid only slightly more than minimum wage. Often no promotions or career ladders exist for these aides, and therefore the turnover rate is great and the care given is of uncertain quality. Nursing homes must deal with high absenteeism rates among nurse's aides. However, the attendance rate may improve in the future as a result of the Omnibus Reconciliation Act of 1987, which decreed that all nurse's aides must undergo 70 hours of training and be registered. Turnover rates for nurse's aides across the country are approximately 50% per year. In Texas the turnover rate is about 250% per year. Therefore it is not surprising that most lawsuits involving Alzheimer's patients occur in nursing homes.

In an attempt to provide security and a higher quality of life for the second-stage or early third-stage patient, specialized Alzheimer's disease units have been set up in some nursing homes. These units provide areas for continuous walking or passage of wheelchairs. Two interesting lawsuits originated in this type of setting.

In the first case the patient managed to get to an infrequently observed outdoor area in his wheelchair. He then fell asleep and sustained severe sunburn on his bald head before he was discovered by a nurse's aide. The patient eventually died of resultant sepsis that began as an infection in the burn area. The nursing home was successfully sued.

In the second case two patients with late second-stage Alzheimer's disease were permitted to have play-type dough as a part of their occupational therapy program. For some unknown reason both patients decided to eat the dough, and they became asphyxiated when it lodged in their throats. This accident brought about a lawsuit over surveillance of patients in the nursing home, even though a nurse's aide was only 15 feet away at the time. At this writing the case is still in court and the outcome is in doubt.

Another source of nursing home problems involves conflicts between nurse's aides. As a result of a personal vendetta, in one instance an aide accused another aide of abusing a patient with Alzheimer's disease. The police and the department of health abuse investigation exonerated the accused nurse's aide, but the patient's family sued the nursing home.

Special equipment such as air beds with intermittently inflating channels can cause problems. Many types of these beds and mattresses are currently on the market to aid in the treatment of patients with decubitus ulcers.

In one interesting case a patient on such a mattress had the head of the bed elevated several degrees because of reflux esophagitis. The patient had third-stage Alzheimer's disease and was in the semifetal position. He was left unattended in the bed in one position for only a few minutes. When the aides returned, they found the patient on the floor. Because there was a conflict between the director of nurses and the nurse in charge of the patient, it was assumed by the administrator and the staff that someone had left the patient on the floor to make this nurse "look bad." Six days later, however, when the patient was left in the same position with the air supply to the bed running, the patient again slid off the bed. This time his head became caught in the siderails and he was asphyxiated. The local newspapers became aware of this incident and gave it wide publicity. A lawsuit ensued against the nursing home and the manufacturer of the bed. Because the nursing home had provided no in-service training for the personnel who operated the bed, even after the first incident, it was impossible for the defending lawyers to plan a useful defense for the nursing home.

In the preceding case the siderail restraints were an integral part of the problem, but in another case different restraints were the focal point of a lawsuit. The second case involved a patient with early third-stage Alzheimer's disease who was frequently restrained in a geriatric type of chair with a seat belt. The patient began to escape from this restraint frequently. Although the escapes continued for several months, the physician made no adjustment to the orders for restraints or medication. One day, approximately 20 minutes after being left alone, the patient was found dead, having been strangled by the seat belt as he tried to escape. The family sued the nursing home, which in turn sued the physician. The physician's malpractice insurance settled the case out of court. In many instances poor nursing care combined with poor physician care can create a bad outcome that results in a lawsuit.

Nursing homes are also responsible for preventing ambulant patients from escaping from the facility. In San Antonio, Texas, a nursing home patient with dementia who had escaped wandered onto a train track and was killed by a train. The family filed a lawsuit, claiming that the nursing home's efforts to confine the patient had been inadequate for his personal safety.

SUMMARY

To avoid increasing numbers of lawsuits against nursing homes, individual caregivers, and physicians, several changes need to be made. These changes include education of both caregivers and relatives, a better understanding of the limitations of institutional care, and improved reimbursement—all of which would enhance the quality of care in nursing homes. As every insurer of physicians and institutions knows, the key to prevention of lawsuits is good communication between care providers and care recipients or their family.

24

Stress in caregiving

Zebbie C. Tipton and Patrick Sloan

Caregivers are often referred to as "hidden victims" because they commonly experience more psychological and health problems than do people who are not caregivers. It has been estimated that for every disabled patient in a nursing home there are two or more impaired elderly living with or being cared for by their relatives.

In 1987 the Office of Technology estimated that for every American suffering from dementia at least three times as many family members are affected by the emotional, physical, social, and financial burdens of caring for these individuals. Symptoms of stress, depression, and chronic immunosuppression were found to be three times more common in caregivers when compared with a community sample of noncaregivers. Similarly, caregivers reported more health problems and used prescription medication and health care facilities more often than did noncaregivers. Furthermore, caregivers had limited social activities, fewer planned vacations, and fewer visits from friends; they attended church less often and were less satisfied with their quality of life than were noncaregivers.

Family members of persons with Alzheimer's disease often have been struggling with the problems of caregiving for months or years before seeking professional help. It is usually when the family can no longer deny or cope with the situation that they seek help. Although they or others may have suspected for a long time that Alzheimer's disease was the problem, the diagnosis often comes as a shock. It is common for the family to experience a gamut of feelings—denial, depression, anxiety, anger, and guilt—before and after the diagnosis is made. The family may have unrealistic expectations, for example, that the diagnosis is incorrect or that the patient can be cured.

Caregivers may be confused because the patient's condition may appear to improve at times before it worsens.

Formal diagnosis has the impact of making tangible the fears and concerns felt but often not fully realized by many caregivers—terminal illness, mortality, loss of the relationship with the person as he was known, and changing roles in the family (since the affected person can no longer function in his previous role). Often the diagnosis is made when the person requires more supervision, is no longer able to operate a motor vehicle safely, and when the family begins to realize that major changes in life-style or responsibilities are needed. It is at this juncture that professionals have an opportunity to make important interventions and establish a helping relationship with the patient and the caregivers because, as the disease progresses, the patient's impairments will diminish his abilities in self-care and will offer more challenges to the caregivers. These changes will be extremely stressful for the patient and his caregivers.

It is difficult for the family to adapt to the changing situation as the patient's disease progresses. The most common pitfalls encountered by families of persons with dementia include not allowing the patient to do what he is able to do, protecting the patient by limiting his activities, always putting the patient's needs first, using logic and reason to excess, and having overall expectations that are unrealistic.

STAGES OF ACCEPTANCE

Through our experience we have noted that most families go through various stages of acceptance of the diagnosis and the disease process, just as patients with terminal illness and their families go through the various stages associated with death and dying described by Kübler-Ross. Therefore we have found it helpful to use a model of stages of acceptance in describing the reactions of caregivers. We must keep in mind, however, that these stages may occur in varying lengths, will not necessarily take place in sequence, and may not have a clear demarcation.

Denial

The first stage, denial, is characterized by disbelief and minimization or avoidance of the diagnosis and its implications. Some families may remain in a state of denial for long periods until either the patient's symptoms or the persuasion of others (i.e., family members, friends, or professionals) helps the caregivers to finally accept the diagnosis. It is wise not to discourage caregivers from obtaining second opinions on the diagnosis, unless the patient has been evaluated several times and all the evaluations concur.

Resistance

At some point the patient and the caregivers may assume the attitude that they will not be affected by or let the disease "get to" them. This attitude is not unusual since fighting disease is a natural reaction for many people. This phenomenon commonly occurs among those individuals who enjoyed good health most of their lives or were particularly vigorous or active people. Professionals must encourage hope and determination but also must confront resistance tactfully. After the stage of resistance has been resolved or worked through affirmation can take place.

Affirmation

In this stage the caregivers accept help and begin to discuss their feelings openly. They start to address the difficulties involved in adjusting to their relative's disease and its ramifications. During this stage families become more interested in obtaining information about the disease and support services.

Acceptance

Acceptance occurs when the family and the caregivers learn to come to terms with the illness and its problems and go about living their daily lives. The attitudinal and emotional adjustment of the caregivers is usually obvious: they become more settled and matter-of-fact in dealing with the day-to-day struggles of caregiving. They also appear to be more accepting of the fact that their relative is not going to improve.

Growth

Personal growth and a renewed sense of hope and determination to carry on commonly follow the stage of acceptance. This process is reflected when caregivers begin to talk about the future beyond the patient's death, resume their lives or seek new directions, and show signs of having learned and grown from their experience. In working with caregivers for an extended time, professionals have the opportunity to assist them through these stages, helping them to communicate and deal with the subtleties of this process and providing a consistent source of information and support throughout the journey.

THE CAREGIVER BURDEN

A spectrum of potential negative effects of caregiving on the family is commonly referred to as "caregiver burden." Clinical experience, empirical research, and anecdotal reports have revealed that the burden of care is a complex and multifaceted problem in which stress arises from several aspects of caregiving and changes over the course of the disease. Areas of stress include health concerns, psychological well-being, financial problems, effects on social life, and the relationship between caregivers and patient. The patient's level of cognitive impairment or the length of time a caregiver has been giving care does not adequately predict the sense of burden.

Caregivers have reported physical and mental strains on their health. Physical demands include difficulties in feeding, inconsistency in the patient's sleep patterns, coping with wandering behavior, and cleaning up the results of urinary and fecal incontinence. The mental strains reported most often were financial problems, lack of support, and no personal time.

A number of burden scales have been developed that focus on health status, financial strain, social activity, and distressed feelings. It is interesting that one study using such a scale found that the burden was not related to the degree of the patient's impairment but to the frequency of visits to the patient by other family members.

Caregiving is typically a 24-hour-a-day job with little respite, and caregivers tend to ignore the physical and psychological signs of stress. Caregivers who were wives and daughters experienced higher levels of stress than caregiver husbands, regardless of whether the patient lived at home or in a nursing home. The highest burden scores were for children, siblings, or nonrelated individuals who lived with the patient, followed by wives who lived with the patient or cared for patients who were in a nursing home. The lowest burden scores were for husbands with wives in nursing homes.

Different sources of stress were reported by wives, husbands, and daughters. Wives caring for their husbands in the home said that they were more affected by changes in personality and aggressive behaviors in the patient. Husbands caring for their wives experienced sources of stress related to memory loss and wandering, personal hygiene, and conflicting demands on their time by others living in the same residence. Daughters who were caring for a parent at home were subject to high levels of stress, particularly in two conditions—when the patient was the father and when the disease progressed rapidly. Daughters' levels of stress also were associated with less life satisfaction, being employed full-time or part-time, or caring for others in the residence. Daughters caring for fathers were more burdened than daughters caring for mothers. It seems that women who are expected to care for others while caring for the patient are especially vulnerable to high levels of stress.

CHARACTERISTICS OF CAREGIVERS

Caregivers are most commonly female. They have sometimes been referred to as the "sandwich generation" because they care for both their aging parents and their children and family. In addition, they are often employed outside the home.

Caregivers have reported that the explanations given to them by helping professionals were too brief. They felt uninformed about likely future problems related to the disease, such as personality changes, pacing, and the inability to read or write. Many families stated that they were not prepared for these changes or for the extent of deterioration that would occur.

NURSING HOME PLACEMENT

Placement in a nursing home is more strongly associated with the caregivers' perceived burden than with the severity of the patient's dementia. Caregivers reported the following reasons for selecting nursing home placement: (1) being overwhelmed by full-time caregiving, (2) their own illness or declining health, (3) financial difficulties, (4) having no assistance with care, (5) no longer being recognized by the patient, and (6) the effects of the patient's disruptive behavior.

Caregivers' stress does not necessarily cease when the patient is placed in a nursing home. Their decision to refer their relative to a nursing home often has been made only after they have experienced considerable stress, guilt, and financial strain. When the family has negative attitudes about nursing homes in general or when the patient has expressed opposition to being placed in a nursing home, the guilt that ensues following placement is a significant stressor for the caregiver. Sometimes the family has even gone so far as to promise their loved one that they would never place him in a nursing home.

The caregiver also may experience the stress of feeling useless or inadequate after relinquishing the caregiver role. There is usually less guilt felt by the caregiver if the patient is admitted to a nursing home directly from the hospital or if the physician has expressed concern for the caregiver's declining health. A small proportion of former caregivers expiate their guilt by visiting the nursing home several times per week and essentially continue to assume the care of the patient. Nursing home costs place an extreme financial burden on caregivers, often resulting in depletion of retirement or other income that helps support the family. Professionals should be prepared to help caregivers cope with the physical and psychological consequences of caregiving both before and after nursing home placement.

CHANGING FAMILY ROLES

Helping families through the stages of diagnosis, acceptance, and long-term care requires that health care professionals recognize the ramifications of this traumatically stressful disease process and its effects on family communication. It is most helpful to approach the patient, the caregivers, and the disease process with an active interdisciplinary team effort that begins at the cognitive and emotional levels of the patient and family (see box, pp. 316 and 317).

Families vary considerably in how they cope with stress. Some families draw together, whereas others separate and avoid interaction, a process referred to as "disengagement." The most stress-resistant or balanced families are described as "cohesive." They interact without rancor, support one another, and are neither "enmeshed" nor "disengaged." The enmeshed family appears cohesive on first appearance, but later interviews reveal that one individual is making all the decisions and the others are passively agreeing without dissent.

PATIENTS AS SURVIVORS

The various stages of coping and intervention described in this chapter are directed toward the goal of reducing caregivers' stress. Researchers have not yet found a cure for Alzheimer's disease and most other forms of dementia. Patients, caregivers, and professionals are profoundly aware that those afflicted with this disease will not

STEPS IN HELPING FAMILIES

Family Network

Understanding the family network, which includes identifying the major decision-maker, financial resources, and major concerns, is important. Sometimes relatives who live far away can have a major negative impact unless they are included in the patient's care. A question such as "Are you sure there is no one else in the family who needs to be consulted?" from the professional can yield important information.

Education

Providing accurate information and educating the family about the disease process cannot be overemphasized. Although absolute predictions about the progression of the illness cannot be made, specific findings about the patient's medical condition, neuropsychological test findings, and the relative strengths and weaknesses of the patient and family need to be addressed.

Follow-up

Most families are overwhelmed when first confronted with the information that their relative has Alzheimer's disease. The professional who recognizes this situation will leave avenues open for follow-up by a statement such as "I realize that this is a lot to absorb today. I know you will have further questions. I can be reached during the day at this phone number."

Literature

There are a number of well-written pamphlets and booklets available from the Alzheimer's Association. These publications are designed to amplify and reinforce the professional's information since frequently relatives forget most of the salient points raised in the initial discussion.

Support Groups

Many families coping with the stress of caring for someone with Alzheimer's disease isolate themselves. The professional can assist them by explaining the vital role played by friends, religious organizations, and, in particular, Alzheimer's disease support groups.

Respite Care

Respite care refers to temporary assistance for caregivers so that they can rest. This rest can be done within the home setting, at a day care center, or in a nursing home. There are pros and cons to each choice. Caregivers who avail themselves of such services report an increased sense of well-being in comparison to those who do not.

Steps in Helping Families—cont'd

Psychological Therapy

Some families who are observed to be dealing poorly with the increased demands of having a relative with Alzheimer's disease will need psychological or psychiatric help. The rare instance in which a family member becomes highly disturbed will require individual referral. Most often, however, a problem-oriented approach is appropriate. This approach includes some self-disclosure on the part of the family members, but, more important, it involves identifying specific stressors and potential solutions. Working out a solution may be as simple as extracting a commitment from each adult child in the family to assume some level of responsibility for aspects of the patient's care. On the other hand, it may be as complex as having to analyze how one family member dominates, bullies, or belittles the others.

---

ultimately survive. Unlike the patient with a terminal illness, for whom some degree of prediction about time until death is possible, a patient with Alzheimer's disease often lives for a long time after the diagnosis has been made. This unpredictability is a major source of family stress and needs to be addressed within each family. Family members should be reminded that help is usually only a phone call away and that knowing whom to call is important. Those who have made the journey to acceptance and growth attribute survival to various factors–personal and spiritual strength, supportive families and friends, community resources, and professional consultation.

BIBLIOGRAPHY

All about Alzheimer's, *Newsweek*, Dec. 18, 1989.

Bamgarten M and others: The psychological and physical health of family members caring for an elderly person with dementia, *J Clin Epidemiol* 45:61-70, 1992.

Brody EM: Women in the middle and family help to older people, *Gerontologist* 21:471-480, 1981.

Chenoweth B, Spencer B: Dementia: the experience of family caregivers, *Gerontologist* 26:267-272, 1986.

Corelick E, George LK: Predictors of institutionalization among caregivers of patients with Alzheimer's disease, *J Am Geriatr Soc* 34:493-498, 1986.

Dellasega C: Caregiving stress among community caregivers for the elderly: does institutionalization make a difference? *J Community Health Nurs* 8:197-205, 1991.

Given CW, Collins CE, Given BA: Sources of stress among families caring for relatives with Alzheimer's disease, *Nurs Clin North Am* 23:69-82, 1988.

Gwyther LP, George LK: Caregivers for dementia patients: complex determinants of well-being and burden, *Gerontologist* 26:245-247, 1986.

Harper S, Lund DA: Wives, husbands, and daughters caring for institutionalized and noninstitutionalized dementia patients: toward a model of caregiver burden, *Int J Aging Hum Devel* 30:241-262, 1990.

Kiecolt-Glaser JK and others: Chronic stress and immunity in family caregivers of Alzheimer's disease victims, *Psychosom Med* 49:523-535, 1987.

Killeen M: The influence of stress and coping on family caregivers' perceptions of health, *Int J Aging Hum Devel* 30:197-211, 1990.

Kübler-Ross E: *On death and dying,* New York, 1972, Macmillan.

Lawton MP, Brody EM, Saperstein AR: A controlled study of respite service for caregivers of Alzheimer's patients, *Gerontologist* 29:8-16, 1989.

Lundervold D, Lewin-Lewis M: Effects of in-home respite care on caregivers of family members with Alzheimer's disease, *J Clin Exper Gerontol* 9:201-214, 1987.

Office of Technology: Losing a million minds: confronting the tragedy of Alzheimer's disease and other dementias, Pub. No. OTA-BA-323, Washington, DC, 1987, Government Printing Office.

Reifler BF, Wu S: Managing families of the demented elderly, *J Family Pract* 14:1051-1056, 1982.

Russell CS, Olson DH: Circumplex model of marital and family systems: review of empirical support and elaboration of therapeutic process. In Bagarozzi DS, Jurich AP, Jackson RW, editors: *Marital and family therapy: new perspectives in theory, research and practice,* New York, 1983, Human Sciences Press.

Zarit SH, Ory NK, Zarit JM: *The hidden victims of Alzheimer's disease: families under stress,* New York, 1985, York University Press.

Zarit SH, Reever KE, Bach-Peterson J: Relatives of the impaired elderly: correlates of feelings of burden, *Gerontologist* 20:649-655, 1980.

Zarit SH, Todd PA, Zarit JM. Subjective burden of husbands and wives as caregivers: a longitudinal study, *Gerontologist* 26:260-266, 1986.

25

Stress in nursing care

James M. Turnbull

Stress has been defined in a number of ways. Hans Selye, probably the most famous writer on the subject, referred to stress as a physiological state that results when an organism is influenced by a stressor. Stressors include both physical stimuli (e.g., noise, heat, cold, pain) and psychosocial stimuli (e.g., death of a relative, moving into a nursing home, changing jobs).

Human response to stressors is mediated, or influenced for good or ill, by personality, coping skills, and awareness of what is happening (insight). Thus the stress of the job of caring for a patient with Alzheimer's disease is influenced by a variety of factors. A nurse's resistance to the stressors of the job depends on what is happening in her own life. Marital squabbles, problems with children, and a death in the family all influence the nurse's ability to do the task at hand.

The following stressors in the daily care of the patient with Alzheimer's disease are associated with the patient: uncooperativeness, incontinence, heavy lifting, aggressiveness, failure to communicate needs, death, wandering, insomnia, and mood swings.

Most stressful of all is the lack of a time frame in which to make plans. With most other diseases there is a clear prognosis or course, but in Alzheimer's disease this certainty is lacking. A patient may live for 1 year or 20 years after the diagnosis has been made, and this uncertainty is very stressful.

Worker "burnout," which is the direct result of stress, is fairly common among people who care for patients with dementia. Burnout is a process that consists of three stages.

The first stage involves an imbalance between the resources and the demands placed on the resources. In other words, whether the individual is a health care worker or a family member, the demands placed on him exceed that person's ability to deliver.

For example, a nurse who is also the single mother of two teenage children undergoing their own life crises is suddenly faced with the illness of a co-worker who is unable to stay on the job. Doing the work of two while a replacement is being sought, she spends extra hours at work and is unable to attend to the needs of her children, and their surliness and uncooperativeness increase. The nurse finds herself experiencing demands beyond her ability to meet them.

The second stage is the immediate (short-term) emotional response, which is characterized by tenseness, anxiety, and feelings of exhaustion.

The third stage consists of several changes that the nurse undergoes, such as a tendency to treat the patient in a detached and mechanical fashion or a cynical preoccupation with having her own needs met.

Burnout is a transactional process. In other words, it is an interaction among many different factors—in this example, job stress, the strain on the nurse, and the way the individual accommodates psychologically to the whole process. What happens is that a previously committed person disengages from her work and develops a series of signs and symptoms.

Nurses are often unaware of their own health risks, despite being able to identify the major stressors in the workplace and at home, ethical conflicts about appropriate patient care, team conflicts, role ambiguity, workload, organizational deficits, marital and family disputes, and financial concerns. Young, recently graduated nurses, more than their experienced peers, relate that their number one stressor is the disparity between the ethical and practical values acquired in nursing school and the limits set by their daily routine, for example, not having sufficient time to listen and talk to a patient, having different priorities than the physician involved, and being left alone while feeling responsible for the well-being of every patient on the unit. Role ambiguity and role blurring also concern young registered nurses, who often view experienced aides, nursing assistants, and licensed practical nurses as more competent than themselves despite the fact that they have had less training.

INSTITUTIONAL SETTINGS

In an institutional setting, the signs and symptoms of burnout can be summarized in the following way:
- A highly resistant attitude toward going to work every day characterized by frequent tardiness or even absenteeism

- A feeling of being overwhelmed by the thought of going to work when getting up in the morning
- A sense of failure
- Anger and resentment, directed particularly at supervisors, the institution itself, and sometimes residents

These feelings are followed by guilt and blame, discouragement and indifference, social isolation and withdrawal, and negativism toward life in general.

Individuals who are burned out spend time watching the clock during the day and feel tremendously fatigued after work. They come home and are unable to engage with their own families in any meaningful way. Some individuals I have treated for burnout who worked with patients with Alzheimer's disease simply went home to bed and lay down for several hours, refusing to get involved with the family, meal preparation, or daily chores.

Another sign of burnout is a loss of positive feelings toward patients and a tendency to group them all together. The nurse is unable to concentrate on or to listen to what the patient is trying to say. Instead, the nurse has a feeling of immobilization, of being unable to do anything about the situation. The nurse then becomes cynical and blames the patients, as if it were their fault that they are in the institution. The burned out professional demonstrates a tendency to go by the book, to follow instructions in a mechanical way, and to do the very minimum.

A series of psychosomatic complaints follows, including insomnia, avoidance of discussing work with colleagues, and self-preoccupation. The nurse develops frequent colds, viral infections, headaches, and upset stomachs. She becomes rigid in her thinking and resistant to change.

Some individuals even become paranoid about their co-workers and the administration. At this stage the health care professional may use drugs and alcohol, begin to have marital and family conflicts, and show a heightened rate of absenteeism.

STRESS AND PERSONALITY

Individuals respond to the stresses of their job according to their own personality traits, what they want to do with their lives, what sort of experiences they have had, and the quality of their life outside work. Individuals who have an external locus of control are more vulnerable to burnout than those who have an internal locus of control. Individuals with an external locus of control project all problems onto the environment and see themselves as victims. This attitude applies to their whole life. These people are not self-motivated but require tremendous amounts of support to continue doing their job. Individuals who start out being extremely humanitarian tend to burn out in institutions such as nursing homes because they do not see their work resulting in changes for good.

On the other hand, individuals with an internal locus of control consider themselves the masters of their own destiny and require much less positive feedback to feel good about themselves. The person with an internal locus of control feels much less stressed about caring for a patient with Alzheimer's disease than his counterpart with an external locus of control.

Patients with Alzheimer's disease are rarely, if ever, openly appreciative of the tremendous amount of work done for them by family members and nurses. If being thanked, praised, complimented, and rewarded in some way is of paramount importance to a nurse's well-being, the professional will be sorely disappointed in caring for these patients.

Worker burnout always affects patient care. It is well known in psychiatric hospitals, on inpatient units, that high rates of suicide attempts, high rates of elopements from the unit, high rates of depression, and general misery among patients occur when the staff members are demoralized. This patient reaction, in turn, increases the degree of stress that the staff feels, and a vicious cycle has begun. Attempts to improve staff morale can turn this situation around. As staff members begin to feel better, patients begin to do better.

JOB SATISFACTION

Nurses who care for patients with dementia expect a certain degree of job satisfaction. Traditionally, nursing homes have not been high-prestige work locations; little glamour is attached to working in such institutions. In fact, sometimes the relatives of residents are abusive toward and demanding of staff members who are working as hard as they can. Although this type of abuse reflects guilt and shame, it is difficult for staff members not to take it personally. Therefore it is important for nursing homes to be able to attract professionals who are content to work with chronically ill individuals and who are not burned out and cynical about their job.

Much of the job satisfaction experienced by nurses comes from the professional endorsement they receive from their colleagues and the fact that they like their co-workers. The friendships that nurses make at work can create an important and highly sustaining support system.

PREVENTIVE MEASURES

How can burnout be prevented in people who care for patients with dementia? There are two aspects of prevention, individual and organizational. Interventions designed to alleviate burnout include the following measures:

1. Reduction or elimination of excessive job demands (people must not be expected to do more than they can reasonably accomplish)
2. Change in personal goals and preferences to meet the reality of the situation
3. Increase in the resources for meeting the demands of the task
4. Provision of coping substitutes for the withdrawal characteristics of burnout

Burnout in an institution is a highly contagious disorder and requires tremendous efforts to achieve reversal. Such efforts are often met with resistance by a pessimistic and thoroughly demoralized staff. In almost no other situation is the adage "an ounce of prevention is worth a pound of cure" so appropriate.

Since work overload is a common cause of burnout in many human service agencies, one of the simplest solutions is to hire more staff. However, the tendency to define the solution solely in terms of more resources has some very serious flaws. Researchers have suggested that tremendous changes in staff-patient ratios are necessary before any substantial change can occur if this is the only step taken. Burnout has many other causes, such as role conflict, ambiguity of the definition of work, lack of variety, lack of autonomy and control over one's work, and destructive norms. These factors have nothing to do with the number of people hired.

STAFF DEVELOPMENT

One of the first ways in which intervention is possible and necessary is staff development, which has three main objectives.

The first objective is to reduce the demands that workers impose on themselves by encouraging them to adopt more realistic goals. The second is to encourage the people who work in an institution to adopt new goals that might provide alternative sources of gratification. The third objective to help the workers develop new monitoring and feedback mechanisms that reflect short-term gains—for example, reporting regularly to someone who listens to what a person has been able to accomplish and getting positive feedback. Staff development should also seek to provide frequent opportunity for in-service training designed to increase role effectiveness. It should attempt to teach staff members coping strategies such as time-study and time-management techniques.

In my early work with patients, one thing that I learned was to be pleased with relatively small gains. New staff members frequently expect to be "world shakers" and to make tremendous gains with patients very early in their careers. Nurses who work with the elderly, particularly those with Alzheimer's disease, do not make many gains. Nurses must learn to work with patients' relatives, who may give some positive feedback. In-service training provides opportunities to learn new techniques for working out problems with patients or to redefine old techniques.

WORKLOAD

Another way in which burnout can be prevented is to change job and role structures. This type of change can be made by limiting the number of people for whom staff members are responsible at any one time. This approach is particularly important for settings in which nurses work with groups of ill patients. For example, suppose a program has 12 patients and 3 staff members. Either the staff members can share the responsibility for all 12 patients, or they can each take responsibility for 4 patients. Researchers have found that overload is lessened when responsibility is divided. Even though the patient-staff ratio is no different, there is less stress when the group is divided into three smaller groups, with certain staff members assigned to each one. The staff members also feel a greater sense of personal responsibility and control when they are solely responsible for a smaller number of patients.

It is important to select the mix of patients assigned to staff members carefully. In general, the most difficult patients should not be assigned to any one staff member. Newly hired staff members are often given the most difficult patients, but patients who are repugnant, resistant, abusive, very withdrawn, or severely disabled should not be assigned to new staff members who have had limited training.

TIME-OUT

Most jobs in the human service industry allow little opportunity for reflection and thought. Yet both are vital to effective coping. Time-outs, which allow staff members to escape temporarily from the demands of their role and to think about what they are doing without interruption, reduce overload and strain.

One way of ensuring that time-outs will be available is to use auxiliary workers such as volunteers or part-time employees. Vacation time policies also can be used to provide relief. Sometimes employees need to be encouraged to take frequent vacations. The tendency to allow vacation time to accumulate and to regard this time as a kind of status symbol should be discouraged. Flexibility must be maximized so that people can take vacations on short notice whenever they need to. At one mental hospital where I worked, one staff nurse boasted to me that during 3 years she had taken no vacation time and therefore had accumulated over 8 weeks. Although she probably thought that always being present made her a better nurse, this was not true.

Another difficulty arises over the matter of part-time workers. I think that part-time workers are extremely beneficial to an institution. Unfortunately, most institutions do not provide fringe benefits, such as medical leave, medical coverage, and insurance, for part-time workers.

COGNITIVE RESTRUCTURING

Women, more often than men, invoke self-induced stress by striving for perfection. The "type E" woman tries to be everything to everybody. Although difficult, it is possible to change this type of self-concept through repeated practice and affirming self-talk. This personality type is characterized by the following three features:

1. Seeing the world in terms of all black or all white. The person reasons: "I failed to prevent this patient's pressure sore. Therefore I am a total failure as a nurse." The antidote is to think in percentages. "I'm not a complete failure. Of the patients I am caring for, 85% to 90% have *not* developed sores."

2. Mind-reading or drawing conclusions about what other people are thinking based on supposition and minimal data. For example: "The administrator hasn't spoken to me for 3 days now. I must have upset her. She'll probably fire me." The antidote is to check the validity of the conclusions reached and change to a hypothesis that can be tested. For example: "I have no direct evidence that the administrator

is deliberately avoiding me. There may be any number of reasons that she hasn't talked to me. I'll break the ice myself and approach her."

3. Overuse of imperatives such as "should," "must," and "ought to." Imperatives signal the presence of inflexible and often unreasonable demands. Rules and expectations that involve demanding words require reexamination and challenge.

ADMINISTRATIVE SUPPORT

Administrators of institutions need to think about ways to make life more pleasant and work more enjoyable for their staff members. One such approach is career ladders. Lack of career ladders has been identified as a major source of dissatisfaction among people who are not professionally trained. Career stages do alleviate burnout by enhancing the individual's vicarious sense of competence.

Competence is one of the most important factors leading to self esteem on the job. However, human service work is expected to be more than just a job. It is considered a calling in the truest sense of the word. A nurse who prepares to work on an Alzheimer's unit or in a nursing home must do more than someone who wants to become a factory worker, bartender, or postal employee. The greater preparation is emotional as well as financial and intellectual. Yearly merit raises that are given automatically are not enough to reinforce a nurse's confidence. A true career ladder requires advancement in the form of meaningful increases in responsibility, privileges, and status.

Administrators and managers must know how to do their jobs properly. They must make their goals clear, develop a strong and distinctive guiding philosophy, and make education and research a major focus of the program in which they are involved. Most of all they must make the people who are working for them and with them understand that they are doing a good job. Although supervisors may feel uncomfortable saying "thank you" or acknowledging that their staff members are working hard in unusually trying circumstances, offering such support is one of their most basic and vital responsibilities.

PERSONAL SUPPORT

The value of friends who sustain a nurse outside the job is commonly underestimated. Yet the nurse's relationships with the key people in her life require time, attention, and cultivation. Sometimes outside guidance may be necessary to help the nurse develop and maintain these relationships. One of the most encouraging recent developments related to this goal is the use of cognitive therapy, in which individuals change the way that they define themselves by thinking differently.

BIBLIOGRAPHY

Chappel NL, Novak M: The role of support in alleviating stress among nursing assistants, *Gerontologist* 32(3):351-359, 1992.

Hein E: Job stress and coping in the health professions, *Psychother Psychosom* 55:90-99, 1991.

Kunkler J, Whittick J: Stress-management groups for nurses: practical problems and possible solutions, *J Adv Nurs* 16(2):172-176, 1991.

Monderine MA, Brown MC: A practical, step-by-step approach to stress management for women, *Nurse Pract* 17(7):18-28, 1992.

Selye H: *Stress in health and disease,* Sydney, 1976, Butterworths.

26

Elder abuse

Curtis B. Clark and Lynda Weatherly

THE "UNENDING FUNERAL"

Caregivers have referred to Alzheimer's disease as an "unending funeral." Cognitive function does not improve, and a general decline that may take 7 to 10 years can be expected, although some individuals have been known to survive as long as 20 years.

This disease does not discriminate according to race, religion, or socioeconomic status. Caregivers or the middle-aged children of the "sandwich generation" are caught between the competing demands of their own lives, such as responsibilities to their spouse, children, and work demands, and the burdens of caring for a frail elderly parent with dementia. Although a caregiver's intentions may be good, the strains of a relationship may develop over a long period and result in abuse. The theory of the stressed caregiver emphasizes the importance of stress in triggering abusive behavior and reinforces the idea that the care of a family member with Alzheimer's disease is, indeed, a "36-hour-a-day" burden.

Fulmer and Wetle suggest that 500,000 to 1.5 million cases of abuse and neglect occur annually in the United States. The incidence of elder abuse is difficult to determine, but it seems to lie somewhere between 4% and 10% of persons older than 65 years. The persons abused and the criteria used are not universally accepted, and this disparity may account for the variation in the prevalence of elder abuse from investigator to investigator. Unfortunately, the problem of elder abuse is likely to grow as the percentage of those afflicted with Alzheimer's disease increases along with population growth.

In addition to the theory of the stressed caregiver, the increase in dependency by patients who suffer from Alzheimer's disease seems to be a crucial factor in elderly abuse. Both abused and nonabused patients tend to have a similar degree of physical impairment; however, abused victims seem to have significantly greater cognitive

328

impairment. Thus recent onset of an increased dependency state places a patient with Alzheimer's disease at much higher risk.

Only recently has attention been focused on abuse of the elderly. In a 1981 report the U.S. House of Representatives Select Committee on Aging said that elder abuse was "alien to the American ideal." The report further stated that "the abuse of our elderly is at the hands of their children and, until recent times, has remained a shameful and hidden problem."

Elder abuse was not given attention until the 1960s, and significant work in this area was not begun until about 1978, when several investigators began studying the problem. Pillemer focused on 42 physical abuse cases, and researchers found that 64% of the abusers were financially dependent on their victims and 55% were dependent on the victim for shelter. Abusers are most likely to be close family members, usually an adult child of the patient. Sons more often than daughters are prone to feel that their parents should continue to support them in their old age, even though these parents may have developed mental impairment or physical disabilities. Since such sons continue to expect parents to provide the nurturing and parental role, they may be having difficulty accepting the fact that their parents are aging and failing in health.

DEFINITION OF ELDER ABUSE

Although definitions of the problem vary widely, the American Medical Association has proposed the following definition of elder abuse:

Abuse shall mean an act or omission which results in harm or threatened harm to the health or welfare of an elderly person. Abuse includes intentional infliction of physical or mental injury, sexual abuse, or withholding necessary food, clothing and medical care to meet the physical and mental health needs of an elderly person by one having the care, custody, or responsibility of an elderly person.

A number of terms have been used in an attempt to define and describe the phenomenon of elderly abuse. Elder mistreatment, elder miscare, old age abuse, nonaccidental injury, granny bashing, and granny battering have all been used by various researchers and writers. Regardless of the term that one chooses to describe this phenomenon, it must be remembered that elder abuse is a form of family violence that has some similarities with child and spouse abuse. Elder abuse and neglect are forms of family violence that have been addressed by elder abuse reporting laws in at least 30 states. Although child and spouse abuse have been recognized and addressed by the courts for many years, the same type of abuse of an elder citizen has only recently been recognized as significant, worthy of reporting, and requiring appropriate treatment, care, and prevention. One significant difference in the handling of child abuse and elder abuse cases is that the elder patient, if competent, can refuse protective services. At times the moral and legal aspects of abuse may be in conflict. If the elder person is incapable of giving consent, the physician should contact the adult protective services or local law enforcement for assistance. Individual rights must be honored at all times, and such a conflict is well suited to an interdisciplinary approach for resolution.

Examples of abuse are active physical assault, verbal and psychological assault, denial of rights, inadequate nutrition, misuse of drugs, financial exploitation, sexual abuse, and withholding of basic life resources. There may be a pattern of intrafamilial violence with reports to the authorities of children and wives also being abused.

Although uncommon, sexual abuse of the elderly does occur. Cases have been described in which a son who had previously been the caregiver of his mother was discovered sexually abusing his mother in a nursing home. In another case a male orderly in a nursing home who was responsible for feeding a cognitively impaired female, was observed fondling the patient at feeding time.

RECOGNITION OF ABUSE

Abuse of the elderly can be a most difficult diagnosis to make. Such behavior is not only problematic to determine; it is even more difficult to prove. There is a fine line between the normal deterioration of a patient and what can be a "bona fide" abuse situation. Physical signs of abuse, such as bruises, welts, and cigarette or rope burns caused by involuntary confinement, may be difficult to evaluate adequately because patients with Alzheimer's disease who have cognitive dysfunction are poor historians. Lacerations are more straightforward indications of abuse. Neglect can be subtle and more difficult to determine than gross physical abuse. Many abused elders are at home, and the caregiver who has charge and custody can keep the elderly person's injuries from becoming apparent to outside individuals. In addition, the person may be denied medication or even basic medical care. Since the abused elderly may have physical disabilities, he may be kept as a prisoner and not allowed to have any contact with the outside world.

Many times abusers are family members who have a fixed income and may transfer the funds of the patient to their own personal account for expenditures. Diversion of funds to the caregiver may sometimes result in denial of life-saving medications for the patient. In some instances such diversion results in a situation in which there are no funds to purchase the basic necessities. Such circumstances have been known to result in the death of the patient.

Gradually, but certainly, patients with Alzheimer's disease lose the capacity to perform any activity of daily living. The period of total disability and the need for total care may continue for years, and, contrary to popular belief, most of these patients are not placed in nursing homes. As patients become more dependent, they are more likely to be abused in some manner.

ABUSER PROFILE

Estimates suggest that 40% of abusers of persons with Alzheimer's disease are spouses and 50% are children or grandchildren. Since this disease is such a devastating and prolonged illness, caregivers play an extensive role in the day-to-day care of these patients. In abusive situations the average length of time that the relationship has existed is approximately 9.5 years. Studies have shown that the least socially active individual in the family is usually given the responsibility of caregiving.

The family members who are responsible for the care of the patient may not realize the tremendous time, effort, financial burden, and exhausting activity involved in the responsibility that they have accepted. Early in the illness caregiving that seems to be simple may develop into a complex, time-consuming, and stressful situation. There is evidence that abusers of women and children frequently perceive themselves as being powerless. Being perpetrators of abuse gives them a feeling of power and assists them in compensating for their feelings of inadequacy. This situation also may be true for elder abuse and neglect because the adult child is aware that he is not fulfilling the expectations of society. Striking out or inflicting abuse may make the person feel powerful again. In their book *The 36-Hour Day*, Mace and Rabins provide an excellent guide for families who struggle with the frustrations involved in caring for a family member with Alzheimer's disease and related dementia illnesses.

Caregivers find themselves not only caring for an elderly parent but also having the continuing responsibility of rearing and nurturing their children. The many demands made on their time and finances can bring great stress and exhaustion. Furthermore, many times there is only one parent in the family (due to divorce or death of the spouse), who becomes not only the breadwinner but also the care giver of several individuals in the family. The average woman can expect to spend at least 17 years of her life in nurturing and caring for her children and an equal number of years caring for her parents and or the parents of her spouse. Today men who are caregivers comprise about 30% of the caregivers, and this figure is gradually increasing. Women remain the caregivers of approximately 70% of the elder parents.

As the need for assistance with activities in daily living increases so does the danger for abuse and neglect. Caregivers may be experiencing other problems in the family, such as an unwanted pregnancy drug abuse, or another stressful situation that adds to the likelihood that they will become overstressed and strike out at the dependent parent. Role reversal can cause considerable difficulty in a relationship since the parent may not wish to give up the authoritarian role. The dependent child may find this conflict stressful and experience difficulty in accepting his role as the decision maker in the family. In such situations the relationships between parent and caregiver/child may have never been satisfactorily defined. The children may take on the responsibility of caregiving because of guilt, or they may be fearful that they will be harshly judged by family or acquaintances if they do not assume this role.

VICTIM PROFILE

The overwhelming majority of victims of elder abuse are women. The typical abused patient is a white widowed female over age 75 who is financially, physically, or mentally unable to live alone. She is more dependent on the caregiver for assistance with activities of daily living than her nonabused counterpart.

Abused patients have considerable difficulty accepting the fact that someone they have reared and nurtured is now abusing them. In addition, many barriers exist that prevent elderly citizens from asking for help. These victims may fear retaliation from the abuser. They also may feel shame, guilt, and failure and may blame themselves for the abuse. Since they feel guilt and embarrassment in admitting to society that this abuse is occurring, they may choose to suffer in silence. Many times patients stay in an abusive situation because they are fearful of the unknown. If institutionalized, they fear that they will be alone and are uncertain about the care they might receive. In other situations persons have grown up in an abusive environment and consider abuse to be a normal behavior.

With elder abuse being subtle and difficult to diagnose, it is made more problematic because many physicians do not take the time necessary to extract a detailed medical history. Although data obtained from the nurse's history may indicate possible abuse, the attending physician may choose to ignore or explain away the nurse's assessment by indicating that such injuries were most likely caused by an accident. Evaluating and diagnosing abuse can be a time-consuming and delicate process that requires a great deal of detective work. If a health care team member feels that abuse is likely, it is recommended that the individual be firm and kind but professionally persistent in communication.

Abused patients are likely to have special problems, such as incontinence, nocturnal shouting, wandering, or symptoms of paranoid delusions. Some of the traits generally thought to be prevalent among elders, such as stubbornness, hypercritical attitudes, and somatization, which may represent attempts by the patient to deal with his new dependency role, are also irritating to caregivers.

Rarely will the elderly patient be able to assist in the diagnosis of abuse. Patients with cognitive dysfunction or short-term memory loss cannot give an adequate history and may suffer from fear or emotional blocking. If abuse is suspected, the health care professional may find it necessary to initiate legal actions that are contrary to the wishes of the patient and family. The professional must be prepared to deal with abuser hostility, threats, or harassment. At times, even the patient may manifest such behavior.

In evaluation of suspected abuse, it is important to assess the patient for social and/or environmental isolation. For example, is the patient not allowed to have outside contact through visits to family and friends or even telephone calls? Such control by an abuser can be successful in keeping family, friends, and other contacts out of the home, ensuring continued isolation of the patient and very little likelihood that the abuse will be detected.

It is also important to assess the interaction between the patient and the caregiver. The caregiver's behavior can be evaluated by obtaining answers to two main questions: Is the caregiver overprotective or unwilling to leave the patient unattended with medical, paramedical, or nursing staff? Does the caregiver try to "shadow" the patient closely at all times to prevent appropriate questioning?

In addition to assessing the caregiver's behavior, it is important to note the patient's behavior, especially in front of the caregiver. The patient may appear to be nervous, fearful, apprehensive, or depressed. He may cringe, back off, or dodge as if expecting to be hit. The non-verbal communication between patient and caregiver also should be observed closely. If the caregiver manifests a disinterested attitude toward the patient by not obtaining medications or not securing adequate care at appropriate time intervals, this attitude may also be an indication that the patient is being abused.

PHYSICAL INDICATORS OF ABUSE

Injuries that have not been appropriately and timely treated and fractures that have not been set as necessary should arouse suspicion. Pallor, sunken eyes and cheeks, dry lips, excessive weight loss, and extreme dehydration may be indicators of abuse or neglect. All these factors must be closely monitored to achieve the appropriate index of suspicion that the patient is failing to receive the care that is necessary to serve his best interests. Many times it is necessary for the physician to see the patient on repeated occasions in order to establish a rapport. This approach reassures the patient that the physician is compassionate and caring and is willing to serve as an advocate for him without betraying his confidentiality.

Physical indicators that are particularly important to evaluate include bruises on the face, shoulders, or arms, burns from cigarettes or rope, lacerations, human bites, and fractures that have been left untreated. Bruises may be noted in different stages of the healing process. Welts may be observed, often inflicted by the use of belts or other objects used for corporal punishment. Rope burns, which are commonly found around the wrist or ankles, can arise from the use of crude restraints.

Although any member of the health care team can obtain a history, some individuals are better at investigating abuse than others. A calm, unhurried, persistent, empathic approach that is balanced with skepticism of stories told by the family is essential. Interviewers who have problems with confrontation and tend to believe everything that they are told should not be the investigators of cases of suspected elder abuse.

Severe head injuries have occasionally been inflicted by the caregiver, but unless an appropriate history is obtained, this type of injury can be easily explained as an accident. Emergency technicians and ambulance drivers are an asset in providing valuable information for evaluating the circumstances of injuries, as noted when they arrived at the scene. Repeated trips to the physician's office or emergency department should create suspicion of abuse, particularly if there is a pattern of going to a different physician on each occasion.

Food and fluid deprivation that result in malnutrition and dehydration are more subtle forms of elder abuse. There is a fine line between expected deterioration of the patient and failure to feed the person appropriately, either at home or in a nursing home. Therefore, before either condition is attributed to abuse, it is important to evaluate the patient adequately since many disease states can be responsible for malnutrition and dehydration.

AGEISM

In our youth-oriented society, the elderly are experiencing a great deal of ageism. Ageism can be defined as systematic stereotyping of and discrimination against people because they are old. It is comparable to racism and sexism, which are forms of stereotyping and discrimination based on skin color and gender. Older people are commonly categorized as senile, rigid in thought and manner, garrulous, and old-fashioned in morality and skills.

Many advertisements and cartoons depict the elderly as being roleless and useless to society. Such stereotyping may cause some persons to be inconsiderate of the elderly. Physicians and nurses can aid the elderly by understanding both their capabilities and their limitations and by acting as enlightened advocates for them.

Ageism encourages professionals to adopt a paternalistic attitude toward older people. Such an attitude prevents professionals from allowing elders the privilege of making their own decisions. Ageist attitudes are often shared by elderly people themselves and may help to explain their greater acceptance of abuse than would be expected.

A poor understanding of the process of aging and negative attitudes toward aging may lead to abusive and neglectful behaviors. Education is the key to dispelling the ignorance and negative attitudes associated with the process of aging and elder abuse. Many potentially explosive situations can be defused if knowledge of the existence and the causes of elder abuse is provided to society.

GERIATRIC ABUSE INTERVENTION TEAM

The geriatriatric abuse intervention team (G.A.I.T.) team was or
ganized in 1980 in a family practice setting. It consisted of member
from the community with interest, skills, and dedication to the service
of the abused elderly. The original team consisted of a medical edu
cator, a family practice resident, a medical student, a social services
student, two nurse clinicians, a pharmacist, a social service director o
the local department of human services, a psychologist, and a family
practice physician who served as both member and coordinator.

The assessment process of G.A.I.T. was very effective, providing
evaluations that proved to be accurate in diagnosis. The primary fo
cus of the team was the needs of the patients. No problems arose to
elicit intraprofessional conflict that could have defeated the purpose
of G.A.I.T. Professional services of the team members included accom
panying the client to court, when necessary, in order to serve as a
witness.

The composition of G.A.I.T. has changed over time since various
team members have completed their training, changed employment
status, or relocated to other communities. Three members of the orig
inal team are still active in the G.A.I.T. organization. However, the
team is now under the control of the local and state adult protective
services. It currently serves in a consultation role for an 11-county
area and becomes involved only in those cases in which there is no
apparent solution for the resolution of adult protective cases.

Although all cases of abuse and neglect may not be resolved, the
overwhelming majority of them can be stopped or reduced to livable
circumstances. Every geographical area has enough caring, moti
vated, and knowledgeable persons to form an effective team that will
care for the abused and neglected individuals.

The case examples presented in the boxes below and on p. 337 are
illustrations of abuse or potential abuse. These case histories, which
are composites of patients and families, are intended to reinforce the
significance of elder abuse as a social problem and to dispel the myths
associated with this problem.

PHYSICAL NEGLECT

A 93-year-old woman was brought to the emergency room in the early evening
hours. She was suffering from severe dehydration, had multiple decubitus ulcers on
her hips, shoulders, and heels, and was in a comatose state. Bruises were also noted

Physical Neglect—cont'd

on both breasts. Her son, who had her brought to the hospital, identified himself as the primary caregiver but admitted that he was gone a lot of the time since he worked. When asked why he had neglected to obtain medical care for his mother for so long, he stated, "She never complained. I never noticed anything wrong until my own son said, 'Dad, Grandma smells bad and looks really sick.' "

G.A.I.T. was never able to determine whether any of the injuries had been inflicted by this patient's caregivers. However, this case was one of the most severe examples of neglect that the abuse team had ever seen. After consultation between the police officers and the team, it was concluded that G.A.I.T. could not prove beyond reasonable doubt that intentional abuse had occurred. No criminal charges were filed.

UNINTENTIONAL MEDICAL NEGLECT

Mr. J. was a 67-year-old man who was admitted to the nursing home because he could no longer care for himself and had no available person who could assume responsibility for his care. The patient came to the attention of the nurse practitioner and physician team while they were making routine visits in the nursing home. Mr. J. was noticed because of the loud noises that he was making. On investigation, it was discovered that he was restrained but persisted in asking to go to the bathroom. The nursing home staff reported that the patient was suffering from agitation and had been given antipsychotic medication for sedation. It was soon discovered that his bladder was distended to a severe degree because of a nonfunctional indwelling catheter. When the bladder was drained, the patient became calm.

FINANCIAL ABUSE

A 65-year-old widower who lived alone was seen in the dementia assessment unit after referral by an interested neighbor. The patient was determined to be suffering from early dementia, but much of his conversation made perfect sense. He repeatedly said, "My kids are ripping me off. I don't know how, but I can sense it." When the unit social worker visited his house, she discovered that the man had written several checks for groceries in the past month, some amounting to $200, but there was no food in the house. It was learned that since the man could no longer drive a car, his son and daughter-in-law did all the shopping for him. However, they gave him only a fraction of the groceries that he was paying for and used the rest themselves.

SUMMARY

Elder abuse is not uncommon and may be perpetrated, sometimes unintentionally, by people who would not be suspected of such behavior toward their own loved ones. Often the circumstances that lead to abuse evolve insidiously and imperceptibly. As the relationship between the patient and the caregiver gradually deteriorates, a breaking point may be reached and abuse occurs. A seemingly trivial incident may elicit a disproportionately violent reaction from the caregiver and lead to abuse. Such an incident, however, must be viewed in the context of many other ones that may have irritated and frustrated the caregiver to the point of exasperation. Many of these incidents may be totally unrelated to the patient but may have increased the caregiver's level of stress.

This type of catastrophic reaction and resulting abuse can be prevented by encouraging caregivers to share their problems, thoughts, and concerns with professionals. Relief services are also recommended because they provide caregivers with an opportunity to have time for themselves and to be free to do as they wish without having to worry about their loved ones. Such services are available in most communities through the Alzheimer's Association, Area Agency on Aging, local social services, or local churches.

If the potential for abuse is to be minimized, the caregiver must be supported in his role. The burden of caring for patients with Alzheimer's disease should not be confined to the caregiver. It should be shared with other family members and with society as a whole.

BIBLIOGRAPHY

American Medical Association: *Elder abuse and neglect: diagnostic and treatment guidelines*, Chicago, 1992, The Association.

Bosker G: Elder abuse: patterns, detection, and management, *Resident Staff Physician* 36(3):39-44, 1990.

Bourland M: Elder abuse from definition to prevention, *Postgrad Med* 87(2):139-144, 1990.

Clark-Daniels C, Daniels RS, Baumhover L: The dilemma of elder abuse, *Home Healthcare Nurse* 8(6), 7-12, 1990.

Council on Scientific Affairs: American Medical Association white paper on elderly health, *Arch Intern Med* 150:2459-2469, 1990.

Forte D: Elder abuse: myth or reality? *Nursing the Elderly* 2(2):14-15, 1990.

Fulmer T, Wetle T: Elder abuse screening and intervention, *Nurse Pract* 11(5):33-38, 1986.

Mace N, Rabins PV: *The 36-hour day*, Baltimore, 1981, John Hopkins University Press.

Quinn MJ, Tomita SK: *Elder abuse and neglect,* New York, 1986, Springer Publishing.

Ross M, Ross PA, Ross-Carson M: Abuse of the elderly, *Can Nurse* 81(2):36-39, 1985.

US House of Representatives Select Committee on Aging: *Elder abuse: an examination of a hidden problem,* 97th Congress, Committee Pub No 97-277, Washington, DC, 1981, US Government Printing Office.

COMMUNITY SUPPORT

27

Caregiver education and support

Mary M. Lancaster

The outstanding memory I have is of being abandoned by the institutions I had formerly had a great deal of respect for. I had no information from the doctor or the nurse in his office. I inadvertently heard of the Visiting Nurses from the alternate doctor in the office. They saved what was left of my sanity by giving me information, as well as three days help a week. I was reassured that I was "doing it right." However, by the time I received this kind of help, I was seriously near the breaking point myself. I had also had eye surgery during this period. The medical and nursing profession seem to have an important gap in their education. Emotional and informational support seems to me of equal importance with medical help. I received absolutely no informational support. I stumbled onto what I needed accidentally, and who knows what was available that I never did hear of.

Sommers T, Zarit S: *Seriously near the breaking point,* Generations *10:30, 1985.*

In this age of increasing information about the needs of caregivers for education and support regarding their caregiving role, the preceding scenario should never occur. Although a cure for Alzheimer's disease is not yet known, there is an abundance of management information for the disease that caregivers need to carry out their role. Each member of the health care team must take it upon himself or herself to become involved in the educational process and to lend knowledge, expertise, and support to the caregiver.

Education of the caregiver is the basis of day-to-day management of Alzheimer's disease. Armed with the necessary information, the caregiver will have the sense of support and competence needed to continue as the primary caregiver. This information is vital for both family caregivers and health care personnel. To properly educate caregivers of persons with Alzheimer's disease, health care professionals must keep in mind the overall objectives of their educational efforts (see box, p. 344).

EDUCATIONAL OBJECTIVES

To provide information on the disease itself
To teach the fundamentals of day-to-day care and management
To offer information on relevant community resources

As educators, health care professionals must be knowledgeable about the burden of caregiving. In general, this burden first takes its toll on the free time (i.e., leisure and recreation) of the caregiver. As the disease progresses and the affected person's difficulties increase, the demands of caregiving begin to interfere with homemaking and work outside the home. Isolation follows, shrinking the caregiver's support system and adversely affecting his life satisfaction. In addition, the person with Alzheimer's disease may take out his own frustrations on the caregiver, making the task of caregiving more difficult and emotionally burdensome. In many ways the presence of an impaired person can severely disrupt the normal functioning of a family. For an in-depth discussion on the effects of caregiving on the family, see Chapter 24.

BASELINE INFORMATION

To address the educational needs of the caregiver appropriately, the health care professional must gather baseline information about the family. This step begins with an assessment of the family's current emotional state. If the family is in emotional crisis, the crisis must be resolved or diffused before learning can take place. Families who are still denying that a problem exists must first be assisted to accept that their loved one is impaired. Any other sources of stress impinging on the family (e.g., unresolved financial or legal matters) also must be handled. In addition, family members should be assessed for their ability to adapt to the ever-changing needs of the patient and other family members. If the family members are unable to adapt their daily lives to meet changing roles and demands, they may be unable to use the information provided or to apply it to their own situation.

Family caregivers must be able to understand the information they are given. All too often health care educators use language that is foreign to the caregiver. Asking the caregiver what he knows about the disease is a useful tool for determining the educational level of the caregiver. It is also an excellent way to find out what misinformation and misconceptions the caregiver may have about the disease and its management. Many of the problems and crises that caregivers experience evolve from misinformation or lack of information. Finally, it is important to find out if the caregiver is ready and willing to learn. If the caregiver still denies that the disease exists, he will not be ready to listen to what the educator has to say.

PLANNING

After the baseline assessment has been done, the caregivers must be involved in developing a treatment and education plan. Although many are overwhelmed and confused when they first seek help, their involvement in developing the plan helps them to set realistic goals for themselves and the patient. The gathering of the baseline assessment and the development of the treatment plan are educational in themselves for the caregivers.

During these first two stages (assessment and planning), the family is given small segments of vital information. This information helps to keep the caregivers functioning until they can be involved in more in-depth learning.

ONGOING EDUCATION

Initially, caregivers should be taught about the disease, its course and symptoms, and the available treatment. Since Alzheimer's disease has several stages, educational efforts should concentrate on the problems and behaviors associated with the stage in which the patient currently exists. Information about the later stages, although important and necessary, may not be relevant for the caregivers of a patient who has just begun to develop symptoms. Other topics that will need to be addressed include information about the aging process, common family problems resulting from the stress of caregiving, available community resources, and day-to-day management strategies. All this information should be provided over a lengthy period of time since research has shown that most people can absorb only small amounts of information at any one time.

A critical issue is the health care professional's own limitations as an educator. Each person has an educational style, and some teaching styles are more effective than others. It takes time and practice to communicate with people effectively and to relay information. No one has all the answers to Alzheimer's disease. Health care professionals must admit to themselves and to the caregivers that because of the nature of the disease, the solutions and management trials offered are not going to work in every situation. There will be times when "I do not know but I will try to find out" may be the best response. Getting back to the caregiver with an answer is particularly important for maintaining a good ongoing relationship with the caregiver, one that is centered on trust and honesty.

A continuing relationship with a health care professional offers caregivers a real sense of security. They need to feel that there is someone they can turn to with their questions and problems. Many times this individual will be a member of the nursing or social work staff. Most caregivers tend to have the feeling of not wanting "to bother the doctor with this trivial question," and they will turn to someone else. In general, caregivers need a piece of information or an answer to their question quickly; waiting until the next appointment with the physician may be too late. Caregivers should be encouraged to keep a notebook on hand for jotting down questions, incidents, and problems. This notebook can then be taken to the physician's office or to a support group meeting for review.

CRISIS PREVENTION

Anticipatory education, or information before the facts, is vital. It may help to alleviate unnecessary emotional conflict and strain if the caregiver has an idea of what the future may hold. Most families function on a fairly even plateau, and since patients with Alzheimer's disease tend to deteriorate slowly, the family usually has time to adapt to the successive stresses. However, as the disease progresses, each additional impairment that the patient develops adds to the overall strain on the caregivers and further reduces the harmony among family members. This situation can continue until at some point even a very minor additional stress (e.g., the patient loses the car keys) makes the situation intolerable and leads to a crisis.

Through anticipatory guidance and education, the caregivers can be assisted to delay or possibly avoid this type of spiraling crisis. When it is noticed that the patient has new problems or difficulties or that his condition is changing, providing the caregivers with information on what behaviors may lie ahead and providing them with management strategies can help allay their fear, frustration, and anxiety.

Caregivers must learn to react to the catastrophic and emotional over-reactions of their loved one by remaining calm and removing the person from the upsetting situation. Having strategies for dealing with problems in advance will help to achieve the desired response from the patient and the caregiver.

Education on behavior management of the patient is probably one of the most important and most difficult tasks because behaviors vary so greatly among patients. Well-meaning caregivers sometimes evoke a severe reaction from the patient through lack of information on how to deal with certain behaviors (see box below).

Caregivers also need to know that they are human, with feelings and emotions like everyone else. They need to know that, despite their best efforts, they may occasionally react to situations based on their own emotions instead of remaining calm. They need to know that this is a natural reaction to stress so that their guilt feelings about how

---

REACTION CAUSED BY CAREGIVER

Mrs. M. was diagnosed as suffering from Alzheimer's disease 4 years ago. She is currently living with her daughter and son-in-law. One Sunday morning Mrs. M.'s daughter instructed her mother to get dressed for church. Mrs. M. had always been able to manage dressing herself. Yet 15 minutes before they were to leave, the daughter found Mrs. M. crying in her room. She said that she did not want to go to church. The daughter, feeling rushed, insisted that her mother get dressed and go with the family. The daughter tossed three of Mrs. M.'s favorite dresses on the bed and told her mother to hurry. Moments later Mrs. M. began screaming and tearing at her clothes. The daughter, angry at her mother for being so slow and childish, took one of the dresses and began to help her mother get dressed. Mrs. M. immediately began to fight with her daughter.

• • •

Mrs. M. was suddenly faced with her inability to dress herself. If her daughter had been prepared for this event, both mother and daughter might have reacted differently. Instead of rushing her mother, who was already distressed, the daughter could have simply asked her mother what was wrong and if she needed help. In addition, by forcing a choice on her mother (which dress to wear), the daughter added to the stress. The whole situation may have stemmed from Mrs. M.'s inability to decide what to wear. To avoid the confrontation that eventually occurred, it probably would have been most effective to redirect Mrs. M.'s attention to some other task, such as applying makeup or fixing her hair. Once her mother had calmed down, the daughter would have been able to help her get dressed.

they reacted can be minimized. Through anticipatory education and helping caregivers to analyze their interactions with the patient, they can be assisted to see that their behavior may be contributing to the patient's troublesome behaviors.

CORRECT BALANCE

Well-intentioned caregivers can effectively block the patient's competence and capabilities by expecting too little from him. Being too helpful can promote apathy, dependence, and deterioration in the patient. This negative effect can be seen not only in patients with dementia but also in patients who have had a stroke or who suffer from a chronic condition. For example, if the patient begins to have difficulty feeding himself, the caregiver may take over and feed him instead of giving the patient the opportunity to feed himself in an adapted way. Devices that make eating easier are available, and the caregiver must be helped to be accepting about spilled food and soiled shirts and to provide the patient with "finger foods." The caregiver may need guidance about ways to allow the patient maximum self-sufficiency while offering just enough assistance to compensate for his real limitations. A delicate balance between overcompensation and undercompensation must be achieved. Allowing the patient to continue to perform as many functions as possible, even in adapted ways, helps to maintain the patient's sense of self-esteem and pride.

OVERINVOLVEMENT

Overinvolvement in the care of the patient commonly occurs with a caregiver who is trying to compensate for the patient's disabilities and the loss of his role in the family. When involvement with the patient is carried to an exaggerated extent, the caregiver may sacrifice many aspects of his own personal health and welfare. In such a situation the caregiver becomes the "second victim" of Alzheimer's disease. Overinvolvement can lead to emotional and physical breakdown of the caregiver. Educating caregivers about this tragedy and explaining that they must take care of themselves is of grave importance. Becoming emotionally and physically drained can actually hinder caregiving and interaction with other family members and the patient. Offering the caregivers stress management strategies provides them with tools that they can use to keep themselves well balanced.

ROLE REVERSAL

Role reversal and changes in family structure are likely to occur with Alzheimer's disease. The caregivers should understand that they may need to assume some of the roles of the person who has the disease. Assuming the patient's role and place within the family can be very difficult and emotionally charged. Some caregivers may need to learn how to manage the day-to-day business of cooking, cleaning, washing, and running a household. Others may need to be educated on financial and legal business, taking care of the car, or finding a job. Through education caregivers can be helped through these changes and instructed in ways to lessen the impact of these changes on the patient and the other family members.

INFORMAL VERSUS FORMAL TEACHING

Education can be carried out both informally and formally. Family meetings with health care professionals are good mechanisms for informal teaching. These meetings offer a good way to identify the specific behavior that is most troublesome, how the family members explain the behavior, what solutions they have tried, and the effectiveness of their solutions. Family meetings are also an opportune time to discuss more sensitive issues such as legal and financial matters, wills, burial arrangements, and advance directives. These matters must be discussed, and the assistance of the health care team makes the discussion much easier. Informal education also can be carried out at the bedside, in the home, over the telephone, or walking down the street. Role modeling is an excellent way to provide this type of education. Having staff members and caregivers work side by side, for example, a public health nurse in the home or a staff nurse in a hospital or nursing home, affords each the opportunity to learn from the other. It must be remembered that education is a two-way process. For instance, the caregivers may be able to provide information about the best way to gain the patient's cooperation, and nursing personnel can teach caregivers how to incorporate exercise into the patient's daily activities. Usually the caregiver has taken care of the patient at home for quite some time and is very knowledgeable about the idiosyncrasies of the patient. Health care professionals must be accepting of the caregiver's knowledge and experience and apply this information to care planning. The caregivers should be encouraged to contribute to care plans. Frequently they have already discovered a solution to a problem that may be perplexing to staff. It must be remembered that the treatment and management of Alzheimer's disease are still in the early stages of research and that much of what is accomplished in these areas is done through trial and error.

Formal education can take place in support group meetings, seminars, training classes, and in-service programs. Many of the same topics are covered in formal classes; however, these classes do not generally allow as much demonstration, feedback, and interaction as informal teaching. A critical area of education is continuing education about aging in general and other problems or diseases that the patient might have. Caregivers will need instruction about how to assess the patient for acute problems such as infections, pain, constipation, or fractures. They must be taught that the cognitively impaired person may not be able to relate signs and symptoms of acute conditions and that therefore continuing physical assessment of the patient is vital.

WRITTEN INFORMATION

Education can be accomplished through verbal interaction, that is, by sitting and talking. However, verbal information must be supplemented and reinforced with written information. Numerous pamphlets and books are available through the local Alzheimer's Association, and this information should be provided to the caregivers. These resources are another vehicle for presenting necessary material, and they provide hands-on information that the caregiver can take home. For the caregiver, written material such as a pamphlet serves as a reminder of the information that was presented verbally and can be used as a step-by-step guide.

Written information can be individualized to meet the patient's and the caregiver's needs by adding specific instructions and information in the margins of the pamphlets and books. Research has shown that much of the initial information the caregiver receives from the physician or other health care professional is lost because the individual is overwhelmed and confused by the diagnosis and his attention is not focused on learning. Pamphlets and books allow the caregiver and other family members to review the information at home when they are more attentive and can absorb the information at their own rate.

Education of caregivers goes beyond learning about day-to-day management of the patient and the disease. It also must involve education about what can happen to the caregiver and other family members and the impact of caregiving on family roles. Caregivers are often very interested in possible cures and treatments and there fore are susceptible to media coverage of "breakthroughs" and "cures." Caregivers need to recognize that the media frequently sensationalize this type of information. Caregivers must be informed that some people will take advantage of their desperate situation. It is vital to encourage caregivers to investigate any advertisements carefully and to discuss them with the patient's physician. They should be made aware of side effects that can result from experimental treatments and the quality-of-life issues involved in the treatments. Caregivers need to know that it takes many years for research to be completed on a new drug and for that drug to be approved by the Food and Drug Administration and available to the public. However, there are legitimate research programs in progress throughout the country, and frequently subjects are needed for these studies. Caregivers and patients should have the option of becoming involved in such studies if they meet the criteria. Involvement in these programs offers the caregiver a sense of doing something to help his loved one and others who may be afflicted with Alzheimer's disease in the future.

SUPPORT GROUPS

Education and support should not be separated. They are currently the backbone of patient and caregiver management. Caregivers need the support of others to be able to assimilate the information they have received and to put it into practice. Research has demonstrated that providing information alone, without meeting the needs of caregivers for support, is not nearly as successful as a combined approach. A study conducted at Duke University in the early 1980s demonstrated that the mere *feeling* of being supported had a greater impact on reducing caregiver strain than the amount of actual outside help (support) the caregiver received. Support groups have a long history of providing mutual aid to their members through the sharing of common experiences and problems. Members of support groups develop ties with one another based on the commonality of their emotions and experiences. If caregivers, through the use of support groups, can openly discuss their problems and share their emotions, the physical and mental stress of providing care can be eased and may allow the family to provide in-home care for a longer period.

Most support groups develop from the caregiver's need to receive information and emotional assistance. Because no one person possesses all the knowledge or answers to Alzheimer's disease, the support group serves as an open educational forum for both caregivers and interested health personnel. The informal format of most support groups allows everyone to learn from one another. For example, I have gained a great deal of knowledge about caring for victims of Alzheimer's disease and the associated stresses on caregivers from leading a support group for the last 10 years. Support groups provide the time needed for relaxed discussion and problem-solving.

The members of a support group have varying roles within their community and their family. They may be spouses, adult children, grandchildren, health care personnel, and friends of persons with Alzheimer's disease. However, the common interest and caregiving experience place the group members on a similar level. A technical aspect to be considered in developing or participating in a support group is the caregiver-patient relationship. The varying relationships give rise to different needs, viewpoints, and emotions on the part of the caregiver and the patient. Separate groups may be necessary to meet the needs of the various members adequately. Having separate groups can help avoid a potentially disturbing situation, such as having the spouse and the adult child of a patient attend the same meeting. In this situation the freedom to express true feelings and emotions may be hindered by the presence of the other family member. In one of the support groups I was involved in, the daughter of a patient was attending the same group as her father (the mother was the patient with Alzheimer's disease). One day the daughter came to me to express her concern about attending the group. She felt unable to discuss her feelings and emotions openly and honestly within the group because they differed from those of her father. Since her father was the primary caregiver, she felt that she had to let him do what he considered best. After a lengthy discussion, she decided that she would attend another support group for herself and also attend the one with her father in order to keep the lines of communication with him open.

Health care personnel, who may or may not have personal experience with family members who have Alzheimer's disease, often become involved in support groups. These individuals can provide informational and administrative support to the group. They can lend their expertise and knowledge of various fields at the meetings. Some health care personnel attend groups to share their own frustrations and problems in providing care to Alzheimer's patients in the institutional setting. These health care personnel face many of the same problems that family caregivers do, in addition to different ones. It must be remembered that, regardless of education and experience in caring for Alzheimer's patients, no one "knows it all" or is immune to the stresses and strains of caregiving.

Participants of support groups work through various stages of involvement in the group. Initially, the interactions may be superficial and may center around telling one's own story. Most often, new members attend a group session because they are in need of an immediate solution to a problem or some information. However, after attending the meetings several times, they begin to develop a basic trust and understanding with the group. As this process takes place, the members grow and mature and begin to recognize and discuss their personal feelings, emotions, and needs. Eventually this type of discussion enables the members to assist one another in identifying and resolving problems and conflicts. This aid is the ultimate goal of a support group. While receiving support and guidance from one another, the members are also lending support and guidance to others.

Support groups provide caregivers a time to bring before the group a new problem that they have encountered. Frequently someone in the group has experienced the same situation and suggests a solution. Support groups also offer a time for socialization for the caregivers. Isolated by the necessity to be with their family member 24 hours a day, caregivers rarely have an opportunity to visit with other people. In addition, if the patient is in an advanced stage of the disease, his ability to carry on a real conversation has been lost. Therefore the caregiver may have little chance to make conversation. I frequently hear caregivers say: "I went so stir crazy that I was talking to pictures, the walls, anything that would stay still and listen. If it had not been for this group, I don't know if I could have held out much longer." The support group offers a time to meet new people, to develop friendships, and to "get away." In addition, having the meeting revolve around the care of the patient can help ease the guilt caregivers may feel about having taken time for themselves.

Although support groups have been shown to increase the caregiver's sense of support and knowledge about Alzheimer's disease and community resources, there are potential dangers associated with support groups. Of primary concern is that some support groups may begin to view themselves as a replacement or substitution for professional psychotherapy. Lay support groups cannot provide professional counseling or psychotherapy. However, through a caregiver's interactions and participation in a group, individuals who are experiencing a great amount of stress or difficulty in coping can be identified and referred for professional help.

A second potential danger is one of dependency, either on the group itself or on the leader of the group. In the event that the group disbands, caregivers who have become totally dependent on the group for information, social interaction, and support may find themselves at a great loss. This sort of dependency also can focus on the group's leader. Because of their high visibility in the group, their interest in combating Alzheimer's disease, and their knowledge of the disease, leaders are primary targets to take on the responsibility of the other group members. Many group leaders have said that a great deal of their time and energy are expended on the problems and needs of the group members. This situation can be especially dangerous if the group leader is also a caregiver, one whose time and energy are already stressed to the maximum. This additional responsibility can lead to burnout for the leader, which leaves the group members stranded. Through careful guidance, group members can be helped to find additional sources of support outside the group.

Sometimes group members become so familiar with the behavior, problems, and symptoms of the disease that they tend to forget the individual nature of the disease and start "packaging" information and solutions. Yet this type of packaged information may not apply to another person's situation. Along with this familiarity comes the potential for diagnosing friends and relatives and recommending treatment plans without the proper medical evaluation, diagnostic workup, and advice.

When a group has been meeting for a long time, a great deal of freedom, trust, and understanding develops among the group members. They can talk openly about their problems and what may be ahead for them. They are able to discuss life and death issues, funeral plans, and autopsy. This openness is one of the goals of the group, but it must be kept in mind that newcomers may be present at any meeting. New members of the group, especially if their family member has been diagnosed only recently, become easily frightened when they hear about the problems that caregivers and patients face in the last stages of the disease. They may become so overwhelmed with fear and distaste for the group that they never return. One solution is the development of a group for newcomers. If this approach is not reasonable, new group members can meet with an especially sensitive caregiver while the regular group members continue with their discussions. There is a delicate balance in trying to meet all the needs of caregivers who are experiencing various stages of the disease at the same time.

It is important for group leaders to have training in group dynamics and process. Situations arise that can be highly disruptive to the group. Some individuals talk so much that they monopolize the entire time, whereas others never get the opportunity to speak. The group leader will need to know how to draw a very shy, quiet individual into the conversation. Arguments can develop, and some members may appear particularly hostile or abusive. Involving group leaders in workshops on group process can help them feel more comfortable with their role and more assured in handling difficult situations. In addition, professionals who are experienced in group process can be called on to assist in the meetings.

Developing, implementing, and leading support groups can be stressful and time-consuming. Yet there is great satisfaction to be found in taking this responsibility. Support groups are for all the members. Involving caregivers in a useful and meaningful interaction with one another yields personal rewards for everyone.

SUMMARY

Environmental press theory suggests that persons adapt and cope with situations based on their knowledge and experience. If the amount of environmental press (stress and demands) outweighs the competence (knowledge and experience), the person is likely to be unable to handle the situation. This inability to cope for a long time can result in the physical or psychosocial breakdown, or burnout, of the individual. However, if the person possesses the competence to handle the situation, his stability can be maintained and tragic results can be prevented. This theory parallels the lives of many caregivers and the current management strategy for the disease. Through education, experience, and support, caregivers can be provided with the competence needed to handle the various problems and situations that arise within their lives and the lives of their loved ones. All members of the health care team must work together to provide caregivers with the information and support they require to continue their job as the number one providers of care to victims of Alzheimer's disease.

BIBLIOGRAPHY

Anderson KH and others: Patients with dementia: involving families to maximize nursing care, *J Gerontol Nurs* 18(7):19-25, 1992.

Buckwalter KC, Abraham IL, Neundorfer MM: Alzheimer's disease: involving nursing in the development and implementation of health care for patients and families, *Nurs Clin North Am* 23:1-9, 1988.

Davies HD: Dementia and delirium. In Chenitz WC, Stone JT, Salisbury SA, editors: *Clinical gerontological nursing: a guide to advanced practice*, Philadelphia, 1991, WB Saunders.

George LK: The burden of caregiving: how much? what kinds? for whom? *Adv Res* 8(2):2, 1984, Duke University.

Given CW, Collins CE, Given BA: Sources of stress among families caring for relatives with Alzheimer's disease, *Nurs Clin North Am* 23:69-82, 1988.

Gwyther L: Caregiver self-help groups: roles for professionals, *Generations* 53:37-38, 1982.

Hayter J: Helping families of patients with Alzheimer's disease, *J Gerontol Nurs* 8(2):81-86, 1982.

Katzman R, Jackson JE: Alzheimer's disease: basics and clinical practice, *J Am Geriatr Soc* 39:516-525, 1991.

Kuhlman GJ and others: Alzheimer's disease and family caregiving: critical synthesis of the literature and research agenda, *Nurs Res* 40:331-335, 1991.

Lawton MP: Competence, environmental press, and the adaptation of old people. In Lawton MP, Windley PG, Byerts TO, editors: *Aging and the environment: theoretical approaches*, New York, 1980, Garland STPM Press.

Ory MG: Families, informal supports, and Alzheimer's disease: current research and future agendas, *Res Aging* 7:623-644, 1985.

Powell L, Courtice K: *Alzheimer's disease: a guide for families*, Reading, Mass, 1986, Addison-Wesley.

Roberts BL, Algase DL: Victims of Alzheimer's disease and the environment, *Nurs Clin North Am* 23:83-93, 1988.

Shibal-Champagne S, Lipinska-Stachow DM: Alzheimer's educational/supportive group: considerations for success—awareness of family tasks, preplanning, and active professional facilitation, *J Gerontol Soc Work* 9(2):41-48, 1985-1986.

Simank M, Strickland K: Assisting families in coping with Alzheimer's disease and other related dementias with the establishment of a mutual support group, *J Gerontolog Soc Work* 9(2):49-58, 1985-1986.

Smith CW Jr: Management of Alzheimer's disease: a family affair, *Postgrad Med* 83:118-120, 125-127, 1988.

Sommers T, Zarit S: Seriously near the breaking point, *Generations* 10:30-33, 1985.

Stolley JM, Buckwalter KC, Shannon MD: Caring for patients with Alzheimer's disease: recommendations for nursing education, *J Gerontol Nurs* 17(6):34-38, 1991.

Tanner F, Shaw S: *Caring: a guide to managing the Alzheimer's patient at home*, New York, 1985, Alzheimer's Resource Center.

Zarit S, Todd P, Zarit J: Subjective burden of husbands and wives as caregivers: a longitudinal study, *Gerontologist* 26:260-266, 1986.

28

Social services

Patricia S. Brown

Because Alzheimer's disease is a slow, insidious disease, caregivers often become so involved in caring for their patient that they forget to look to the social support system provided by their community. As the patient with Alzheimer's disease gradually deteriorates, the demands on the caregivers gradually increase until the situation becomes unbearable. Often, caregivers are embarrassed to seek the help that may be available. They may have had no experience with social services and may equate them with "being on welfare." Also, they may resent having strangers enter their homes or may feel that by involving a public agency they are being disloyal to their loved one.

It is imperative for health care professionals to know about the social services and benefits available to the elderly. Much has been said about the "fragmented" systems that abound, and often when people do seek help, they are confused about where to go. This situation is especially true for caregivers of the patient with Alzheimer's disease.

One readily available resource is the Area Agency on Aging (AAA). The federal agency, the Administration on Aging (AOA), distributes money provided through Title III of the Older Americans Act to each state based on its number of residents 60 years of age or older. The state units on aging then distribute the funds to each AAA with the proviso that the money be used solely for the benefit of people 60 years of age or older, with emphasis on serving those in the greatest social and economic need. There is no charge for programs offered under the Older Americans Act; however, everyone is encouraged to contribute to the programs so that more people can be served. Although each AAA is autonomous, certain services for the homebound elderly are available in most communities. These include home-delivered meals, a homemaker program, personal care and chore services, minor home repairs, transportation, legal assistance, a long-term care ombuds man, respite care, adult day care, hospice, and senior center services such as telephone reassurance and friendly visiting.

Most AAAs use a social model of case management as the entry point for Title III services for the frail, health-impaired elderly. A case manager will make a home visit and, through the use of an assessment tool, will determine what services are necessary to enable that person to remain at home. A care plan is developed and approved under the guidance of a case manager (usually a health professional with an M.S.W. or an R.N.), services are ordered, and a follow-up phone call is made to determine whether the service(s) is being received. Reassessments are conducted every 3 to 6 months, depending on the condition of the client, to verify continued need. The Title III case management program also provides information and referral services to assist older people in finding the solutions to their problems. In some states the AAA directly provides case management, whereas in other states the AAAs are required to contract with other agencies.

For information on how to access senior services in any area of the country, there should be a telephone listing under "Area Agency on Aging." If there is no such listing, the local senior citizens center should be called. For those areas having neither of these agencies there is a national toll-free number, sponsored by the Administration on Aging, called Eldercare Locator. To receive information on senior services in a specific zip code area, the toll-free number is: 1-800-677-1116.

NUTRITION PROGRAM

A few years after the Older Americans Act was passed in 1965, a nutrition program for the elderly was started. Since that time the nutrition program has become the largest funded service delivered through the AAA network. Both congregate and home-delivered meals which operate out of senior citizens centers and other community buildings, must provide one third of the required daily dietary allowance for older people. In addition to the nutritional benefits, the congregate meals program provides seniors the opportunity to socialize with their peers. The focus of the home-delivered meals program is to enable the frail elderly person to remain at home as long as possible.

Programs may vary from state to state, but most Title III nutrition programs provide meals 5 days a week, usually at noon. In larger metropolitan areas breakfast, evening, and weekend meals also may be available. Low-sodium menus are usually provided, and in areas with large populations of ethnic elderly, the menus there will reflect those tastes. Special diets are sometimes available.

Eligibility for the nutrition program is the same as for all Title III programs, with the added eligibility requirement for home-delivered meals being that the person must be defined as "homebound," according to each state's definition of that term. A complete assessment is performed to establish the need for home-delivered meals. These meals are also available to the caregiver as a form of respite from the many duties that the caregiver has assumed in caring for a spouse or relative. The Administration on Aging also has approved home-delivered meals for the growing number of adult dependent children of frail, homebound elderly people who receive meals.

Various ways have been devised to provide home-delivered meals to as many seniors as possible. For those who live in remote areas or where delivery is not readily available, a packet of five frozen meals may be delivered once a week or every 5 days (if the person also receives weekend meals). Sometimes toaster ovens are provided to the homebound person if there is no oven in the home.

Other nutrition programs are available in many communities. Probably the best known ones are those sponsored by church groups, generally referred to as "Meals on Wheels." The aging network usually coordinates with these programs to avoid duplication. There are also numerous agencies and programs that sponsor "food pantries" or "food banks" that provide food on an emergency basis.

HOMEMAKER, PERSONAL CARE, AND CHORE SERVICES

Like home-delivered meals, this group of in-home services is one of the most important in enabling frail, health-impaired elderly to remain at home. The homemaker may do housecleaning, laundry, grocery shopping, and meal preparation and run errands. Personal care may be provided by homemakers, depending on their level of training. Most Title III homemakers can provide assistance in bathing, dressing, and hair care.

Chore services may include heavy cleaning and outdoor work such as bringing in wood or coal and doing yardwork. Minor home repairs may be available, often through the use of volunteers. Repairs to steps, construction of wheelchair ramps, and replacement of window and door screens are examples of eligible minor repairs. Probably the most difficult request received is for roof repairs, and usually only minor repairs can be made. If the roof should need replacing, the individual is referred to a reputable company in the hope that the firm will perform the work at a reduced fee.

Closely related to home repairs is the weatherization program, which is federally funded under another entitlement. This program provides income-eligible people with storm windows and insulation for their homes to cut down on their energy losses.

Eligibility for the Title III programs is based on age and need. However, it is unusual to find programs for this range of services without a waiting list. Contributions are encouraged so that more people can be served. In communities that use volunteers to provide similar services, there are organizations such as Shepherd Centers, Good Samaritans, and Carpenter's Helpers.

RESPITE, ADULT DAY CARE, AND HOSPICE

According to the Brookdale Foundation's guide to starting a respite program for people with Alzheimer's disease and their families, a respite program is a service that provides family caregivers with intervals of relief from the demands of their caregiving roles. However, respite is not a new idea. Informal respite has been provided for many years through the informal support system—relatives, friends, and neighbors who are willing to come in and "sit" with the patient while the caregiver runs errands, goes to the doctor, or takes time for himself.

Today there is a growing need for structured respite services. Some hospitals and nursing homes provide overnight, weekend, or longer respite care in their facilities. This service allows the caregiver to go out of town or have some free time. Other programs, sometimes referred to as sitter/companion services, are usually "private pay" and can be expensive. The Alzheimer's Association has provided numerous grants to area chapters to establish in-home respite care programs. Some of these programs use trained volunteers, and others use paid staff, but both are designed to provide a sitter for the patient with Alzheimer's disease in the patient's familiar surroundings.

SAFETY DEVICES

One of the greatest fears of many elderly people is that they will fall and break a bone and that no one will find them until it is too late. However, several safety devices are available that enable frail, elderly people to remain in their homes with a certain degree of reassurance that someone will be checking on them. For example, there are several emergency response systems on the market. With most of these systems the individual buys a unit to be placed in the home, pays a monthly fee, and is linked by phone to a base station, which is usually located in a hospital. The individual can alert the base station by pressing a "panic button." Many hospitals provide the unit placed in the home and require payment of a small monthly fee. Some security businesses have response systems in addition to burglar systems. There is a Red-Eye Alert program operated by local fire departments that will provide, on request, a "red-eye" sticker that is placed on the door or front of the house. If a fire should occur, the firefighter is alerted to the fact that there is an invalid in the house who will need assistance.

Another program, the Vial of Life, is a project of the American Association of Retired Persons. It will furnish anyone with a plastic container in which to place pertinent medical information. The container is placed in the refrigerator, and a sticker is placed on the front door indicating that there is a Vial of Life container in the home.

In the Carrier Alert program, participating individuals have a sticker on their mailbox. If the postal carrier notices that mail is not being picked up, he notifies his supervisor, who then calls the senior citizens center to send someone to check on the individual. Similarly, the Gatekeeper program alerts utility meter readers to notice conditions around the home of an elderly person that might indicate that the person is experiencing difficulties. Most senior citizens centers will make daily telephone calls, if requested, to be sure that a homebound person is all right. In addition to these emergency services, most cities now have a 911 telephone emergency number that receives and handles distress calls.

ADULT DAY CARE

Adult day care, geriatric day care, dependent day care, and therapeutic adult day care are some of the names for community-based programs in which impaired elderly can be cared for during the day. Whatever the title, there are two distinct models of day care—social and therapeutic. There are some similarities between the two models: both may accept clients on a drop-in basis or may require that the person be enrolled for a minimum number of days each week; both may provide meals and transportation; both should provide activities and supervision; and, most important, both should have adequate facilities and staff to provide a safe environment for the participants. Social models may supervise medications, but the therapeutic model may administer medications. The therapeutic model, which is supervised by a registered nurse, may provide health services not available in the social model. The social model often will not accept people who are incontinent.

In some communities there may be no adult day care programs in place, whereas in other communities there may be only one social model. In most metropolitan areas a variety of community-based adult day care facilities are available. In 1990 the National Council on Aging's National Institute of Adult Day Care (NCOA's NIAD) drafted standards and guidelines for adult day care. Unfortunately, many states have not adopted these standards and have no licensure requirements, except for compliance with local and state fire, health, and safety building codes, making the selection process difficult for the caregiver. In a community or state that has no adult day care standards, it is advisable for the caregivers to make unannounced visits to the centers at various times of the day (e.g., during mealtime, at midmorning and midafternoon, and at various times to observe the quality of meals provided or activities offered or lack of activities). Attention also should be given to the ratio of staff to participants. NCOA recommends a minimum of 1 staff person per 6 clients, but a study of adult day care done by NCOA'S NIAD shows that national averages range from 1 staff person per 12 to 25 participants.

Hospice care is primarily a comprehensive program of care delivered to someone who has been diagnosed as having a terminal illness and whose life expectancy is 6 months or less. It is customarily provided in the patient's home. Hospice care provides all the reasonable and necessary medical support services for the management of the illness. When a person receives hospice services from a Medicare-approved hospice, Medicare Hospital Insurance (Part A) pays almost the entire cost. More specific information can be obtained by calling the National Hospice Organization's toll-free number: 1-800-658-8898.

HOME HEALTH CARE

Probably one of the fastest-growing industries in this country during the past 10 years has been home health care. This service provides in-home nursing care; physical, occupational, or speech therapy;

medical social services; home health aide or homemaker services; and medical supplies and appliances. Some of these services are reimbursable by Medicare, Medigap insurance, Medicaid, or private health or long-term care insurance.

HOUSING ALTERNATIVES

Sooner or later most caregivers are faced with the situation of no longer being able to cope with the demands of the patient who is living at home or residing with the caregiver. At this juncture a decision must be made about alternative housing arrangements. There are several types of facilities that provide different levels of care. Continuing care communities, which will accept a person who is well and able to live independently, offer congregate dining, housekeeping services, and eventually a nursing home bed. Assisted living facilities have private or semiprivate rooms. Services include three meals a day in a group setting, laundry, housekeeping, and supervision of medications. Both types of services usually offer some form of transportation.

It may be time to consider nursing home placement in a health care facility under the following circumstances: (1) when the patient with Alzheimer's disease requires 24-hour care, has violent outbursts or exhibits other dangerous behavior, or requires help with needs such as bathing or going to the toilet or (2) when the caregiver suffers from exhaustion, stress, or isolation. Although nursing homes are alike in many ways (e.g., having similar purposes and regulations), there are differences that make one nursing home better suited to a particular patient than another would be. This situation is especially true for the patient with Alzheimer's disease because many nursing homes are not equipped to care for the patient with this condition. Also, Medicaid will not pay for the level of care provided in Alzheimer's disease units. If the private-pay patient in an Alzheimer's disease unit should reach the stage where custodial care is needed, the nursing home will transfer that person to a regular nursing home bed. If the nursing home has Medicaid beds, when the patient becomes income eligible, Medicaid will start paying the costs.

The most important step for the caregiver is to select the right nursing home. In fact, the same steps that are recommended for selecting an adult day care program should be the starting point in nursing home selection. Comprehensive guides to nursing homes are available in many states.

TRANSPORTATION

In nearly all assessments conducted to determine the needs o older people, transportation is at the top of the list. However, th kinds of transportation available are as diverse as the communitie themselves. Some districts have rural mass transit programs tha are based in the senior center in each county. Two-way radio enable the dispatchers to operate vans in an efficient manner. Rea sonable fares are charged to riders, regardless of age. Most of th vans are equipped with wheelchair lifts, and the drivers are traine in transporting people with disabilities for medical appointment and other necessary errands. It should be noted, however, that th vans do not carry oxygen and are not a substitute for ambulances Some agencies and organizations also provide transportation. Fo example, the Department of Health and Human Services pays fo Medicaid rides for health purposes. The American Cancer Societ and the American Kidney Foundation provide volunteer transporta tion to treatment centers. Information on these programs can b obtained from the pertinent treatment centers, from the local office of the Department of Health and Human Services, or from the loca senior citizens center.

INSURANCE

One of the most confusing issues an elderly person or his care giver must contend with is health insurance. The main types o health coverage available for older people today are briefly de scribed in the following sections. It should be noted that thes change often.

Medicare Hospital Insurance (Part A)

This insurance program provides hospital coverage for peopl who are 65 years or older and for certain disabled people. Any persor who has paid into the Social Security system or is the spouse of some one who has paid into this system is automatically eligible upor reaching age 65. This insurance will pay all approved hospital charge after deductibles have been met.

Medicare Supplementary Medical Insurance (Part B)

This insurance plan is available to the same groups noted for Par A. The monthly premium, which was $31.80 in 1992, is deducted fron the person's Social Security check. For those who work beyond age 65 and do not receive a Social Security check, the beneficiary is billed quarterly. Part B pays 80% of approved medical expenses after deductibles for services such as outpatient visits, doctor's office visits, and home health care. As one might expect, there are exceptions to these guidelines. Further information about Medicare can be obtained by calling the organization's toll-free number (1-800-638-6833) or from its pamphlet called *The Medicare Handbook.*

Medigap Insurance

As of July 1992, the government requires that any health insurance policy sold as a supplement to Medicare Part B conform to at least one of ten policies. Policy A provides very limited coverage, whereas Policy J provides extensive coverage beyond Part B. Insurance companies are required to provide information about all policies so that the consumer can more easily make a decision on the type of insurance he may need.

Warning: There is an open enrollment period for both Medicare Part B and Medigap. Anyone approaching age 65 should contact his local Social Security office 3 to 4 months before that time to avoid penalties.

Qualified Medicare Beneficiary (QMB)

This program requires state Medicaid programs to pay the Medicare premium as well as the deductibles and coinsurance payment for seniors with incomes below the federal poverty line. To be eligible in 1992, single seniors needed to have incomes below $7056 and assets of less than $4000; married seniors had to have incomes below $9432 and assets of less than $6000. It is generally agreed that a person who receives both Medicare and QMB insurance or a person who receives Medicaid needs no other health insurance. The local Department of Health and Human Services can be contacted for more information.

Medicaid

Medicaid, which is funded by both the federal and state governments, provides health care coverage for seniors and certain disabled or low-income people. The federal government defines what services may be provided, with some being mandatory. However, it is up to each state to decide what services it will provide, in addition to the mandatory ones, and to whom those services will be provided. In certain states Medicaid is the only method of financing custodial nursing home care for low-income people. In other states, under a waiver system, Medicaid also covers in-home care for low-income people. To file for Medicaid, the individual must call the local Department of Health and Human Services to set up an appointment. As a rule of thumb, any person eligible for Supplemental Security Income or Aid to Families with Dependent Children is eligible for Medicaid. If a single person has assets over $2000, he is not eligible for Medicaid. However, the person may "spend down" his assets to become eligible. This process must be done within certain guidelines to avoid being charged with fraud. The purchase of an irrevocable burial trust as part of the spend-down process is a wise choice for a person with limited resources. More information on Medicaid is available through the local Department of Health and Human Services.

The box on p. 367 contains information that will help to clarify the requirements for and benefits of Medicare and Medicaid.

Long-Term Care (LTC) Insurance

Long-term care can be very expensive. A 1-year stay in a nursing home can cost anywhere from $25,000 to $50,000. In-home care can be equally expensive or even more expensive when the costs of homemaker, personal care, aides, sitters, and health professionals are needed on a daily basis in addition to the normal costs in maintaining a home. LTC insurance is best primarily for those aged 65 to 75 who have significant disposable income and who believe that peace of mind is more important than a good investment decision. An LTC policy should be chosen only after a comparison of information from several companies.

Some things to look for are: Does the policy provide coverage in a home setting as well as in a nursing home or extended care facility? Does the policy limit the number of years of coverage; if so, how many? Does the policy have a built-in factor to offset the inflationary increases in the costs of care? What, if any, are the restrictions on preexisting conditions? Are there any restrictions on the types of conditions that are not covered? Does the policy begin paying on the first day of a nursing home stay? Another factor to be considered in purchasing LTC insurance is the age of the individual. All these factors will affect the amount of the premium.

The Health Insurance Association of America offers a very informative pamphlet entitled "The Consumer's Guide to Long-Term Care

MEDICARE AND MEDICAID

Medicare is a federal health insurance program not related to income, resources, or medical bills.

Medicaid is a state-operated health insurance program, but it is funded by both the state and federal governments, with eligibility based on income and resources.

Medicare pays full cost for skilled care in a nursing home for 20 days and all but $81.50 per day for an additional 80 days.

Medicaid pays for skilled care, level I, and intermediate care, level II, when one cannot afford to pay.

Unlike Medicaid, Medicare requires a 3-day stay in a hospital before entrance into a nursing home.

Medicare will pay for home nurse visits up to three times a week, under a physician's orders.

Medicaid will pay for 60 home nurse visits per year, under a physician's orders.

Neither Medicare nor Medicaid will pay for eyeglasses, dentures, or hearing aids.

Nursing home Medicaid is entirely different from other coverage groups of Medicaid and has different qualifying criteria.

Preadmission evaluations are completed by the nursing home and sent to the state Medicaid office for determination of medical need for nursing home Medicaid.

Financial eligibility for nursing home Medicaid is determined through the local office of the Department of Health and Human Services.

One's homestead is totally excluded from consideration as a resource, regardless of its value.

Penalties will be imposed for transfers of property or money for less than fair market value within 30 months of applying for Medicaid.

Any amount in an irrevocable burial trust agreement is not counted toward the $2000 resource limit.

Half of total resources (with a minimum of $13,740 and a maximum of $66,480) held by a married couple at the time of institutionalization can be retained by the spouse who remains at home.

Nursing homes admit patients on a first-come, first-served basis. All nursing homes have waiting lists. Certain exceptions can be made for persons being discharged from a hospital.

Nursing homes cannot discriminate against individuals who receive Medicaid or who are applying for Medicaid when admitting from their waiting list.

Nursing homes cannot make a "third person" (e.g., spouse or child) responsible for payment of a bill for a Medicaid recipient.

Medicaid denials can be appealed.

Insurance." This organization also has another helpful booklet called "The Consumer's Guide to Medicare Supplemental Insurance" (see Bibliography for the association's address).

BENEFITS
Social Security

Although we think of Social Security as a retirement benefit, many people receive Social Security payments because (1) they are disabled, (2) they are dependents of someone who receives Social Security, or (3) they are widows, widowers, or children of someone who has died. The basic principles of Social Security have remained essentially unchanged since it began more than 50 years ago. However, since that time Congress has passed laws intended to help Social Security keep pace with changes in society. In addition to new legislation, several "built-in" changes tied to economic factors help Social Security benefits keep up with the cost of living and with workers' average wages. Under the current system, in 1992 employers and employees shared equal parts of 7.65% of the employee's wages, with a cap of $55,500 annual income that can be taxed. For self-employed people, the tax was 15.3% of earnings. Retirees under the age of 70 who still wished to work were limited to earning no more than $10,200 per year in 1992. After age 70 there are no caps, and a retiree can draw the full benefit due him regardless of earnings. More information can be obtained by requesting SSA Publication No. 05-10024, January 1992, from the nearest Social Security office.

Veterans Affairs Benefits

Veterans Affairs (VA) benefits are available to any veteran who did not receive a dishonorable discharge. Dependents and survivors of veterans also may be eligible for certain VA benefits. When an individual applies for these benefits, he is asked to provide birth and death certificates, marriage licenses, insurance policies, and record of military service. Having all these documents on hand at the time of application will speed the process. VA hospitals give priority to providing medical care to veterans (1) with service-connected disabilities, (2) who receive a VA pension, (3) who are eligible for Medicaid, or whose condition is related to exposure to radiation from participating in nuclear tests from September 11, 1945, to July 1, 1946. Medical care in VA facilities may be provided on a space-available basis to non-service-connected veterans who meet certain income requirements.

The VA provides, on a limited basis, skilled or intermediate-type nursing care for related medical care in the VA facility or private nursing homes for convalescents or persons who are not acutely ill and not in need of hospital care. Domiciliary care may be provided on an ambulatory self-care basis for veterans disabled by age or disease who are not in need of hospitalization for an acute illness.

Disability compensation is paid monthly to veterans with disabilities incurred through, or aggravated during, military service. The amount of the compensation is based on the severity of the veteran's condition. If the veteran is rated 30% or more disabled, additional amounts can be paid for dependents. For those veterans who are totally and permanently disabled and whose income from all sources is within prescribed limitations, pensions are available. Additional benefits may be available for veterans who are permanently housebound, in nursing homes, or in need of regular aid and attendance.

ALZHEIMER'S ASSOCIATION

The Alzheimer's Association, a national voluntary organization that was founded in 1980, is designed to help families affected by Alzheimer's disease. The national office is located in Chicago, and there are more than 200 nonprofit voluntary chapters throughout the country. The association and its affiliate chapters have four major goals: support, research, education, and advocacy. Each chapter develops its services based on these goals. Support groups (see Chapter 27) are of great help to caregivers, reflecting the words in the Alzheimer's Association's national logo: "Someone to Stand by You." Fifteen percent of all money raised by local chapters goes to the national office, with most of that money being targeted for educational literature and research into the causes, cures, or treatment of Alzheimer's disease. Chapters, for the most part, must raise all their funds locally. One fundraiser that has become the main source of income for chapters is the annual Memory Walk. Most chapters have this walk-a-thon on the same day in October each year. Donations and memorial gifts are also crucial in helping chapters with their operating expenses.

Another function of both the local chapters and the national office is the dissemination of information related to the diagnosis, treatment, and management of patients with Alzheimer's disease. Seminars for both lay and professional people are also sponsored by the chapters. Advocacy efforts include increasing the public's awareness of the devastating effects of Alzheimer's disease on families, communities, and the nation and working for legislative action to help ease the burden on the family caregiver. Although each chapter is operated locally with its own board and director, most chapters provide essentially the same services: information and referral, support groups, respite programs, monthly or quarterly newsletters, educational packets, lending library, wanderer's and safe return program, and sometimes, day care. The association's national toll-free number (1-800-272-3900) can provide information about the nearest chapter.

SENIOR CITIZENS CENTERS

No report on services for the elderly would be complete without mention of senior citizens centers. Although these centers have been referred to throughout this chapter, it must be emphasized that they are recognized as community focal points for information about services for the elderly. Some centers are directed toward serving active independent older persons in the community. Others have a comprehensive program that provides services for both well and frail older people. Its members not only receive services; they also provide services by visiting the homebound or making daily phone calls to be sure that homebound persons are all right. Since all centers are informed about the availability of services for senior citizens, they should be used as a source when determining how to meet the needs of frail, health-impaired elderly and their caregivers.

SUMMARY

Some people view the service delivery system for older people as fragmented, and certainly there are numerous agencies and businesses involved in serving this client population. However, the actual process of getting elderly people and their families to agree to seek help may be even more difficult than locating the needed services. This process requires not only a great deal of patience, understanding, and compassion but also a thorough working knowledge of the services available. For information on what services are available and how to access those services, a call to the local senior citizens center, the Area Agency on Aging, or the local chapter of the Alzheimer's Association (any one of which should be listed in area telephone directories) is advised.

BIBLIOGRAPHY

Advocates Senior Alert Process: special report on the QMB program, Washington, DC, 1992, Advocates Senior Alert Process.*

Commonwealth Fund Commission on elderly people living alone, Baltimore, 1987, Commonwealth Fund Commission.

The consumer's guide to long-term care insurance, Washington, DC, 1992, Health Insurance Association of America.†

The consumer's guide to Medicare Supplement Insurance, Washington, DC, 1992, Health Insurance Association of America.†

A guide to nursing homes in Tennessee 1991-1992, Nashville, 1991, Tennessee Health Care Association.

How to start and manage a group activities and respite program for people with Alzheimer's disease and their families: a guide for community-based organizations, New York, 1991, The Brookdale Foundation, The Brookdale Center on Aging of Hunter College.

Medicare, Medicaid, and Medicare supplement insurance: what you need to know to protect yourself, Nashville, Tenn., 1992, Legal Services of Middle Tennessee, Nashville Legal Aid Society.

A profile of older Americans, Washington, DC, 1986, American Association of Retired Persons.

Social Security update 1992, Department of Health and Human Services, Social Security Administration, SSA Pub No 05-10003, Washington, DC, Feb. 1992.

SSI-supplemental security income, Department of Health and Human Services, Social Security Administration, SSA Pub No 05-11000, Washington, DC, Jan 1991.

Standards and guidelines for adult day care, Washington DC, 1990, The National Institute on Adult Day Care (The National Council on the Aging).

Statewide study of the needs of senior Tennesseans, Nashville, 1986, First Tennessee District, Tennessee Commission on Aging.

A summary of Department of Veterans Affairs benefits, VA Pamphlet 27-82-2, revised March 1991, Washington, DC, 1991.

Understanding Social Security, Department of Health and Human Services, Social Security Administration, SSA Pub No 05-10024, Washington, DC, 1992.

Weissert WG and others: *Adult day care: Findings from a national survey*, Baltimore, 1990, Johns Hopkins University Press.

---

*Advocates Senior Alert Process, 1334G St NW, Washington, DC, 20005.

†Health Insurance Association of America, 1025 Connecticut Ave NW, Washington, DC, 20036-3998.

29

The Alzheimer's Association

Nancy Erickson

In the late 1970s, "Alzheimer's" was a name few people knew. The general public and most health care professionals equated this disease's symptoms with senility and believed that its occurrence and course were common elements in the aging process.

In an attempt to find definitive information about the disorder affecting their loved ones, to learn how to cope with its progression and to gain hope for the discovery of its cause and cure, seven independent caregiver groups joined together in 1980 to form the Alzheimer's Disease and Related Disorders Association. From a handful of dedicated family members with an initial annual budget of $85,000, this association has become the nation's leading nonprofit health organization (with a combined national chapter budget of more than $40 million) serving patients with Alzheimer's disease and their families.

This charity organization is anchored by a 60-member volunteer board of directors representing family members of individuals with Alzheimer's disease, health care professionals and practitioners, and business leaders in addition to a Medical and Scientific Advisory Board of physicians, scholars, and researchers in the clinical, social, and biological sciences, who oversee the research programs and scientific information projects.

The foundation of this association is its chapter network of more than 200 chapters in all 50 states. Each chapter is guided by a volunteer board of directors and operates with a budget that may range from less than $25,000 to over $1 million. More than 35,000 volunteers nationwide participate in providing services, such as leading one of the 1800 support groups, raising scarce dollars for the association's research programs, providing respite care, and educating the public about the effects of Alzheimer's disease. As the network has evolved and chapter operations have become more sophisticated, state councils have been formulated for the primary purpose of addressing the legislative and regulatory concerns of the individual with Alzheimer's disease.

Many chapters began in the living room of a caregiver who was answering phone calls from other caregivers who desperately needed help in caring for a memory-impaired spouse or parent. Although many chapters have now moved their operation from a home to an office, their focus on the needs of the patient and family has not wavered.

The Alzheimer's Association mission declares its dedication to research for the prevention, cure, and treatment of Alzheimer's disease and related disorders and to providing support and assistance to afflicted patients and their families. This mission is carried out in the following ways:

- Supporting research into the cause, prevention, treatment, and cure for Alzheimer's disease and related disorders
- Educating the public and disseminating information to health care professionals
- Forming chapters to provide a nationwide family support network and other programs in local communities
- Advocating for improved public policy and promoting needed legislation
- Offering patient and family services to aid present and victims and caregivers

A synopsis of key areas suggests the breadth of the programs, services, and resources offered by the association and its chapter network. Research, patient and family services, public awareness and education, and public policy form a nucleus for the defense and support of the patient and family member fighting this devastating disease.

RESEARCH ACTIVITIES

In July of 1989, President George Bush officially declared the 1990s the "Decade of the Brain." This designation signified a pledge by the federal government to focus vital resources on brain research. This pledge stems from the needs of more than 50 million Americans with disorders and disabilities of the brain, 4 million of whom suffer from Alzheimer's disease.

The remarkable advances that have occurred in brain research in the past decade, coupled with this timely support from the federal government, promise exciting opportunities for Alzheimer's research in the 1990s.

The Alzheimer's Association began the "Decade of the Brain" by funding 67 new studies. These projects and other continuing research investigative activities cover a broad range of topics in Alzheimer's disease research. Investigation of the role of amyloid and the study of abnormal proteins continue to be in the forefront of research. In addition, genetic studies are bringing scientists closer to understanding the role of chromosome 21 and chromosome 19 in the development of the disease.

Other projects are breaking new ground in understanding how the brain controls certain cognitive abilities (e.g., comprehension, speech and language, reasoning) and what happens to these abilities when the brain undergoes degeneration. These research projects will enhance our knowledge of the full spectrum of Alzheimer's disease.

The association's research grants program relies on the strength of the Medical and Scientific Advisory Board, a group of 40 internationally recognized scientists representing many fields of study, including neurology, psychiatry, molecular neurobiology, and research on nursing and caregiver burden issues. The expert advice of this board enables the Alzheimer's Association to fund a well-balanced group of research projects that are likely to increase our understanding of Alzheimer's disease.

Through its research grants program, the association has built a sound research investment portfolio. As a short-term investment, studies of patient care, caregiver respite services, and behavioral interventions will make the lives of patients with Alzheimer's disease more comfortable and the burden of the disease on families more bearable.

As a long-term plan, research into basic functions of the brain, chemical reactions, and genetics will improve our understanding of the processes that occur in both the normal brain and the brain of patients with Alzheimer's disease.

This knowledge creates a firm foundation for future research to find the cause(s), effective treatments, and, eventually, methods of preventing Alzheimer's disease. Along the way, we can expect large dividends from our midrange investments in the form of better diagnostic techniques and drugs to help relieve symptoms of this disorder.

Research Programs

The association's research programs began in 1982 with the goal of encouraging more and better research into the cause, treatment and management, prevention, and cure of Alzheimer's disease and related disorders. By the end of 1992, 500 grants and awards totaling more than $27 million were funded by the association through these programs.

Structured to complement the United States Public Health Service funding programs, the research program is designed to encourage investigators to enter research on Alzheimer's disease and related disorders.

Proposals are solicited for biological, clinical, and social research relevant to generative brain diseases such as Alzheimer's disease. The proposed research need not directly involve Alzheimer's disease but must have the potential to add to knowledge about issues relevant to the disease.

Pilot Research Grants

The Pilot Research Grant Program provides 1-year $25,000 grants for worthwhile research proposals, with preference given to investigators new to research in Alzheimer's disease and related disorders.

Investigator-Initiated Research Grants

These grants are structured to build on the success of the Pilot Research Grants by providing sustained support for independent research projects. Investigator-Initiated Research Grants provide a maximum of $45,000 per year, usually for 2 or 3 years.

Faculty Scholar Awards

The Faculty Scholar Award Program provides sustained salary support for investigators at the junior faculty level who (1) have at least 2 years of prior research experience and (2) have shown a commitment to research in Alzheimer's disease and related disorders. Each award provides $45,000 per year for 3 years.

Targeted Research Grants

These grants are designed to support research in specific areas that the Medical and Scientific Advisory Board considers vital. They can be for either 1-year pilot grants ($25,000) or 2-year grants for a maximum of $45,000 each year.

Zenith Awards

The Zenith Awards program is the newest of the research grant programs. The awards are granted to talented scientists who have already contributed substantially to the advancement of Alzheimer's disease research and who are likely to continue to make significant contributions for many years to come. Awardees receive a grant of $100,000 per year for 1, 2, or 3 years, with a provision for possible competitive renewal.

In addition to providing research support to the scientific community, the association has a commitment to communicating the results of this research and working with scientists and government agencies to accelerate research. In cooperation with the Food and Drug Administration (FDA) and the pharmaceutical industry, the association prepared a position paper on clinical drug trials for Alzheimer's disease called "Clinical Drug Trials in Alzheimer Disease: What Are Some of the Issues?" Authored by members of the Medical and Scientific Advisory Board, this paper was published in *Alzheimer Disease and Associated Disorders: An International Journal*.

PATIENT AND FAMILY SERVICES

Alzheimer's disease is often called the "family disease" because the caregiving provided by families is overwhelming. Family members give most of the care at home. One of every three families is affected by this progressive disease, and the financial and emotional burdens often make caregivers "second victims" of the disease.

Because the progression of Alzheimer's disease can range from 3 to 20 years, the needs of patients and family members vary with their individual circumstances. Programs, services, and resources—respite programs, support groups, and educational programming—are a few of the key activities that draw families to the Alzheimer's Association. Family physicians, health care specialists, or nursing professionals working with the patient with Alzheimer's disease can take advantage of these resources by becoming familiar with a local chapter's activities.

The Alzheimer's Association provides direct service through varied programs offered at the chapter level. Three significant, nationally-funded demonstration projects have put the association in the forefront of practical, affordable approaches to providing respite for family members. The National Respite Care Demonstration Program, the Dementia Care and Respite Services Program, and the Senior Companion Program have gained nationwide acclaim by responding to pleas for relief from the stress and fatigue of caregiving.

National Respite Care Demonstration Program

As part of its commitment to providing high-quality services to families and caregivers involved with Alzheimer's disease, the association has been the driving force behind the creation of innovative respite care programs. Since 1986, the association has administered and funded this demonstration program in which Alzheimer's Association chapters provide or collaborate with local agencies to test approaches to day care and in-home respite care. The association developed standards for program administration for the chapters. Since its beginning, the 50 chapters have provided more than 70 unique respite care programs for families affected by Alzheimer's disease. The positive outcomes from these programs are emphasized in the association's evaluation report compiled in April 1991:

- Three out of four caregivers reported that their health had improved as a result of respite.
- Seventy-six percent of those surveyed felt they could manage their lives and their impaired family member better.

Dementia Care and Respite Services Program

The association, in cooperation with and jointly funded by the Robert Wood Johnson Foundation and the federal Administration on Aging, has been testing the financial and programmatic viability of providing specific services for patients with Alzheimer's disease in a day care setting. The program encompasses 19 projects. An example of the success of this program can be found at St. Elizabeth's Day Care Center, which is affiliated with the St. Louis Chapter of the Alzheimer's Association. In 1990 this center became the first site to achieve financial self-sufficiency, and, as a result, St. Elizabeth's was able to shift its Robert Wood Johnson funding to create a third site.

Senior Companion Program

With the support of a grant from the federal Older American Volunteer Program's (ACTION) Senior Companion Program, the association's chapters trained senior volunteers to provide in-home care relief for full-time caregivers of patients with Alzheimer's disease.

More than nine communities were served by 144 volunteers, who supported 432 families with relief from their daily caregiving. The following excerpt from the association's evaluation of the Senior Companion Program (Alzheimer Care Evaluation Report, April 1991) testifies to the need of this service: "...without the SCP [Senior Companion Program] and Alzheimer's Association Respite Program, I don't know what would have happened to me. I do know I would never, never have been able to handle my husband's illness without their help." Jarvik and associates (1990) noted another family's reaction to the program: "At the time we received the Senior Companion services, it was a lifesaver for both my wife and I. The companion was well trained to help Alzheimer patients. My wife's response was uplifting for both of us."

Autopsy Assistance Network

The association's network of 40 volunteer autopsy representatives responds to the needs of family members who make the difficult decision to request an autopsy. These volunteers provide information, counsel, and support in this decision to perform the procedure that still provides the only definitive diagnosis of Alzheimer's disease.

Support Groups

The association's chapter network offers support group opportunities for many special people—the patient with early-stage Alzheimer's disease, the caregiving spouse, the teenage grandchild, and the Spanish-speaking friends of the family. Innovative programs can be found in units such as the Metro Denver Chapter, where the early-stage patient can examine issues about diagnosis, financial and legal concerns, and planning for long-term care. The Eastern Massachusetts Chapter offers support and a forum for sharing concerns that affect the teenage caregiver. Spanish-speaking support groups have been meeting through the auspices of the Los Angeles (California) Chapter and have provided educational programming in community churches with Spanish-language videotape materials.

National Alzheimer's Safe Return Program

One of the most alarming and potentially life-threatening behaviors that accompanies memory impairment is wandering. In relationship to dementia, wandering has been defined as "aimless frequent ambulation." With memory impairment, this behavior puts the wanderer at risk of becoming lost, unable to request or seek assistance, and unable to find his way home. In 1992 the Alzheimer's Association received funding through the U.S. Justice Department to create the Alzheimer's Association Safe Return Program, which plans to use a central registry of information to help identify and locate missing memory-impaired persons. Components include a national toll-free hotline to access the registry and a Fax Alert system to set the search process in motion.

PUBLIC AWARENESS AND EDUCATION

During the course of 1 year, the coast-to-coast Alzheimer's Association's network responded to calls from approximately 200,000 family members asking for direction, help, and counsel. To answer these care management and support inquiries, the association has developed an extensive catalog of more than 50 publications that is available through local chapters.

This catalog represents a stark contrast to the sparse listings of articles and information on Alzheimer's disease in 1979. In the early years, the association joined forces with organizations such as the American Health Care Association to publish a much-needed chronicle about caring for the patient with Alzheimer's disease, *Care of Alzheimer's Patients: A Manual for Nursing Home Staff*; distributed the caregivers' guidebook, *The 36-Hour Day*; and published a comprehensive review of the effects of Alzheimer's disease and management techniques, *Understanding Alzheimer's Disease*.

The range of educational materials produced by the association includes topical brochures, such as "Alzheimer's Disease: Services You May Need" and "When the Diagnosis Is Alzheimer's," and videotape training curricula, such as the "Caregiver Kit" and "An Orientation to Alzheimer's Disease." Spanish-language resources feature pictorial formats (fotonovelas), "Hechos y Realidades," a kit of caregiver fact sheets, two videotapes, and several topical brochures. Other educational products focus on training manuals for Respite Care Services, the Senior Companion Training Program, and support group development.

Products specifically designed to answer queries involving drug development or research include:
- Fact sheets on specific drugs being tested for treatment of Alzheimer's disease

- A report on current research projects funded by the Alzheimer's Association
- A summary of the research update program at the Alzheimer's Association annual meeting

"From Theory to Therapy: The Development of Drugs for Alzheimer's Disease" is the newest specialized product. This information kit, written for a lay audience, highlights drug development, drug testing participation, the effects of drugs that are being developed to treat symptoms of Alzheimer's disease, and the usefulness of drugs currently available to patients.

In 1991 the Alzheimer's Association proudly dedicated the Benjamin B. Green-Field Library and Resource Center, the first privately funded facility specializing in information about Alzheimer's disease for the lay and professional publics. The collection includes patient education materials, Alzheimer's Association products, training materials, and scientific articles, to name a few examples. The materials are found in a variety of formats, such as print, videocassette, audiocassette, slide, and CD-ROM, with equipment available for using them.

Two professional health sciences librarians provide assistance to meet users' information needs, including basic reference services such as finding statistical information, referral to other information resources within or outside of the association, and literature search and extended reference services. The preparation of literature searches is facilitated by access to over 400 on-line databases available through the National Library of Medicine, the BRS Search Service, and Dialog Information services. Bibliographical searches using local sources— the library's computerized catalog, print indexes, and periodical indexes in CD-ROM format—are provided without charge. Charges are requested for certain services.

The public may use materials in the library or borrow materials via interlibrary loan through their local hospital, university, or public library. A description of the library's collection is stored in a computer database, which is readily available from anywhere in the United States by using a microcomputer with a modem and the appropriate software.

Professional Educational Programming

In 1990 the Alzheimer's Association launched a multiyear series of scientific lectures by prominent Alzheimer's disease researchers, titled the Sigma Tau Lectures. Sponsored by the Sigma Tau Foundation of Rome, Italy, these lectures are offered in locations throughout the country, in conjunction with a local Alzheimer's Association chapter.

For 2 years the association has cosponsored the International Symposium on Alzheimer's Disease, an educational forum that attracts 800 of the top scientists in this field.

In July 1992, the Alzheimer's Association presented "Alzheimer Care Strategies: Practical Approaches, Professional Alliances," a national conference on Alzheimer's disease for health care professionals. An audience of more than 1000 nursing home administrators, directors of nursing, social workers, adult day care administrators, home health agency directors, and allied health professionals attended. Five tracks—Care Management Issues, Education and Training Trends, Legal and Ethical Dilemmas, Public Policy and Legislative Issues, and Special Care Environments and Programs—offered more than 60 interactive sessions featuring Alzheimer's disease experts and practitioners from throughout the country. The Second National Conference, scheduled to be held on July 25-28, 1993, in Chicago, will highlight research and practice trends and focus on the association's *Guidelines for Dignity*, a comprehensive guide to quality care for patients with Alzheimer's disease in a residential setting.

Federal, state, and local advocacy efforts have helped to emphasize the urgency of the needs of the patient with Alzheimer's disease in the legislative and regulatory arenas. Through lobbying efforts of association advocates at the annual public policy forum, federal funding for Alzheimer's disease research reached a record level of $295 million in fiscal year 1993.

Summary

For the past 12 years, the Alzheimer's Association has struggled to ease the burden of the Alzheimer's disease patient and caregiver. In its second decade it will continue to strive to stand by all family or professional caregivers who serve the person with Alzheimer's disease—to fight to help him or her retain personal dignity and to maintain existing special abilities. The Alzheimer's Association provides practical approaches to caregiving and caring approaches to service.

For a referral to a local chapter of the Alzheimer's Association or for information about educational programs and materials, call 1-800-272-3900; for the hearing impaired, use the TDD 1-312-335-8882.

BIBLIOGRAPHY

Alzheimer's Association: *National Respite Care Demonstration Program research summary,* Chicago, January 1991, The Association.

Alzheimer's Association: *Alzheimer care evaluation report,* Chicago, April 1991, The Association.

Alzheimer's Association: *Alzheimer's Association materials catalog,* Public Catalog, Chicago, March 1992, The Association.

Jarvik and others: Clinical drug trials in Alzheimer disease: what are some of the issues? *Alzheimer Dis Assoc Disord* 4(4):193-202, 1990.

30

Dementia care units

Larry Hudgins

In the United States there are approximately 20,000 nursing homes with a total bed capacity of 1.6 million. Since older people are frequent users of hospitals, and since their hospital stays are longer than those of any other group of users, nursing homes are viewed as alternatives to prolonged hospitalization. Many individuals who are admitted to a nursing home stay for a relatively short length of time. Nursing home facilities in the community are seen as a bridge between hospital discharge and final disposition to care. Thus these facilities offer a rehabilitation resource for postoperative orthopedic patients and stroke patients and a recuperative resource for patients during the recovery phase of acute medical illness. Nursing homes have become, in large measure, an extension of the hospital. Their staff structure and function are similar to the hospital care model.

Of all nursing home admissions, 30% occur because the family is unable to care for the older person at home rather than as a result of medical reasons. The length of stay generally is indefinite. Of the population above age 65, 5% to 6% are institutionalized, and the average age of nursing home residents has risen to what is considered the "old-old," specifically those individuals who are over age 75. Twenty-three percent of these chronic care patients ultimately die in a nursing home. Many of these individuals are disabled by various forms of dementia, an illness that present-day custodial nursing homes are poorly equipped to handle. When the traditional role of the nursing home began to change, patients with dementia were judged to be difficult to care for and inappropriate candidates for rehabilitation programs. More recently, specialized dementia care units have been proffered to fill this void.

During the early stages of the development of dementia care units, there has been some controversy about whether such units are needed. One concern is that creating more bed space for elder care would add redundancy to a system that is working fairly well. Is it not possible for patients with dementia to receive acceptable or better care in a general care nursing home? The consensus of opinion on this question is that they could not. The main disadvantages of caring for these patients in a custodial nursing home setting include difficulties in coping with wandering patients and intolerance of behavioral disturbances. In addition, other patients in the custodial nursing home setting may be recuperating from an acute illness or from orthopedic or other surgery or may be receiving poststroke rehabilitation. The probability of interference with the care of these patients would be high if wandering patients with dementia were housed within the same unit. The different care requirements for each of these groups result in such divergent goals that the staff may find it difficult to divide their attention between caring for both categories of patients at the same time.

The advantages of having all the patients with dementia in one unit include the same goal orientation and expectations of the unit by staff and families. The unit staff and family caregivers are likely to have developed similar and unified coping skills to care for these patients. The separately contained dementia unit setting offers a better opportunity to develop a flexible activity schedule for the patients. With proper architectural structure, those patients inclined to wander can do so at will without requiring constant staff attention.

The concerns about having all patients with a diagnosis of dementia in one unit are threefold. First, morale tends to be low among staff members who, on a daily basis, must deal with a population of patients who are not expected to recover. Second, such facilities have created a closed community in which turnover is minimal and close relationships develop between family caregivers and staff; this situation often leads to opposition by families when the need arises to move the patient to another facility because of further deterioration of his condition. Third, experience in these units has demonstrated that when the permanent staff are sick or on vacation, other staff members are reluctant to work on the unit that houses "those demented folks."

Currently, there is a consensus that the better option is for specialized dementia care units to be attached to the existing larger custodial nursing homes structurally but to maintain a separate identity. The advantage of the plan is that the staff is not so isolated from general nursing home care and that the patients, once progressive disability ensues to the point that they require custodial care, can be moved easily into the custodial care unit. The family should understand this mechanism for continuity of care for their relative with dementia before admission to the dementia care unit. This care plan arrangement alleviates some of the problems of what to do with the patient who becomes acutely ill, less mobile, and ultimately bedridden. Obviously, a team care approach is of tremendous help to the staff, family, and patient in discussing when a patient should be considered for transfer to another unit. Should the transfer be accomplished when the patient has a noticeable decrease in ambulatory status, or should the dementia unit attempt to help the patient who requires total care and is bedridden? To settle these problems, some bargaining between the staff and the family eventually will be required. However, it should always be kept in mind that the specialized dementia unit is not designed to handle total care patients.

Dementia care units are defined as living areas that are largely self-contained and self-sufficient in terms of services, staffing, and congregate space. The unique offerings of specialized dementia care units are their ability to respond appropriately to each resident's needs and to plan innovatively according to each resident's individual situation. The items of utmost importance in accomplishing this type of inclusive care are staffing, physical plant, and family-patient interaction. Such an organized treatment in carefully planned specialized dementia care units addresses the complex and ever-changing links among staff, resident, family, and institution. This team approach to care is critical to a successful outcome in dementia care.

What criteria should be used to decide which patients are best candidates for these specialized units? The ideal candidates for care in specialized dementia care units include those patients who, despite severe memory problems, are ambulatory and can feed themselves, do not need extensive medical care, are able to follow simple instructions, and can manage to perform some activities of daily living with the help of the staff.

Two decades of experience with special dementia care units has demonstrated a decrease in wandering, agitation, screaming, depression, and psychotic behavior. Other positive benefits include a decrease in (or elimination of) drugs to control behavior, weight gain, improved behavior, greater ability to sleep through the night, and reduced incontinence. Catering to the patient's needs, habits, and uniqueness rather than the dementia is the best service that the specialized dementia care unit can provide.

STAFFING ROLES

In specialized dementia care units, the staff/patient ratio is much higher than in traditional nursing homes or custodial settings. Such a situation does not necessarily mean that the patient directly requires more care but that more staff-patient interaction allows the patient to participate as fully as possible in the unit, thus helping to define his own limits and increasing his level of activity as much as practical. Staff development programs aimed at improving interpersonal communication skills, emphasizing concise documentation of medical records, and fostering respect for individual rights and dignity are basic to the unit concept.

Good patient-staff interaction and communication are central features in the day-to-day management of such a unit. Staff members invest time and energy in learning about the interests of their patients both before they come to the unit and during their stay there. This approach helps the staff to see the patients as being less dependent. Such detail in patient care may not be possible in custodial nursing home units because of time and staffing constraints. Furthermore, in custodial care units, a tremendous amount of staff energy is required to take care of the physical needs of patients. This need is precipitated by a low staff/patient ratio and the complexity of care required for recuperating, but not yet well, patients. While in this situation, nursing home staff might know what to do for their patients but have little time or inclination to get to know them. To suggest that the nursing home custodial care staff change their approach to patient care may be interpreted as saying that they are not doing enough or are doing their job poorly. The challenge to extended care setting nursing staff is to change from custodial care to a team approach since no single discipline can meet the particular needs of the elderly with dementia. Communication in such a setting must be multidirectional so that most of the decision-making is shared and decisions are rendered by consensus rather than by directives. Such a model of residential living requires integrating the staff structure and understanding the needs of residents. The staff should have the ability to interact with residents according to each patient's needs and behavior in various stages of their illness. The staff should be able to seek out what capacities remain in severely impaired individuals since these capacities can be used to improve the quality of life of these patients.

The attitudes of staff and facility administrators should not promote the stereotype of patients with dementia as being mentally ill and totally incapable. It is wrong for the staff to assume that people with dementia are no longer aware of or sensitive to their surroundings or that they have lost all capacity to function. Such stereotyped attitudes are noted when staff or caregivers use methods and assumptions that treat dementia as mental retardation (amentia) rather than as dementia. With dementia, a person is deteriorating from a previously higher level of cognitive functioning; with amentia, the person did not previously have a higher level of functioning. In amentia, a caregiver or staff member frequently takes the role of a teacher of new skills. In dementia, the teaching of new skills is generally not done. In patients with dementia, the ability to do the task is very often intact. It is the ability of the brain to tell the body what to do or the ability to recognize that this is the appropriate time to do the task that is impaired. The differences between the two disorders may seem to be subtle, but, in fact, they call for very different approaches in terms of intervention, goals, and caregiver roles. For the most part, the distinctions between amentia and dementia are not appreciated in nursing home custodial units. Therefore the remaining capacities, still intact in the person with dementia, are never recognized or utilized.

Professional persons cannot serve effectively if they do not understand older people; nor can they serve older people when they have negative beliefs about the elder population.

Specific training must be available for nurse's aides, who probably spend the most time with the patient, and their skills must be reinforced periodically. Training in basic nursing, personal care, social needs, basic restorative services, and resident rights should be part of the continuing education of nurse's aides. Specific topics that should be included in these training sessions are an overview of dementia that explains the stages of the illness and describes the emotional and behavioral problems that may occur with this disease. Therapeutic and recreational services offered in the dementia unit should be reviewed. Staff members should be made aware of the importance of changing staff roles to encompass continuing periodic patient evaluation—how to assess patient needs and their strengths and abilities. Other important topics that must be included are mechanisms that are helpful in responding to difficult behavior problems, the importance of the physical environment of the unit, techniques used to involve families, and ways of compensating for sensory loss in old age. This emphasis on staff development and specific programs is also geared to addressing the staff's needs. Teaching staff caregivers how to deal with patients with dementia also helps to curtail staff burnout. Adequate staff leave programs and switching staff assignments to take care of different residents at various stages of dementia illnesses helps to lessen the impact of personal emotional involvement by the staff. Continuing interaction with the custodial nursing home staff helps to improve dementia unit staff morale. As indicated earlier, this interaction is facilitated if the specialized dementia care unit is structurally attached to the custodial nursing home but still able to develop its own separate identity.

One of the ways in which the dementia unit can be made more viable, to both patients and staff, is to add a day care center. This type of center serves the community, allows for periods of rest during the day for family caregivers, and enriches the activities planned for the unit (see Chapter 20).

Behavioral abnormalities are some of the more frequent and more difficult disturbances that need to be dealt with effectively in people with dementia. There are several simple mechanisms that the staff may use to help with the behavioral problems that can arise in patients in a dementia unit. For example, staff members may be able to intervene by providing a diversion or a distraction before a resident becomes extremely agitated. They can often help the patient avoid strong reactions. Items of interest (e.g., photographs or furniture) to the patient can be incorporated into the physical environment to provide meaning and to serve as a diversion when needed. Joking and lighthearted talking sometimes help to reduce tension; however, it is important that this maneuver in no way belittle or ridicule the elderly person. Touch is a very important method of communication with the elderly person with dementia. It may be used to focus the attention of the patient on a specific task to be accomplished and to have a calming effect on the patient. Touch alone may be the best intervention for diffusing agitation and providing distraction during behavioral problems. Touching is one of the most beneficial therapeutic actions for combating the sensory isolation that the elderly experience. Touch can relate warmth and a genuine concern for the elderly patient with dementia that no other action can accomplish. However, it should be remembered that not all patients like to be touched.

Explanation and discussion are also valuable tools in behavior adjustment, even in cognitively impaired patients. Unit staff should not assume that persons with dementia will not understand even simple explanations or instructions. Similarly, they must make an effort to give residents choices when they resist certain activities so that the patients feel that they have at least some control over their own lives.

Conspicuous visual cues are used to orient the person with dementia (e.g., symbols for dining room, garden room). These cues should be simple and not arranged to overload the patient. For example, at dinner a patient may eat his dessert after eating nothing on his plate. Since only the dessert is placed in front of the patient along with the eating utensil, the cue is easy for the patient. On the other hand, having several items on one dish might be overwhelming to the patient, and therefore he feels unable to cope (i.e., eat). Alternatively, the patient may need time to process the cues in order to act appropriately.

Avoiding fixed schedules and making allowances to individualize schedules for people with dementia will help to control stress and anxiety for both the patient and the staff. This approach allows the patient to follow his own life-style or current mood. For example, setting bath schedules, which often can be followed only if the staff uses coercion, can cause much anger and resistance on the part of residents and can result in frustration and stress for the staff. Giving the patient a choice between bathing or eating a meal may be more productive regardless of the proximate scheduled event.

Chemical restraints continue to be overused as a means of behavior control in custodial nursing. In general, there is too great a reliance on high-dose administration of sedatives and hypnotics and antipsychotic drugs to achieve behavior control. Side effects associated with these particular drugs are common (see Chapter 14). In interactive dementia care units, overuse of psychoactive drugs is avoided because the staff knows the patient's moods and capacities and works within these limits, learning how to bargain with the patient. When preventive mechanisms are used to deal with patients with dementia on their own terms, the need for chemical restraints should diminish.

The staff caregiver can use certain strategies to help the patient in a given task and simultaneously use them to evaluate the resident's remaining capabilities to perform the task. The following strategies are listed from the least intrusive to the most intrusive: (1) waiting, (2) slowing down, (3) asking if the patient wants help, (4) prompting the patient verbally or nonverbally, (5) encouraging the patient, (6) providing the patient with feedback, and (7) doing all or part of the task for the patient.

ARCHITECTURAL DESIGN

Another important consideration in establishing a dementia care unit is the development and construction of the physical plant and architectural design of the building. The architectural layout should avoid the use of "institutional cues," reminiscent of the hospital set-

ting. Dementia care units should, as far as possible, resemble a home
In the most basic sense, specialized dementia care units should b
user friendly and user protective.

In order to make patients feel comfortable, dementia units in
clude mirrors, pictures, and items of interest to the residents. The
provide adequate lighting and avoid shadows, glare, and loud back
ground noise. Fenced exterior gardens may be planned as an integra
part of the facility.

In general, egress control devices should be used in lieu of lockec
doors. For example, magnetic electrical door catches can be used t
signal door openings, which alert the staff when someone is exitin
from the facility. These signals can be monitored from a centra
station. Stress levels of the staff and the family are noted to b
remarkably lower when these persons do not need to watch exi
doors constantly. Accommodations for the wandering patient witl
dementia require additional innovative approaches. A racetrack de
sign has been tried in some situations so that residents can wande
endlessly. Some experts believe that aimless wandering reflects i
resident's desperate effort to leave or an impoverished environmen
that provides no other stimulation for the resident. Wandering i
probably important as a primal activity, but it also provides needec
exercise. Although it is an energy-depleting activity, wandering i
productive in the sense that it is likely to lessen the need fo
sedatives and hypnotics because the patient tires from the exercise.

The general attributes of the architectural environment shoulc
encompass the following: a noninstitutionalized (homelike) image
more negotiable environment (user friendly), sensory stimulatior
without stress (mirrors, paintings, gardens), positive visitor space
(affording some privacy), and opportunities for meaningful wander
ing. Clear signs that incorporate both words and pictures should b
used for concise and precise cueing to identify restrooms, dining area
TV lounge or game areas, and walking spaces.

Additional requirements to reduce environmental stressors include
dampening of extraneous stimuli by using sound-absorbing material
eliminating intercoms, and "painting out" doors to storage areas. This
"painting out" technique serves as a subtle camouflage; for example, a
door that does not color contrast with the wall is not easily recognized
Alternatively, some units have curtains to cover doors that are exits. This
simple maneuver may be a very cost-effective egress control device.

Facility design should be architecturally stylized to reduce pa
tient stress. The goal of simulating a home environment setting
should include the use of "quiet" colors. Also, the family cluster con

struction approach uses small, private living areas for small numbers of patients and includes a bedroom, sitting area, family area, and bath. The family area helps to provide additional privacy for visitations. Such a design respects the residents' space and allows them to keep meaningful things from the past in their living area. These living areas should be spacious enough to allow some personalization with items known to be of particular importance to the patient, such as mementos, family photographs, and furniture. The presence of personal possessions not only may help patients to maintain their identity but also may aid the staff in developing a sense of each person as an individual with a unique history. These items associated with the resident's personal history allow the staff to be creative and innovative in communication, orientation, and reminiscence.

The architectural plans of the kitchen and all other living areas should be used to create a calm and interactive environment where the demands of the physical setting are not beyond the patient's capacity to function. The staff should continually experiment with different busy activities for the residents. Residents may want to set places for the meals, wash and dry dishes, or prepare simple desserts such as cookies. Such activities provide useful recreation and therapeutic time for patients. However, some residents may choose to do such activities at odd hours of the day, and there should be enough flexibility in the program to handle such differences. These simple kitchen or dining room tasks are not done as a learning technique but as a tool for the patient to spend time in a designated task. Some assistance with kitchen tasks may be required of the unit staff, but only to assist the patient in performing the task, not do it for him.

FAMILY ROLES

Family participation is an integral part of dementia care. Visitation by family members frequently helps in regard to the patient's level of activity and reinforces each patient's unique likes and dislikes to the staff. For example, one patient was reported to spend several hours folding clothes constantly before admission to the dementia care unit. Such a repetitive activity can be used effectively in the unit when there is a need to occupy the patient's attention or to divert him from a disruptive behavior. Most families prefer to remain actively involved in the caregiving process after the patient has been placed in the unit. Therefore the staff should create an atmosphere that ensures positive family involvement. They must be aware of the significant burdens that the patient's family have shouldered before making the decision to institutionalize a relative with dementia. All the research on caring for relatives with dementia has documented that it is a very difficult process that can have severe effects on the mental health, self-esteem, and social life of the caregiver. By the time the decision has been made to institutionalize a relative, the primary caregiver may have devoted years of his or her life to the caregiving process. Therefore the decision can be a very painful one, and it is not necessarily associated with feelings of relief. The families may continue to feel the stress of caregiving even though they are no longer responsible for the day-to-day care of the patient.

The reputation and prestige of any dementia care unit are a direct reflection of the investment made in it by family caregivers. The unit staff that pays close attention to the involvement of families will always benefit.

One of the most important facets of good family-staff relationships is the process for resolving complaints. Family meetings are an important way of orienting and involving families at the outset. Providing the family with information in writing is important since the relatives are usually distracted and upset at the time that the patient is admitted. To help keep problems from progressing to a crisis point between the facility and the family, it should be made clear initially that the family is an active participant in planning treatment.

A family's expectations may be heightened by the guilt they feel about having sent their relative to a nursing home. A "family buddy system" may be a good way of helping to orient new families to a unit and to adjust the family's expectations to a practical level. An excellent method of communication with the patient's family is the care-planning conference. Through this conference, the family commonly feels better about having been consulted and informed. The best decisions about the resident's care can be made when staff and family are in accord and decisions are made by consensus.

In addition, introducing the family members to the staff and the key members of the team that runs the unit is critical in attaining family support. Such an introduction can be done over several sessions to identify staff, their positions, and how they relate to the patient. Family-oriented educational programs offer additional benefits. These educational sessions can be used to review normal aging changes, information about Alzheimer's disease and related illnesses, emotional issues for families, communication techniques, difficult behavior, medications, depression, daily routines in the unit, and successful family visits. One way to establish a good working relationship with the family is to ask for help in putting together a good social/medical/family history of the relative. Such a history will help the unit staff relate to and communicate with the patient in a more personal way.

The family can also be recruited to become more formally involved by attending patient care conferences in which treatment plans and patient activity plans are discussed along with any particular problems that the staff is having. Such intervention planning avoids the crisis-only intervention mindset that is prevalent in custodial care settings. This type of communication among staff, family, and family caregivers optimizes the patient's functional ability to live within and up to the limits of his dementia. Interdisciplinary team meetings allow for direct efforts at trouble-shooting and averting problems that might precipitate patient stress, family anger, and unit staff withdrawal.

Whatever the mechanism used to gain consensus in patient care, there must be a strong psychosocial component to care since the patient cannot make decisions for himself. Dementia care falls somewhere between medical treatment provided in custodial care nursing homes and psychiatric treatment offered in most mental health facilities. Dementia unit care involves an ongoing assessment that allows for continuous remodeling of approaches to patient care. The treatment team can apply whatever intervention is appropriate for the situation, affecting the patient's activities program and physical, social, and emotional environment. Since the primary dementia disorder is progressive, the family's expectations must be adjusted to a realistic level as the goals of patient care become more existential rather than focusing on permanent gains or improvement. Through this process of ongoing reassessment and reevaluation of the patient, it is recognized that, as the dementia progresses, the affected person becomes increasingly dependent on his environment to influence his actions and behavior. A major part of the patient's environment is a responsive unit staff.

BIBLIOGRAPHY

Benson DM and others: Establishment and impact of a dementia unit within the nursing home, *J Am Geriatr Soc* 35(4):319-323, 1987.

Calkins MP: *Design for dementia: planning environments for the elderly and the confused*, Owings Mills, Md, 1988, National Health Publishing.

Cohen U, Weesman G: *Holding on to home: designing environments for people with dementia*, Baltimore, 1991, Johns Hopkins University Press.

Coons DH: *Specialized dementia care units*, Baltimore, 1991, Johns Hopkins University Press.

Coons DH: Training staff to work in special care units, *Am J Alzheimer Care Res* 2(5):6-12, 1987.

Coons DH: Wandering, *Am J Alzheimer Care Res* 3(1):31-36, 1988.

Greene JA, Asp J, Crane N: Specialized management of the Alzheimer's disease patient: does it make a difference? *J Tenn Med Assoc* 78:559-563, 1985.

Hamdy RC: Nursing homes: reducing the impact of institutionalization, *J Tenn Med Assoc* 84(1):13-15, 1991.

Mace NL: *Dementia care: patient, family, community*, Baltimore, 1991, Johns Hopkins University Press.

Mace NL, Gwyther LP: *Selecting a nursing home with a dedicated dementia care unit*, Chicago, 1989, Alzheimer's Disease and Related Disorders Association.

Matthew LP and others: What's different about a special care unit for dementia patients? A comparative study, *Am J Alzheimer Care Res* 3(2):16-23, 1988.

Rubin A, Shultlesworth GE: Engaging families as support in nursing home care: ambiguity in the subdivision of tasks, *Gerontologist* 23(6):632-636, 1983.

Shulman MD, Mandel E: Communication training of relatives and friends of institutional elderly persons, *Gerontologist* 28(6):797-799, 1988.

Turnbull J: The nursing home physician image: time for a face-lift, *Geriatrics* 44(8):83-90, 1989.

FUTURE PROSPECTS

31

Promising areas of research

Kevin F. Gray

Dementia is emerging as a major challenge, not only for health care providers but for society as a whole. Government estimates suggest that up to 4 million Americans suffer from severe dementia and that an additional 1 to 5 million patients have mild to moderate dementia. At least 50% to 60% of these patients have Alzheimer's disease. Given the growing number of elderly persons in the population, the number of Americans with severe dementia is projected to triple by 2040. Currently, the direct and indirect annual costs of dementia total $100 billion. These costs are steadily increasing—as health costs rise, as human longevity is extended, and as the prevalence of dementia increases. Barring some unforeseen military or environmental catastrophe, dementia will be one of the key health problems confronting society in the twenty-first century. Research must lead the way, not only medical and scientific research but also research into efforts for improving delivery of services to those afflicted with Alzheimer's disease, and for optimizing health and support for caregivers of patients with the disease.

DIAGNOSIS

With the refined diagnostic criteria available for Alzheimer's disease, the current level of accurate diagnosis approaches 85% to 90%. These figures indicate that there is still a small but definite level of diagnostic uncertainty even at the best medical centers. Currently, researchers are using brain imaging studies to improve the accuracy of diagnosis of Alzheimer's disease. Structural images of the brain using computed tomography (CT) or magnetic resonance imaging (MRI) demonstrate anatomical changes in the brain but are often unable to distinguish between those changes associated with Alzheimer's disease and those related to normal aging. Functional imaging techniques, using single photon emission computed tomography (SPECT) and positron emission tomography (PET), allow researchers to examine blood flow and metabolism in specific brain regions. These functional techniques reflect brain activity and demonstrate areas affected by Alzheimer's disease at a time when brain structure still appears normal. In some laboratories SPECT and PET use sophisticated radioactive tracers to highlight brain chemicals such as dopamine and acetylcholine. This method allows visualization of nerve pathways known to be affected in Alzheimer's disease. Changes in the production of these brain chemicals may be the earliest sign of Alzheimer's disease, making very early diagnosis and intervention possible.

Other emerging techniques include magnetic resonance spectroscopy (MRS) and quantitative electroencephalography (QEEG). MRS allows noninvasive studies of cellular chemical reactions, including the metabolism and breakdown of brain cells, and the effects of drugs on brain chemistry. Eventually, when MRS is combined with MRI, it will be possible to measure changes in the brain chemistry of specific anatomical structures, and thus it will be a valuable tool for detection of Alzheimer's disease. QEEG, which makes use of computer technology to monitor brain electrical activity, one day may be used to identify specific brain diseases such as Alzheimer's disease. Neuroimaging continues to evolve to higher levels of sophistication. A brand new technique using the superconducting quantum interference device (SQUID) measures tiny changes in magnetic fields caused by the brain's electrical activity and may eventually be used in Alzheimer's disease research. Most of these new techniques are expensive and are available for research only in major medical centers. However, they may become more readily available in the future.

Accurate diagnosis of Alzheimer's disease in the future will be based on learning more about the underlying causes of the disease, understanding the sequence of events as the disease progresses, and eventually understanding the genetics of the disease at the molecular level. Although various risk factors for Alzheimer's disease are being studied, only increased age, a family history of the disease, and, perhaps, a history of head trauma appear to be associated with it. Since studies of identical twins show that both twins develop Alzheimer's disease only approximately 40% of the time, it is thought that genetic factors must interact with environmental factors to produce the disease. However, studies of occupational and environmental exposures (e.g., aluminum) have not shown correlation with development of Alzheimer's disease. To date, there is no confirmed risk factor for Alzheimer's disease that can be modified by intervention or change in life-style.

Researchers studying the progression of Alzheimer's disease have focused on amyloid protein in the brain. One form of amyloid, beta-amyloid, is deposited in the brain to form the plaques seen in the disease. Beta-amyloid is part of a larger protein, the amyloid precursor protein (APP), that is split by enzymes to create the beta fragment. In patients with Alzheimer's disease, this beta-amyloid originally was thought to be the abnormal product of an "incorrect" splitting of APP that was toxic to other brain cells. Over time, accumulation of this "poison" would lead to more incorrect splitting of APP, more beta-amyloid formation, and further damage to brain cells, eventually causing the loss of mental abilities characteristic of Alzheimer's disease. This theory of an ever-worsening cascade of brain damage caused by amyloid has become more complicated recently because new research demonstrates that beta-amyloid is normally found in all cells and therefore may not be as toxic as previously believed. The accumulation of excess amyloid in the brain of patients with Alzheimer's disease could be caused by overproduction of APP or could result from defects in the normal processing and breakdown of amyloid. The trigger mechanism that starts this amyloid buildup is unknown. In fact, since amyloid deposits can be found in the brains of elderly persons without Alzheimer's disease, the question of what causes the disease remains elusive.

The use of genetic manipulations to create animal models with inherited Alzheimer's disease is anticipated, and this approach will greatly help researchers understand the disease process. Much of the current work on the genetics of Alzheimer's disease has centered on amyloid. A handful of families with a form of inherited Alzheimer's disease have a defect on chromosome 21 and produce excess APP. Other rare mutations on chromosomes 19 and 14 also cause inherited Alzheimer's disease. These genetic findings indicate that Alzheimer's disease is not a single disease with a single cause but a complex disorder similar to heart disease. Certain families have rare genetic defects that cause the disease; however, most people with the disease do not appear to have a genetic defect.

Ideally, research will lead to the development of a diagnostic test for Alzheimer's disease that accurately identifies the illness even before symptoms arise. Such a test might allow preventive measures or treatment methods to be tried before the brain damage becomes extensive. Improvements in diagnosis might also allow specific disease subgroups to be targeted for individualized treatment. Current attempts are under way to develop a diagnostic screen for Alzheimer's disease. One promising method uses cerebrospinal fluid obtained from lumbar puncture to detect various amyloid proteins found in the brains of affected individuals. However, since amyloid proteins are also found in normal brains, further refinement of this screen is necessary. Another potential diagnostic test would be based on the theory that Alzheimer's disease is caused by a fundamental breakdown in cellular machinery. The tangles found within nerve cells in the disease are made up of protein fibers that normally form microtubules, key structural elements that help to maintain cell shape. In Alzheimer's disease these protein fibers appear to be abnormally altered. By studying cellular repair mechanisms involving microtubules, it may be proved that patients with Alzheimer's disease have characteristic defects that could be detected via blood test or skin biopsy.

FACILITIES

The future of health care for patients with Alzheimer's disease will focus on the interface between home care and institutional care. Both forms of care are essential and should be viewed as mutually supportive components along a continuum of disability. At present, most funding for long-term care is strongly biased toward institutional settings, with a lack of adequate financial coverage for home care. This situation clearly does not take into account studies showing that families and patients prefer home care and that patients with Alzheimer's disease generally do best in familiar environments. In addition, although $30 to $40 billion are spent annually for the direct care of patients with Alzheimer's disease, if all the families caring for these patients at home were replaced with hired caregivers, the direct care costs would increase by more than $26 billion. The federal government will need to devise a more appropriate long-term care plan, recognizing that home care for patients with Alzheimer's disease is preferable and that institutional care should not be viewed as competitive with home care.

In the future, improved screening evaluations will accurately detect the true extent of the patient's disabilities and remaining functional capacity. Use of these instruments, such as the recently devised

Executive Interview, will be essential for correctly timing the patient's entry into a nursing care facility. Waiting too long to institutionalize the patient with Alzheimer's disease can place undue strain on the family, whereas premature institutionalization can compromise the quality of life for the patient and create unnecessary financial burdens. Long-term care facilities of the future will have special care units for Alzheimer's disease with improved environmental designs that allow the patient to live in a secure, restraint-free atmosphere of "contained freedom." Staffing and supervision will be provided by nurses and physicians with special training in the diagnosis, treatment, and care of patients with Alzheimer's disease. Future research in this area is needed to help determine which programs provide the best patient outcomes, to design the optimal training and deployment of staff personnel, and to set ideal parameters for family involvement with the Alzheimer's disease special care unit.

TREATMENT

Current treatment for Alzheimer's disease is divided into two domains—control of problem behaviors such as delusions and agitation and restoration of lost mental abilities. Problem behaviors, which contribute to caregiver burden and burnout, greatly influence the decision to institutionalize the patient. Medications given for behavioral disturbances often merely sedate the patient rather than affecting target symptoms such as aggression. The drugs classified as neuroleptics (e.g., Haldol, Moban, and Mellaril), are helpful for delusions, suspiciousness, fearfulness, and hallucinations, but they produce potentially harmful side effects, such as muscle stiffness and poor balance, that can lead to falls. The future will see a wave of "gentler" drugs that target specific symptoms. Some currently used drugs, such as trazodone, buspirone, estrogen, and certain drugs used to control seizures, may prove helpful for agitation in patients with Alzheimer's disease. A new group of experimental drugs known as "serenics" is being studied, and these agents show promise in reducing aggressive behavior. In the next 5 years, "atypical neuroleptics" will become available for the treatment of psychotic symptoms without affecting muscle tone or causing tardive dyskinesia. Research into improved techniques for modifying problem behaviors without drugs will help to establish guidelines for care providers. Studies show that simplification of the environment, with an emphasis on predictability and carefully regulated stimulation, improves the behavior of patients with Alzheimer's disease. Other environmental manipulations currently being investigated include orientation strategies, improved furniture design, control of room illumination, and use of room color to provide visual contrast and atmosphere.

Drugs for restoring the mental abilities lost in Alzheimer's disease are in the very early stages of development. Most experiments have focused on enhancing levels of acetylcholine, a brain chemical that plays an important role in memory and is abnormally low in the brains of patients with Alzheimer's disease. The drug tacrine (Cognex) helps to prevent the natural breakdown of acetylcholine. Despite liver toxicity noted in preliminary clinical trials, tacrine shows some promise for slowing down or slightly reversing the mental decline associated with Alzheimer's disease. Unfortunately, recent research has demonstrated that many different brain chemicals are low in affected individuals, making it highly unlikely that any drug affecting the level of only one brain chemical will ever be a cure-all for Alzheimer's disease. Future research will explore combinations of drugs and target multiple brain systems. The drug selegiline (deprenil, Eldepryl) now used in the treatment of Parkinson's disease, helps to prevent breakdown of the monoamine class of brain chemicals and has shown promise in early Alzheimer's disease trials when combined with acetylcholine-enhancing drugs. Future research will also evaluate the use of dietary manipulation and food supplements to help the body manufacture vital brain chemicals. Certain drugs, collectively known as "nootropics" (e.g., Hydergine, piracetam), are reported to improve mental ability, possibly by increasing blood flow to the brain or by aiding nerve cell metabolism. At best, controlled studies have shown only modest effects for these drugs, despite reports of dramatic improvement noted in some individuals. The term "smart drugs" is used in the popular press to describe nootropics, along with various herbs, amino acids, and food supplements. To date, all these substances are of unproven benefit and require further research trials. Nonetheless, it seems inevitable that drugs for enhancing memory and thinking will be available eventually, not only for patients with Alzheimer's disease, but for anyone hoping to improve normal brain function.

In the future, when it is possible to identify persons at risk for developing Alzheimer's disease, another important treatment domain will be prevention, a strategy that will also include treating patients with very early Alzheimer's disease long before any symptoms arise. Many future strategies for combatting the disease will target amyloid. Since substance P, a naturally occurring protein, appears to block nerve cell loss caused by amyloid, it may prove to be a new means of therapeutic intervention in Alzheimer's disease. Research into the use of angiotensin-converting enzyme inhibitors to block the enzymes that split APP could prove helpful in limiting beta-amyloid accumulation. In addition, direct manipulation of the genes that regulate amyloid production is envisioned. Future interventions at the cellular level will include protection strategies whereby potentially toxic substances (e.g., excitotoxins, free radicals) are neutralized by "neuroprotective" drug therapy. Calcium channel blockers, vitamin E, and a group of scavenger compounds ("lazaroids") that inhibit the formation of oxygen free radicals are being tested for their neuroprotective effects. Investigators also speculate that nerve growth factor may protect the brain against the neuronal loss noted in Alzheimer's disease. A better understanding of how brain cells are affected by the aging process is extremely important, and much research is targeting apoptosis, the phenomenon of genetically programmed cell death. Control of apoptosis could conceivably result in the creation of "immortal" nerve cells, grown in tissue banks for eventual transplantation into the damaged brains of patients with Alzheimer's disease. Transplantation of fetal brain tissue might one day play a role in the treatment of the disease since experiments involving the transplantation of fetal nerve cells into the brains of aged rats appear to show that this method can improve memory function.

FAMILY SUPPORT AND SERVICES

Alzheimer's disease is truly a family affair, and families today provide more care to a greater number of elderly over longer periods of time than ever before. In the future the pressures on family caregivers will continue to increase because of several important trends in our society: (1) with the decline in the birth rate, there will be fewer young potential caregivers as the number of elderly requiring care increases; (2) the increased mobility of our society, which tends to disperse the family, will decrease the number of available caregivers; (3) economic pressures will continue to create more two-career families, and therefore women, the traditional caregivers, will be less available for caregiving; and (4) the increasing divorce rate means that fewer caregivers will have emotional and financial support from a spouse.

Future research into caregiving will aim at predicting family members who are at risk for burnout, allowing interventions such as respite care to be made in a timely fashion. To date, caregiver morbidity has been correlated with depression and medical illness in the caregiver. Caregiver burden has been correlated with excessive patient dependency on the caregiver, with caregiver fears that the patient will decline further, and with a "lack of time for self" reported by the caregiver. More frequent supportive visits by other family members alleviate the caregiver burden.

In the future, Alzheimer's disease caregivers will have improved access to information and referral services. The National Institute on Aging sponsors an Alzheimer's disease education and referral center (1-800-438-4380). The Alzheimer's Association sponsors an information service that allows families to learn about drug studies that are currently recruiting patients with Alzheimer's disease (1-800-272-3900). Future programs will provide case managers and improved transportation services for underserved populations such as minority caregivers or those living alone or in rural areas. It is hoped that federal long-term care insurance will become universally available to those in need, operating along a continuum from the time the diagnosis of Alzheimer's disease is made until the patient's eventual death.

BIBLIOGRAPHY

Chafetz PK: Structuring environments for dementia patients. In Weiner MF, editor: *The dementias: diagnosis and management*, Washington, DC, 1991, American Psychiatric Press.

Cummings JL, Benson DF: *Dementia: a clinical approach*, ed 2, Boston, 1992, Butterworth-Heinemann.

Mace NL, Rabins PV: *The 36-hour day*, Baltimore, 1991, Johns Hopkins University Press.

Matsuyama SS, Jarvik LF: Hypothesis: microtubules, a key to Alzheimer's disease, *Proc Natl Acad Sci* 86:8152-8156, 1989.

Royall DR, Mahurin RK, Gray KF: Bedside assessment of executive cognitive impairment: the executive interview, *J Am Geriatr Soc* 40:1221-1226, 1992.

Schultz R, Visintainer P, Williamson GM: Psychiatric and physical morbidity effects of caregiving, *J Gerontol* 45:P181-P191, 1990.

Selkoe DJ: Aging brain, aging mind, *Sci Am* 267:134-142, 1992.

Selkoe DJ: Amyloid protein and Alzheimer's disease, *Sci Am* 265:68-78, 1991.

Stern RG, Davis KL: Treatment approaches in Alzheimer's disease: past, present, and future. In Weiner MF, editor: *The dementias: diagnosis and management*, Washington, DC, 1991, American Psychiatric Press.

US Congress, Office of Technology Assessment: *Losing a million minds: confronting the tragedy of Alzheimer's disease and other dementias*, Washington, DC, 1987, Office of Technology Assessment.

US Department of Health and Human Services: *Progress report on Alzheimer's disease,* NIH Pub No 92-3409, Washington, DC, 1992, National Institute on Aging.

US Department of Health and Human Services: *Report of the advisory panel on Alzheimer's disease,* DHHS Pub No ADM-89-1644, Washington, DC, 1989, US Government Printing Office.

Whatley SA, Anderton BH: The genetics of Alzheimer's disease, *Int J Geriatr Psychiatry* 5:145-159, 1990.

Zarit SH, Reever KE, Bach-Peterson J: Relatives of the impaired elderly: correlates of feelings of burden, *Gerontologist* 20:649-655, 1980.

Glossary

If you would converse with me, you must first define your terms.

—*Voltaire*

abscess   Accumulation of pus caused by infection.

abstracting ability   Ability to shift voluntarily from one aspect of a situation to another. A characteristic of Alzheimer's disease and other psychiatric disorders is the inability to shift readily from the concrete to the abstract and back again as demanded by circumstances.

abulia   Loss or impairment of the ability to perform voluntary actions or to make decisions.

acetylcholine   Neurotransmitter that is deficient in patients with Alzheimer's disease.

agnosia   Inability to recognize various objects. Although agnosia often is present in the early stages of Alzheimer's disease, it may be so subtle and slight that it goes unnoticed. In the early stages of Alzheimer's disease, this condition can be recognized only through detailed psychological tests.

akathisia   Syndrome characterized by an inability to remain in the sitting position because of motor restlessness and a feeling of muscular quivering.

akinesia   Absence or loss of the power of voluntary motion.

amitriptyline (Elavil)   Tricyclic antidepressant commonly given at bedtime. It has both sedative and anticholinergic side effects.

amnesia   Memory impairment.

amyloid deposition   Deposit of an abnormal protein (amyloid) in the brain of a patient with Alzheimer's disease.

analgesics   Medications used to relieve pain; painkillers.

angina   See **Anginal pain.**

anginal pain   Chest pain experienced by a patient with coronary artery disease. Typically the pain occurs during exercise and is relieved by rest or appropriate medication. If such measures do not relieve the pain within a few minutes, the patient may have developed a myocardial infarction.

anhedonia   Loss of pleasure in things that normally interest the individual.

anomia   Difficulty in finding the correct word for an object. For example, the patient may recognize a pencil and may know what it is used for but may be unable to think of the word "pencil." Often the patient uses a sentence to describe a particular word. For instance, instead of "pencil," the patient may say "the thing you use to write with," or instead of "key," he may say "the thing used to open a door." Anomia is one of the first manifestations of Alzheimer's disease. Usually the patient initially has difficulty naming objects that he does not deal with in everyday life.

anosognosia   Failure to recognize a disease or deficit.

antacids   Drugs given to reduce the acidity of the contents of the stomach.

antibiotics   Group of drugs used to combat infection. For severe infections, antibiotics usually are administered intravenously. In most other cases, they are administered orally.

anticholinergic side effects   Side effects produced by medication that inhibits the parasympathetic branch of the autonomic nervous system (e.g., dry mouth, blurred vision, urinary retention). Medications with anticholinergic side effects include antihistamines, neuroleptic drugs, and antidepressants. These drugs sometimes are combined with antacids.

antihistamines   Drugs taken for allergies and the common cold. Most antihistamines induce a certain degree of drowsiness and may cause sedation. They often are included in sleeping medications bought over the counter.

apathy   Condition in which the patient shows little or no emotion.

aphasia   Impairment in the speech process. *Receptive aphasia* is an inability to comprehend what one hears. *Expressive aphasia* is an inability to express oneself, even though the question has been heard and understood. The two types of aphasia can be differentiated by asking the patient to execute a certain command, such as closing the eyes, sticking out the tongue, or raising the left arm. If the patient hears and understands what is being said, he will execute the command. If he cannot hear or cannot comprehend what he hears (receptive aphasia), he will be unable to comply. When these commands are given, it is important not to mimic the gesture that the patient is expected to perform. For instance, while asking the patient to raise his arm, the examiner must refrain from raising an arm.

apnea   Cessation of breathing. *Sleep apnea* is the cessation of breathing while sleeping, which characteristically occurs in grossly overweight and obese individuals. With apnea, insufficient oxygen reaches the brain, and the individual may wake up distressed.

apraxia   Inability to carry out purposeful movements and actions despite intact motor and sensory systems. Apraxia usually is present early in Alzheimer's disease, but it may be confined to actions that the patient does not routinely perform during daily activities. For example, the patient may not be able to tie a bow tie but may still be able to tie a regular tie. This situation is often attributed to a lack of practice. In the early stages apraxia may be more apparent when the patient faces several choices. He may have no difficulty putting his shirt on, but, when faced with a variety of shirts, ties, underwear, trousers, and coats, he may become confused as to which one to pick first. As the disease progresses, apraxia comes to affect even daily activities, and the patient no longer can dress, feed, or wash himself, even though he has no paralysis.

arteriosclerosis   Condition in which the inner lining of the arteries is coated with cholesterol, triglycerides, and other fatty substances. This deposition, which often also invades other layers of an artery, causes the arteries to become rigid and their lumens to narrow. This change diminishes the amount of blood that flows through these arteries and the amount that reaches the various organs supplied by them. If arteriosclerosis affects the arteries that carry blood to the brain, the blood supply to the brain is reduced and the patient is at increased risk of developing a stroke.

aspiration pneumonia   Pneumonia caused by inhaling gastric contents or food into the lungs.

asthma   Disease in which the trachea and the bronchi (airways) become constricted, reducing the amount of air that reaches the lungs. Asthma characteristically occurs in attacks, with the patient experiencing sudden breathlessness and an inability to breathe comfortably. In many instances asthma reflects an allergic reaction to a number of substances that may contain pollen. Asthmatic attacks also are often precipitated by smoking.

ataxia   Inability to coordinate voluntary actions.

atrophy   Wasting of tissues, organs, or the entire body. One of the characteristic features of Alzheimer's disease is the wasting away of the brain, which becomes much smaller than that of an individual of the same age and sex who does not have the disease.

audiometric testing   Use of an electrical instrument to measure hearing acuity.

autoanalysis   See **Biochemical screening.**

autonomic nervous system   Part of the nervous system that is not under voluntary control. The autonomic nervous system has two main subdivisions: parasympathetic and sympathetic. On the whole, the parasympathetic system takes over while a person is relaxing or sleeping, whereas the sympathetic system is active predominantly when an individual is in an excited state.

benzodiazepines   Class of drugs used to treat anxiety and insomnia. The group includes flurazepam (Dalmane), chlordiazepoxide (Librium), diazepam (Valium), and alprazolam (Xanax). Some patients become addicted to these drugs, and abrupt withdrawal may lead to seizures.

b.i.d.   (L. *bis in die*) Abbreviation designating that a medication is to be administered twice daily.

biochemical screening   Series of laboratory tests for measuring the concentration of various blood substances. The screening often is done on automated equipment and sometimes is referred to as autoanalysis or sequential multichannel autoanalysis (SMA).

bipolar disorder   Mood disorder comprising episodes of both mania and depression; formerly called "manic depressive illness." Patients with bipolar disorder may appear either manic or depressed.

bradyphrenia   Slowing of information processing.

bulimia   Episodic eating binges or excessive intake of food or fluid, generally beyond voluntary control. Although often a condition of young women, it is also seen in patients with Alzheimer's disease.

cachexia   Severe weight loss associated with dehydration.

calculi   (singular, *calculus*) Crystals or very small stones present in the urinary tract system. If a stone is present in the kidneys or ureters, the patient will have very severe flank pain radiating to the groin and will pass blood in the urine. If the stone is located in the urinary bladder, the patient may feel a constant urge to empty the bladder, but only a few drops of urine are passed at a time. A bladder stone also is often associated with pain or scalding. When calculi are present in the bladder, they increase the excitability of the bladder and may be responsible for bouts of urinary incontinence.

cardiac reserve capacity   Heart's ability to increase its output to meet the body's increased demand during exercise.

cataract   Condition in which the lens of the eye becomes opaque. It is frequently seen in old age and is one of the most common causes of impaired visual acuity in older people. In some instances cataracts are caused by specific diseases, such as diabetes mellitus or hyperparathyroidism, but most often the cause is unknown. Patients with cataracts often see better in dim light because the pupils are dilated and a larger portion of the lens is exposed (in bright light, the pupils are constricted and only a small part of the lens is exposed). Cataract surgery is the treatment of choice.

cerebrovascular accident   See **Stroke.**

chlorpromazine (Thorazine)   Neuroleptic agent that belongs to the class of drugs known as phenothiazines. It causes extrapyramidal effects, sedation, and orthostatic hypotension.

cholesterol   Fatty substance present in the bloodstream that is essential for the adequate functioning of a number of body cells. However, if the concentration rises above a certain level, cholesterol tends to be precipitated along the inner lining of the arteries, giving rise to arteriosclerosis. This situation, in turn, is associated with an increased risk of developing coronary heart disease, stroke, and peripheral vascular insufficiency.

cholinergic   Relating to nerve cells that use acetylcholine as their neurotransmitter.

cholinesterase   Group of enzymes capable of breaking down acetylcholine.

chromosomes   Microscopic rod-shaped structures that contain genes and are found in every living cell. The genes transmit the characteristics inherited from the parent cell to the next generation. It has been postulated that Alzheimer's disease may involve some defect in chromosome 21, the same chromosome that is defective in Down's syndrome. All patients with Down's syndrome who survive the third decade of life develop the manifestations of Alzheimer's disease.

circadian rhythm   See **Sleep/wake cycle.**

circumstantial (tangential) thinking   Disturbance in thinking characterized by an excessive amount of detail that is irrelevant.

cognitive functions   Operations of the mind by which an individual becomes aware of objects of thought or perception. Includes all aspects of perceiving, thinking, and remembering.

computed tomography (CT) scan   Special radiological test in which a very large number of x-ray films are taken simultaneously from different angles. The various films are put together by a computer to produce a detailed view of the brain. In advanced stages of Alzheimer's disease, the CT scan often reveals that the brain has atrophied and that the ventricles of the brain are dilated. In early stages of the disease, however, the CT scan is essentially within normal limits. Although there has been a great deal of controversy over whether a CT scan should be done routinely in patients suspected of having Alzheimer's disease, the current consensus is that such an investigation is necessary. It must be emphasized, however, that such an investigation is not necessary to confirm the diagnosis of Alzheimer's disease but to exclude other conditions that may mimic Alzheimer's disease, such as a brain tumor, brain hemorrhage, or stroke. A CT scan may be done with or without contrast medium. The former technique usually is preferred so that the various parts of the brain can be clearly visualized. The main problem with performing a CT scan is that the patient must lie still on the table, which is sometimes difficult for patients who have advanced Alzheimer's disease.

congestive cardiac failure   Condition in which the heart cannot maintain adequate output. The common manifestations of heart failure include swelling of the legs (particularly worse toward the end of the day) and breathlessness on exertion. One of the first signs is awakening several times a night to pass a large amount of urine.

In the early stages the patient tends to wake up in the middle of the night short of breath. This breathlessness usually is relieved when the patient sits up. In the later stages the patient cannot lie flat in bed and must be in a semisitting position supported by two, three, or four pillows.

coronary heart disease   Condition in which the lumina of the arteries supplying blood to the heart are narrowed by deposition of cholesterol along their inner linings. Patients with coronary heart disease may have anginal pain or a myocardial infarct.

cortex   Outer layer of the brain. Alzheimer's disease affects the cortex: The number of brain cells (neurons) is reduced, and certain typical microscopic findings are noted, including neurofibrillary tangles and plaques.

cross-sectional study   Study done at one point in time on several people of different ages. Many such studies have been done in an attempt to examine the aging process, but it now is generally thought that those studies can be misleading because it is inaccurate to compare generation with generation and to attribute changes to the aging process when, in fact, most changes could be the result of alterations in economic, cultural, and social circumstances. Currently, longitudinal studies are preferred because these studies do follow-up on a group of individuals as they age. The main drawback of longitudinal studies is the long period before results become apparent, often exceeding 20 to 30 years. Two major longitudinal studies in progress are the Framingham study and the Baltimore study.

decubitus ulcer   (plural, *decubiti*) Ulcer that develops when a patient is bedridden for prolonged periods. The usual sites for these ulcers are the sacral region, the heels, and, in rare cases, the shoulder blades and the back of the head. To prevent decubiti, foam mattresses or special beds should be used and the patient should be turned regularly while in bed.

delirium   Acute medical condition manifested by disorientation, confusion, and fluctuating levels of consciousness. Unlike Alzheimer's disease, delirium has an acute onset and is associated with semiconsciousness or an impaired state of consciousness. It usually is caused by a reversible condition.

delusions   False beliefs firmly held despite obvious evidence to the contrary. These beliefs are not accepted by other members of the person's culture. Some examples are delusions of being controlled, delusions of grandeur (an exaggerated idea of one's own importance or identity), and delusions of persecution.

dementia   Irreversible mental deterioration caused by a medical condition.

diabetes mellitus   Disease in which the body's utilization of glucose is reduced, resulting in an increase in the blood glucose level. Patients with diabetes mellitus often may experience acute confusion if the blood glucose level reaches a high level or (if the condition is treated) if the blood glucose level is inadvertently reduced to a very low value.

diaphragm   Muscle that separates the chest from the abdominal cavity. The diaphragm plays an important role in breathing. By contracting and relaxing, it pulls on the chest wall, increases the volume of the chest, and facilitates the drawing of air into the lungs.

diazepam (Valium)   Benzodiazepine used to treat anxiety and muscle spasms. It is long-acting and particularly liable to accumulate in elderly patients.

digitalis   Drug often used to treat heart failure, especially when the heart rate is irregular and rapid.

digoxin   See **Digitalis.**

diuretics   Drugs that increase the volume of urine produced. All diuretics increase the amount of sodium and water in the urine, and most also increase the amount of potassium lost in the urine. This effect may be particularly serious if the patient is simultaneously taking digitalis. The incidence of digitalis toxicity is increased if the patient has a low blood potassium level. Some diuretics also increase the amount of calcium lost in the urine.

diurnal pattern   See **Sleep/wake cycle.**

double-blind studies   Research method used to evaluate the efficacy of a drug in which neither the patient nor the physician knows whether the patient is receiving the agent being tested or a placebo.

dysarthria   Difficulty in articulating words.

dysphagia   Difficulty with swallowing.

dysphasia   Mild form of aphasia.

dysuria   Pain or a burning sensation while passing urine. Dysuria often denotes an infection in the bladder.

echolalia   Tendency to repeat a question asked or a word of a question without being able to answer the question.

electrocardiogram (ECG)   Graphic record of the heart's electrical activity. ECGs usually are obtained to detect insufficient blood supply to the heart or cardiac irregularities.

electroencephalogram (EEG)   Graphic record of the brain's electrical activity. In patients with Alzheimer's disease, the EEG shows that most brain waves are of smaller magnitude than those of normal individuals; generalized slowing may also be observed. Currently, an EEG is not necessary in the routine diagnostic workup of a patient suspected of having Alzheimer's disease.

electrolyte   Chemical substance in the blood. Examples include sodium, potassium, calcium, and magnesium. Electrolyte levels can be reduced or elevated by various diseases or medications.

embolism   Development of an embolus.

embolus   Clot or other blockage brought to a blood vessel from another part of the body.

endocrine disease   Disease of the endocrine or hormonal glands, including the thyroid, parathyroid, pituitary, adrenal glands, and gonads.

estrogens   Hormones secreted by the ovaries. Estrogen secretion tends to decrease drastically during menopause; this sudden reduction may be responsible for a number of signs and symptoms, including atrophic vaginitis.

etiology   Study of the causes of a particular disease.

excoriation   Breaking down of the skin's surface; a condition associated with irritation. Excoriation often occurs when urine is left in contact with the skin.

extrapyramidal side effects   Variety of signs and symptoms that includes muscular rigidity, tremors, drooling, shuffling gait, restlessness, peculiar involuntary posture, and motor inertia. Neuroleptic drugs are particularly liable to give rise to these side effects.

fibroblast   Connective tissue cell capable of forming collagen.

flurazepam (Dalmane)   Hypnotic medication that tends to remain in the body for a long period, particularly in elderly patients. This situation may lead to drowsiness and unsteadiness the morning after the drug is taken.

gag reflex   Retching or gagging caused by contact of a foreign body with the mucous membrane of the space between the mouth and the pharynx.

genes   Microscopic structures located on the chromosomes that transmit specific characteristics from generation to generation. Current studies in Alzheimer's disease are focusing on identifying a particular gene that may be defective. This approach would allow identification and accurate diagnosis of individuals with the disease and possible "repair" of the defective gene through genetic engineering. (See also **Chromosomes.**)

genetic markers   Substances produced by abnormal genes. They can be found in individuals possessing these abnormal genes but not in people with normal genes.

genetic pattern   Organization and structure of various genes. It is possible to identify abnormal genes in a number of diseases and to diagnose these diseases by finding the abnormal gene and abnormal genetic pattern.

geropsychology   Psychology of old age.

glaucoma   Condition in which the fluid in the eye is under increased pressure. Glaucoma is a serious condition since, if allowed to persist, the pressure may interfere with the blood supply of the optic nerve and lead to blindness. A characteristic feature of glaucoma is the halos a patient often sees around objects; headaches also are common. Glaucoma can be managed relatively easily by administering eye drops regularly. Surgery also is sometimes used to treat this condition. In late stages, before vision is completely lost, the patient may have tunnel vision.

granulovacuolar degeneration   Microscopic finding describing degenerative changes in the brain cells.

gray matter   Structures in the brain that appear gray when the brain is cut. These include the outer layer of the cortex and a few structures in the center of the brain known as the basal ganglia. The gray matter contains most of the neurons.

gyri   (singular, *gyrus*) Convolutions on the surface of the brain. In Alzheimer's disease the gyri tend to become narrower and less convoluted.

hallucinations   Apparent subjective sensory perception of sight, sound, or smell with no basis in external reality.

haloperidol (Haldol)   Neuroleptic drug that is one of the butyrophenones. A powerful medication that produces severe extrapyramidal side effects, haloperidol should be given only for delusions, hallucinations, or bizarre behavior.

Heimlich maneuver   Emergency procedure designed to clear an airway obstructed by a foreign object, usually food.

hematoma   Collection of blood within an organ tissue or space resulting from trauma to a blood vessel.

Hippocrates   Greek physician who lived on the island of Cos in the fifth century BC and is generally considered to be the Father of Medicine.

histopathology   Study of diseased tissue through microscopic examination.

human immunodeficiency virus (HIV) test   Test performed to detect the virus responsible for acquired immunodeficiency syndrome (AIDS).

Huntington's disease   Genetic neurological disorder, usually appearing in midlife, characterized by involuntary movements and eventually dementia.

hyperinnervation   Excessive nerve stimulation.

hyperthyroidism   Disease in which the thyroid gland is overactive. Patients with hyperthyroidism tend to be overactive and to feel as if they have an enormous amount of energy. They also commonly lose weight and prefer cold weather.

hypnotics   Drugs that are given to induce sleep. Since drugs are metabolized more slowly as an individual ages, the effect of hypnotics may be prolonged in an older individual, causing increased sleepiness. Also, older people may be more sensitive to these drugs.

hypothermia   Condition resulting when the body temperature falls to 35° C or less (compared to the normal temperature of approximately 37° C).

hypothyroidism   Disease in which the thyroid gland does not produce sufficient thyroxin. Patients with hypothyroidism tend to tire easily, to become constipated, to sleep most of the time, and to be oversensitive to cold (preferring very warm environments).

illusion   Misperception of a real external stimulus, for example, a shadow on the wall caused by the moon and a tree outside is perceived as a stranger entering the room.

imipramine (Tofranil)   Drug used to treat depression; it is one of the tricyclic antidepressants. Imipramine is particularly prone to causing anticholinergic side effects.

indwelling Foley catheter   Tube introduced through the urethra into the urinary bladder. A balloon at the end of the tube is inflated to keep the catheter in position. This type of catheter should be used only as a last resort in the treatment of urinary incontinence. Its use is associated with a number of side effects, most importantly urinary tract infections, which often spread from the bladder to the kidneys.

insight   Person's ability to be aware of his problems. In the early stages of Alzheimer's disease, the patient usually has insight into his impaired mental functions, particularly his poor memory. As time passes and the patient's condition deteriorates, this insight is gradually lost and the patient may not realize that he has a poor memory. Lack of insight is particularly useful in differentiating Alzheimer's disease from depression, which sometimes can give rise to apparently impaired mental functions, a condition referred to as pseudodementia. In all but the early stage of Alzheimer's disease, the patient has no insight into his poor memory, whereas with depression the patient usually has this insight and often tends to exaggerate this memory problem. A depressed patient commonly will state that his memory is poor and thus he cannot remember what day of the week it is or cannot recall recent events. A patient with Alzheimer's disease, on the other hand, will maintain that his memory is quite good and readily confabulate, that is, give wrong answers about recent events or incorrectly identify the day of the week.

intramuscular   Within a muscle. Denotes the route of administration of medication by injection into a muscle. The usual sites for intramuscular injection are the buttocks, thighs, and occasionally the shoulders.

intravenous   Within a vein. Denotes the route of administration of medication or fluids into a vein.

intravenous line   Slender tube that is inserted into a vein and kept in position to allow regular administration of medication or fluids.

ischemic attack   Condition resulting from an interference with blood flow.

Kegel exercises   Set of exercises designed to strengthen the pelvic floor and perineal muscles to control stress incontinence. These exercises mainly consist of constricting the external urinary sphincter and some of the perineal and pelvic muscles. The easiest way of knowing when these muscles contract is to attempt to interrupt the flow of urine while micturating. To be effective, Kegel exercises must be repeated as often as possible.

kyphoscoliosis Condition in which the curvature of the thoracic vertebrae (upper part of back) is increased and is associated with a sideways deformity of the spine. This condition often is the result of osteoporosis.

kyphosis Condition involving excessive curvature of the thoracic vertebrae. It often results from osteoporosis because the increased fragility of the vertebrae causes them to become wedge-shaped, thus exaggerating the normal curvature of the thoracic spine.

lacuna Small space or cavity.

laxative Drug taken to increase the bowel motions and to prevent constipation.

lipofuscin Pigment that accumulates in the nerve cells as a person ages. It also collects in muscle, heart, and liver cells. The significance of this pigment is not fully understood.

lithium Lithium carbonate is a salt used in the treatment of acute mania and as a maintenance medication to help reduce the duration, intensity, and frequency of recurrent episodes of bipolar disorder.

logoclonia Repetition of the first syllable of a word that has just been heard.

lumbar puncture Test that involves introducing a needle through the back between two lumbar vertebrae to obtain a sample of the fluid that surrounds the spinal cord (cerebrospinal fluid). Until recently, a lumbar puncture was part of the routine diagnostic workup of patients suspected of having Alzheimer's disease, but it currently is not done routinely in these patients. It is reserved for the diagnosis of infections, tumors, multiple sclerosis, and other conditions affecting the spinal cord or brain.

magnetic resonance imaging (MRI) Specialized radiological test that allows a clear view of various body organs. When MRI is done on the head, the brain can be clearly visualized. This imaging method is not yet used routinely in the diagnostic workup of patients suspected of having Alzheimer's disease.

metabolic diseases Diseases that interfere with the body's metabolism. The concentration of various substances in the blood is maintained within a very narrow range of normality by a number of factors. For instance, glucose is controlled by the amount of insulin produced by the pancreas (in addition to a number of other factors). In metabolic diseases the concentration of these various substances is altered.

mood disorders Group of disorders characterized by prominent and persistent disturbances in mood (depression or mania). The disorders usually are episodic but may be chronic.

morbidity State of being diseased.

mucosal smear Test in which a few cells from the lining of the vagina (mucosa) are smeared on a glass slide and examined microscopically to determine whether enough estrogens (female hormones) are circulating in the blood. By examining these mucosal cells, it is possible to tell whether a patient has atrophic vaginitis.

multiinfarct dementia Condition in which the dementia is caused by repeated small strokes. Often these strokes do not give rise to any paralysis or other neurological deficit. However, as time goes by and more strokes are produced, the number of brain cells gradually diminishes and the patient may slowly manifest a dementia illness. It is important to differentiate multiinfarct dementia from Alzheimer's disease since the incidence of repeated strokes can be reduced and thus the progress of multiinfarct dementia sometimes can be stopped, leading to stabilization of the patient's condition. With Alzheimer's disease, progression of the disorder is usually relentless.

muscarinic   Having a muscarine-like action, i.e., producing parasympathetic stimulation, such as cardiac slowing, vasodilation, salivation, lacrimation, bronchoconstriction, and gastrointestinal stimulation.

mutism   Condition in which the patient does not communicate verbally.

myocardial infarction   Condition that results when the blood flow through the coronary arteries that carry blood to the heart is completely stopped. This usually happens when a blood clot develops in one of the coronary arteries, accompanied by complicating arteriosclerosis. The condition usually is manifested by severe central chest pain that is not relieved by either rest or sublingual nitroglycerin. The patient is apprehensive, is usually sweating, and has a sense of impending death.

nasogastric tube   Tube that is passed through the nasal cavity into the stomach. It usually is used to feed patients who have difficulty swallowing or who cannot feed themselves.

neoplasm   Cancerous growth.

neurofibrillary tangles   Aggregations of neurofilaments and neurotubules in neurons that are noted through microscopy. Neurofibrillary tangles are commonly seen in normal aged brains but usually are few in number. In Alzheimer's disease, however, these tangles are widespread throughout the cortex and are quite dense.

neurofilament   Slender filament present in neurons. Neurofilaments are thought to be involved in intracellular transport of metabolites.

neuroleptics   Drugs used to treat psychotic symptoms. They include phenothiazines (e.g., Thorazine, Mellaril, Stelazine), butyrophenones (e.g., Haldol), and thioxanthenes (e.g., Navane [thiothixene]).

neuromelanin   Pigment within the nerve cells.

neuron   Nerve cell.

neuropathy   Condition resulting from the degeneration of nerve fibers.

neurotransmitters   Chemical substances that conduct electrical impulses from one cell to another and thus enable an electrical impulse to proceed. The main neurotransmitters that are deficient in Alzheimer's disease are acetylcholine, somatostatin, and, to a lesser extent, serotonin and dopamine.

nonsteroidal antiinflammatory compounds   Medications given to patients with arthritis and other painful conditions. These drugs reduce inflammation and relieve pain. Common examples are aspirin and ibuprofen.

nootropics   Class of chemical compounds that help to correct the decline in learning and behavior in patients with dementia by increasing metabolic activity within the neurons.

o.d.   (L. *omni die*) Abbreviation designating that a medication be administered once a day.

oropharynx   Anatomical term referring to the back of the mouth and upper part of the pharynx.

osteoarthritis   Disease affecting the joints—particularly the hands, knees, and hips—that causes pain and stiffness. Characteristically the pain is much worse after exercise and tends to be relieved somewhat by rest. With osteoarthritis the cartilage that lines the bones becomes less efficient at protecting the bones and preventing them from rubbing against each other in the joint. The cartilage gradually becomes frayed, and loose bits of cartilage may become dislodged in the joint. The exact cause of osteoarthritis is not known, although it currently is thought to be mainly a degenerative disease. It usually is treated with analgesics or nonsteroidal antiinflammatory drugs.

paralalia   Any speech defect, especially in the production of a vocal sound different from the one desired.

paranoid disorders   Also called delusional disorders, these mental conditions involve persistent delusions of persecution or jealousy. Schizophrenia, mood disorders, and organic mental disorders have been excluded as causes in these cases.

paraphasia   Sometimes referred to as paraphrasia. A form of speech in which the individual substitutes one word for another or describes an object for which he has forgotten the name. For example, when presented with a key and asked to name it, the person states "something that opens a door."

parasympathetic nervous system   Division of the autonomic nervous system.

paresis   Weakness resulting in a neurological disorder, such as a stroke.

Parkinson's disease   Disease characterized by muscle stiffness and tremors. It is also known as "shaking palsy" or "shaking paralysis." The muscles are not weakened, but the tremors interfere with the patient's daily activities. Parkinson's disease is caused by damage to certain parts of the brain (substantia nigra). Some patients with Parkinson's disease develop dementia, a condition often referred to as a subcortical dementia because the affected area of the brain lies below the cortex. The main biochemical abnormality in Parkinson's disease is a deficiency of the neurotransmitter dopamine. Many drugs can be used to treat Parkinson's disease.

pathognomonic   Characteristic of a disease.

peripheral vascular insufficiency   Disease in which the lumina of the arteries that carry blood to the legs are considerably reduced. As a result the patient may develop intermittent pain in the leg muscles during exercise, but this pain usually is relieved by rest.

phosphorylation   Addition of phosphate to an organic compound.

physostigmine   Chemical substance that decreases the breakdown of acetylcholine in the synapse.

pica   Craving and eating of unusual foods or other substances. Pica is seen in a variety of medical conditions, including Alzheimer's disease. Common examples include eating of paint, paper, or excessive amounts of ice.

placebo   Inactive substance identical in appearance with the material being tested in experimental research.

plaque   Area of unmyelinated neurons, the center of which is made of amyloid.

positron emission tomography (PET)   Highly specialized test that reflects the metabolic activity of the brain. Currently it is not routinely available.

pressure areas   Regions of the body that are under pressure when an individual lies down, including the sacral region, heels, shoulder blades, and back of the head. Patients who are immobile or bedridden for prolonged periods develop a decubitus ulcer.

pressure sore   See **Decubitus ulcer.**

progesterone   Hormone secreted by the ovaries. Secretion of this hormone tends to decrease dramatically during menopause.

prognosis   Forecast of what is likely to happen when an individual contracts a particular disease. In the case of Alzheimer's disease, the prognosis currently is poor because there is no effective cure and the disease is known to have a slow, progressive course. In general, the younger the individual when the disease manifests itself, the worse the prognosis.

prolapse   Displacement of an organ or part of an organ. Uterine prolapse denotes the displacement and descent of the uterus into the vagina. Bladder prolapse denotes the protrusion of the bladder into the vaginal wall. Both conditions are associated with urinary incontinence secondary to the altered architecture and relationship of the urinary bladder, uterus, and vagina.

promazine (Sparine)   Neuroleptic drug that is one of the phenothiazines. Promazine is no longer widely used because of its sedative side effects.

prostatic hypertrophy   Enlargement of the prostate gland, which is present in men at the junction of the bladder and the urethra. An enlarged prostate may compress the urethra and obstruct the flow of urine. When the pressure of urine in the bladder exceeds that of the sphincter, incontinence results; this type of incontinence is called overflow incontinence. Other signs of prostatic hypertrophy include difficulty in starting the flow of urine and a weak stream.

proteolysis   Protein breakdown.

proton magnetic resonance   See **Magnetic resonance imaging.**

pruritus   Itching.

pseudodementia   Condition in which the patient shows impaired mental functions and signs and symptoms of dementia but in which the underlying diagnosis is not dementia but depression.

psychoactive drugs   Drugs that affect the mind or behavior, such as antidepressant, anxiolytic, and neuroleptic medications.

psychological testing   Series of tests performed by psychologists to assess a patient's mental functions. These tests are described in the Appendix.

psychosis   Form of mental illness in which the patient suffers from delusions, hallucinations, and/or bizarre behavior.

psychotropic drugs   Drugs that exert an effect on the mind and modify mental activity. (See also **Psychoactive drugs.**)

q.i.d.   (L. *quater in die*) Abbreviation designating that a medication be given four times a day.

respiratory reserve capacity   Ability of the respiratory system to increase its work to meet the body's increased demands during exercise.

rigidity, muscle rigidity   Condition in which the muscles become rigid and thus movement becomes difficult. Muscle rigidity often is seen in patients with Parkinson's disease and in the late stages of Alzheimer's disease. In the latter condition, the excessive rigidity causes the body to assume a generalized flexed position while the patient is lying in bed.

sacral plexus   Agglomeration of nerve fibers from the autonomic nervous system that is present in the sacral area. This part of the autonomic nervous system partly controls micturition.

schizophrenia   Severe chronic mental disorder characterized by extreme difficulty in thinking and associated with delusions and hallucinations.

sedatives   Medications used to calm a patient. These agents are particularly useful when a patient is agitated, irritable, and violent. Sedatives should not be used routinely in patients with Alzheimer's disease since a major side effect is drowsiness, which may, in turn, worsen the patient's confusion.

senile macular degeneration   Degenerative condition of the retina that occurs in old age and causes diminished visual acuity and eventually blindness. Currently there is no satisfactory treatment for this condition.

senile plaque   Microscopic finding that describes a small mass between the neurons of the brain. Senile plaques are found in many older people, but they tend to be more numerous in patients with Alzheimer's disease.

sensorium   Term used to describe orientation to time, place, and person. Sometimes it also includes an assessment of short-term memory.

sensory information   Information sent to the brain by one of the five senses (sight, hearing, touch, smell, and taste). For instance, when a person sees a pencil, the shape and appearance of the object are transmitted through the eye to the brain, where they are interpreted as a pencil. Similarly, when the ears detect a sound, this information is transmitted to the brain, where it is interpreted and the individual becomes aware of the meaning of the sound. In the late stages of Alzheimer's disease, the patient may not be able to recognize common objects or the people he lives with, such as his spouse, children, or fellow residents in a nursing home.

septicemia   Condition in which an infection spreads to involve the blood. As a result of septicemia, bacteria or other infective organisms circulate in the bloodstream and may reach any organ.

serotonin   Neurotransmitter present in the brain. The concentration of serotonin usually is reduced in patients with Alzheimer's disease.

sleep apnea   See **Apnea.**

sleep/wake cycle   Twenty-four-hour cycle during which individuals tend to sleep at night and remain awake during the day. This cycle often is referred to as the "circadian rhythm" or "diurnal rhythm." Although the sleep/wake cycle generally is related to the presence or absence of sunlight, it also is regulated by a number of hormonal glands, which secrete various hormones at different concentrations at different times of the day. These glands seem to be regulated by an internal clock. Even when people are deprived of sunlight and timekeeping devices, they tend to retain a circadian sleep/wake cycle. Patients with Alzheimer's disease often have a disturbed sleep/wake cycle and tend to be awake and agitated at night and sleepy during the day. They commonly become particularly confused early in the evening, a phenomenon sometimes called the "sundown syndrome." The altered sleep/wake cycle is particularly stressful for caregivers and has been found to be the least tolerated symptom of Alzheimer's disease.

SMA 6, 18, or 29   See **Biochemical screening.**

social judgment   Ability to determine behaviors and actions that are appropriate to any given social situation.

somatic complaints   Body symptoms such as headache, backache, and dizziness. These complaints may be caused by physical or emotional disorders.

somatization   Conversion of feelings (usually anxiety and depression) into physical symptoms.

stroke   Condition in which part of the brain is deprived of blood. It often occurs as a complication of arteriosclerosis. The three most common causes of strokes are thrombosis, embolism, and hemorrhage. In older patients thrombosis is the most common cause and hemorrhage the least common.

subcortical dementia   Dementia caused by abnormalities in the areas of the brain that lie below the cortex. In Alzheimer's disease the cortex (and certain other areas below it) is grossly affected. In subcortical dementia the cortex is generally spared; the structures below the cortex are largely affected. A common example of subcortical dementia is that seen in some patients with Parkinson's disease.

subdural   Space below the dura mater, which is a membrane lining the outside of the brain and spinal cord.

sulci   (singular, *sulcus*) Fissures seen on the outer surface of the brain. In Alzheimer's disease, sulci tend to become shallow.

sundown syndrome   Condition characterized by a period of severe confusion, occasionally associated with agitation, irritability, and sometimes violence, that typically occurs toward the end of the day. The cause of this syndrome is not well understood but probably is related to the concentrations of various hormones in the blood. It has also been suggested that this syndrome may stem from the reduced natural light at the end of the day, which may precipitate a confused state in the patient.

sympathetic nervous system   Division of the autonomic nervous system.

synapse   See **Synaptic cleft.**

synaptic cleft   Space between two nerve cells. The electrical impulses generated in one nerve cell can pass across the synaptic cleft (synapse) by the release of chemical compounds known as neurotransmitters, which, in effect, transmit the electrical impulses from one nerve cell to the other.

tardive dyskinesia   Involuntary movements, generally of the lips, tongue, or jaw but sometimes of other parts of the body, that occur 5 to 10 years after neuroleptic drugs have been taken.

thioridazine (Mellaril)   Neuroleptic drug that is one of the phenothiazines. Although it causes fewer extrapyramidal side effects than haloperidol, thioridazine produces far more sedation and orthostatic hypotension.

thrombosis   Development of a thrombus.

thrombus   Blood clot that forms inside a blood vessel. A thrombus often is precipitated by arteriosclerosis.

thyroid   Gland situated in the neck that secretes thyroid hormone. If the secretion of thyroid hormone is excessive or insufficient, the patient may show a confusional state. Either imbalance worsens the degree of mental impairment seen in patients with Alzheimer's disease.

t.i.d.   (L. *ter in die*) Abbreviation designating that a particular medication is to be administered three times a day.

tranquilizers   Drugs intended to calm an individual without causing undue sedation. These drugs are better avoided or used sparingly in patients with Alzheimer's disease because they tend to cause some drowsiness. Since elderly individuals cannot eliminate most drugs through their urine (or bile) as quickly and efficiently as younger people can, repeated use of a tranquilizer or other drug may cause the medication to accumulate in the body and lead to drowsiness and even sedation.

triglycerides   Fatty substances present in the blood that are essential for the proper functioning of many cells. As with cholesterol, if the concentration of triglycerides is excessive, arteriosclerosis may develop.

tropic functions   Nourishing functions.

urethral stricture   Constriction in the urethra that can lead to obstruction of the flow of urine and overflow incontinence.

urinary sphincters   Two sphincters located on the urethra. One is close to the junction of the urethra and the urinary bladder (internal urinary sphincter), and the other is closer to the surface of the body (external urinary sphincter). The external urinary sphincter can be contracted at will, and its main use is to postpone micturition for a short time. Normally, urine is prevented from leaving the urinary bladder by the constant contraction of the internal urinary sphincter, which is controlled by the autonomic nervous system. The sympathetic division of this system causes the internal urinary sphincter to constrict, preventing the passage of urine. The parasympathetic component causes the internal sphincter to relax, encouraging voiding.

urinary stasis   Presence of urine in the bladder after voiding (also called residual urine). This condition, which frequently is seen in men with prostatic hypertrophy, often invites infection.

urodynamic tests   Series of tests that evaluate the relationship among the bladder, the urethra, and abdominal pressure to determine the cause of urinary incontinence.

venous return   Blood returning from various parts of the body to the heart.

visual spatial skills   Skills that enable individuals to integrate incoming information so that they can orient themselves geographically and find their way. These skills often are impaired in patients with Alzheimer's disease. One of the most common manifestations of this impairment is a tendency to become lost.

vital signs   Pulse, temperature, blood pressure, and respiratory rate.

white matter   Structure of the brain below the cortex that appears white when the brain is dissected. White matter is mainly made up of nerve fibers that connect the neurons in the gray matter to other parts of the brain or the body.

Suggested readings

Adem A: Putative mechanisms of action of tacrine in Alzheimer's disease, *Acta Neurol Scand Suppl* 139:69-74, 1992.

Advokat C, Pellegrin AI: Excitatory amino acids and memory: evidence from research on Alzheimer's disease and behavioral pharmacology, *Neurosci Biobehav Rev* 16(1):13-24, 1992.

Agnati LF and others: Neuronal plasticity and ageing processes in the frame of the 'Red Queen Theory,' *Acta Physiol Scand* 145:301-309, 1992.

Alafuzoff I: The pathology of dementias: an overview, *Acta Neurol Scand Suppl* 139:8-15, 1992.

Albert MS: Parallels between Down syndrome dementia and Alzheimer's disease, *Prog Clin Biol Res* 379:77-102, 1992.

Albert MS, Lafleche G: Neuroimaging in Alzheimer's disease, *Psychiatr Clin North Am* 14:443-459, 1991.

Alexopoulos GS, Abrams RC: Depression in Alzheimer's disease, *Psychiatr Clin North Am* 14:327-340, 1991.

Allain H and others: Therapeutic target for cognition enhancers: diagnosis and clinical phenomenology, *Pharmacopsychiatry* 23(suppl 2):49-51, 1990.

Alperovitch A, Hauw JJ: Neuropathological diagnoses in epidemiologic studies, *Neuroepidemiology* 11(suppl 1):100-105, 1992.

Amaducci L, Falcini M, Lippi A: Descriptive epidemiology and risk factors for Alzheimer's disease, *Acta Neurol Scand Suppl* 139:21-25, 1992.

Amaducci L, Falcini M, Lippi A: Humoral and cellular immunologic repertoire in Alzheimer's disease, *Ann NY Acad Sci* 663:349-356, 1992.

Amenta F, Zaccheo D, Collier WL: Neurotransmitters, neuroreceptors and aging, *Mech Ageing Dev* 61(3):249-273, 1991.

Azmitia EC, Whitaker-Azmitia PM: Awakening the sleeping giant: anatomy and plasticity of the brain serotonergic system, *J Clin Psychiatry* 52(suppl):4-16, 1991.

Azmitia EC and others: S100 beta and serotonin: a possible astrocytic-neuronal link to neuropathology of Alzheimer's disease, *Prog Brain Res* 94:459-473, 1992.

Backman L: Plasticity of memory functioning in normal aging and Alzheimer's disease, *Acta Neurol Scand Suppl* 129:32-36, 1990.

Backman L: Memory training and memory improvement in Alzheimer's disease: rules and exceptions, *Acta Neurol Scand Suppl* 139:84-89, 1992.

Baddeley A: Working memory, *Science* 255:556-559, 1992.

Banner C: Toward a molecular etiology of Alzheimer's disease, *Int Psychogeriatr* 2(2):135-147, 1990.

Barker R: Substance P and neurodegenerative disorders: a speculative review, *Neuropeptides* 20(2):73-78, 1991.

Basun H and others: Metals and trace elements in plasma and cerebrospinal fluid in normal aging and Alzheimer's disease, *J Neural Transm Park Dis Dement Sect* 3(4):231-258, 1991.

Bauer J and others: The participation of interleukin-6 in the pathogenesis of Alzheimer's disease, *Res Immunol* 143:650-657, 1992.

Beal MF: Somatostatin in neurodegenerative illnesses, *Metabolism* 39(9 suppl 2):116-119, 1990.

Beal MF: Does impairment of energy metabolism result in excitotoxic neuronal death in neurodegenerative illnesses? *Ann Neurol* 31:119-130, 1992.

Beats B, Levy R: Imaging and affective disorder in the elderly, *Clin Geriatr Med* 8(2):267-274, 1992.

Bench CJ and others: Positron emission tomography in the study of brain metabolism in psychiatric and neuropsychiatric disorders, *Br J Psychiatry Suppl* (9):82-95, 1990.

Bennett DA, Evans DA: Alzheimer's disease, *Dis Mon* 38:1-64, 1992.

Bergeron C: Alzheimer's disease: neuropathological aspects, *Can J Vet Res* 54:58-64, 1990.

Bergman H: Understanding placement of the demented elderly, *Adv Exp Med Biol* 282:103-112, 1990.

Berkenbosch F and others: Cytokines and inflammatory proteins in Alzheimer's disease, *Res Immunol* 143:657-663, 1992.

Berson BD: Imaging of degenerative brain disorders, *Curr Opin Radiol* 3:51-54, 1991.

Bertoni-Freddari C and others: Structural dynamics of synaptic junctional areas in aging and Alzheimer's disease, *Ann NY Acad Sci* 673:285-292, 1992.

Beyreuther K and others: Mechanisms of amyloid deposition in Alzheimer's disease, *Ann NY Acad Sci* 640:129-139, 1991.

Beyreuther K and others: Amyloid precursor protein (APP) and beta A4 amyloid in Alzheimer's disease and Down syndrome, *Prog Clin Biol Res* 379:159-182, 1992.

Bissette G, Myers B: Somatostatin in Alzheimer's disease and depression, *Life Sci* 51:1389-1410, 1992.

Blass JP, Baker AC, Ko LW: Alzheimer's disease: inborn error of metabolism of late onset? *Adv Neurol* 51:199-200, 1990.

Blass JP, Gibson GE: The role of oxidative abnormalities in the pathophysiology of Alzheimer's disease, *Rev Neurol (Paris)* 147:513-525, 1991.

Blass JP, Gibson GE: Nonneural markers in Alzheimer disease, *Alzheimer Dis Assoc Disord* 6:205-224, 1992.

Blass JP, Ko L, Wisniewski HM: Pathology of Alzheimer's disease, *Psychiatr Clin North Am* 14:397-420, 1991.

Boerrigter ME, Wei JY, Vijg J: DNA repair and Alzheimer's disease, *J Gerontol* 47:B177-184, 1992.

Bonte FJ and others: Single photon tomography in Alzheimer's disease and the dementias, *Semin Nucl Med* 20:342-352, 1990.

Bowen DM: Treatment of Alzheimer's disease: molecular pathology versus neurotransmitter-based therapy, *Br J Psychiatry* 157:327-330, 1990.

Bowen DM and others: Tacrine in relation to amino acid transmitters in Alzheimer's disease, *Adv Neurol* 51:91-96, 1990.

Bowman BA: Acetyl-carnitine and Alzheimer's disease, *Nutr Rev* 50:142-144, 1992.

Braak H, Braak E: Neuropathological staging of Alzheimer-related changes, *Acta Neuropathol (Berl)* 82:239-259, 1991.

Bradley WG: Alzheimer's disease: theories of causation, *Adv Exp Med Biol* 282:31-38, 1990.

Branconnier RJ and others: Blocking the Ca (2 +)–activated cytotoxic mechanisms of cholinergic neuronal death: a novel treatment strategy for Alzheimer's disease, *Psychopharmacol Bull* 28:175-181, 1992.

Breitner JC: Clinical genetics and genetic counseling in Alzheimer disease, *Ann Intern Med* 115:601-606, 1991.

Breitner JC and others: Twin studies of Alzheimer's disease: an approach to etiology and prevention, *Neurobiol Aging* 11:641-648, 1990.

Breitner JC and others: Use of twin cohorts for research in Alzheimer's disease, *Neurology* 43:261-267, 1993.

Breteler MM and others: Epidemiology of Alzheimer's disease, *Epidemiol Rev* 14:59-82, 1992.

Briley M: Biochemical strategies in the search for cognition enhancers, *Pharmacopsychiatry* 23(suppl 2):75-80, 1990.

Brody H: The aging brain, *Acta Neurol Scand Suppl* 137:40-44, 1992.

Brumback RA and others: Dementia: the importance of clinical evaluation, autopsy confirmation, and research, *J Okla State Med Assoc* 83(3):109-118, 1990.

Bucht G, Sandman PO: Nutritional aspects of dementia, especially Alzheimer's disease, *Age Ageing* 19(4):S32-36, 1990.

Buell U and others: The investigation of dementia with single photon emission tomography, *Nucl Med Commun* 11:823-841, 1990.

Bugiani O, Tagliavini F, Giaccone G: Preamyloid deposits, amyloid deposits, and senile plaques in Alzheimer's disease, Down syndrome, and aging, *Ann NY Acad Sci* 640:122-128, 1991.

Burns A: Cranial computerised tomography in dementia of the Alzheimer type, *Br J Psychiatry Suppl* (9):10-15, 1990.

Burns A: Psychiatric phenomena in dementia of the Alzheimer type, *Int Psychogeriatr* 4(suppl 1):43-54, 1992.

Calne DB, Eisen A: Parkinson's disease, motoneuron disease and Alzheimer's disease: origins and interrelationship, *Adv Neurol* 53:355-360, 1990.

Calne DB and others: Theories of neurodegeneration, *Ann NY Acad Sci* 648:1-5, 1992.

Calvani M, Carta A: Clinical issues of cognitive enhancers in Alzheimer disease, *Alzheimer Dis Assoc Disord* 5(suppl 1):S25-31, 1991.

Carmeliet G, David G, Cassiman JJ: Cellular ageing of Alzheimer's disease and Down syndrome cells in culture, *Mutat Res* 256:221-231, 1991.

Ceballos I and others: Parkinson's disease and Alzheimer's disease: neurodegenerative disorders due to brain antioxidant system deficiency? *Adv Exp Med Biol* 264:493-498, 1990.

Celesia GG: Alzheimer's disease: the proteoglycans hypothesis, *Semin Thromb Hemost* 17(suppl 2):158-160, 1991.

Chan-Palay V: Depression and senile dementia of the Alzheimer type: a role for moclobemide, *Psychopharmacology (Berlin)* 106(suppl):S137-139, 1992.

Chan-Palay VL, Jentsch B: Galanin tuberomammillary neurons in the hypothalamus in Alzheimer's and Parkinson's diseases, *Prog Brain Res* 93:263-270, 1992.

Chazot G, Broussolle E: Alterations in trace elements during brain aging and in Alzheimer's dementia, *Prog Clin Biol Res* 380:269-281, 1993.

Chobor KL, Brown JW: Semantic deterioration in Alzheimer's: the patterns to expect, *Geriatrics* 45(10):68-70, 75, 1990.

Cohen GD: Alzheimer's disease: clinical update, *Hosp Community Psychiatry* 41:496-497, 1990.

Cohn JB, Wilcox CS, Lerer BE: Development of an "early" detection battery for dementia of the Alzheimer type, *Prog Neuropsychopharmacol Biol Psychiatry* 15:433-479, 1991.

Coleman PD, Rogers KE, Flood DG: Neuronal plasticity in normal aging and deficient plasticity in Alzheimer's disease: a proposed intercellular signal cascade, *Prog Brain Res* 86:75-87, 1990.

Coleman PD, Rogers KE, Flood DG: The neuropil and GAP-43/B-50 in normally aging and Alzheimer's disease human brain, *Prog Brain Res* 89:263-269, 1991.

Constantinidis J: Hypothesis regarding amyloid and zinc in the pathogenesis of Alzheimer disease: potential for preventive intervention, *Alzheimer Dis Assoc Disord* 5:31-35, 1991.

Cooke K, Gould MH: The health effects of aluminium: a review, *J R Soc Health* 111(5):163-168, 1991.

Cooper B: The epidemiology of primary degenerative dementia and related neurological disorders, *Eur Arch Psychiatry Clin Neurosci* 240:223-233, 1991.

Cooper JK: Drug treatment of Alzheimer's disease, *Arch Intern Med* 151:245-249, 1991.

Corcoran MA: Gender differences in dementia management plans of spousal caregivers: implications for occupational therapy, *Am J Occup Ther* 46:1006-1012, 1992.

Cork LC: Neuropathology of Down syndrome and Alzheimer disease, *Am J Med Genet Suppl* 7:282-286, 1990.

Costall B and others: Biochemical models for cognition enhancers, *Pharmacopsychiatry* 23(suppl 2):85-88 (discussion 89), 1990.

Cotman CW, Geddes JW, Kahle JS: Axon sprouting in the rodent and Alzheimer's disease brain: a reactivation of developmental mechanisms? *Prog Brain Res* 83:427-434, 1990.

Cotman CW and others: Plasticity of excitatory amino acid receptors: implications for aging and Alzheimer's disease, *Prog Brain Res* 86:55-61, 1990.

Court JA, Perry EK: Dementia: the neurochemical basis of putative transmitter orientated therapy, *Pharmacol Ther* 52:423-443, 1991.

Cowburn RF, Hardy JA, Roberts PJ: Glutamatergic neurotransmission in Alzheimer's disease, *Biochem Soc Trans* 18:390-392, 1990.

Crook TH, Johnson BA, Larrabee GJ: Evaluation of drugs in Alzheimer's disease and age-associated memory impairment, *Psychopharmacol Ser* 8:37-55, 1990.

Crook TH, Larrabee GJ, Youngjohn JR: Diagnosis and assessment of age-associated memory impairment, *Clin Neuropharmacol* 13(suppl 3):S81-91, 1990.

Cross AJ: Serotonin in Alzheimer-type dementia and other dementing illnesses, *Ann NY Acad Sci* 600:405-415 (discussion 415-7), 1990.

Crowther RA: Structural aspects of pathology in Alzheimer's disease, *Biochim Biophys Acta* 1096:1-9, 1990.

Davidson M, Stern RG: The treatment of cognitive impairment in Alzheimer's disease: beyond the cholinergic approach, *Psychiatr Clin North Am* 14:461-482, 1991

Davidson M and others: Cholinergic strategies in the treatment of Alzheimer's disease, *Acta Psychiatr Scand Suppl* 366:47-51, 1991.

Davies I: Comments on review by Swaab: brain aging and Alzheimer's disease. "Wear and tear" versus "use it or lose it," *Neurobiol Aging* 12:328-330, 1991.

Davies P: Therapy for Alzheimer's disease: choosing a target, *Clin Neuropharmacol* 14(suppl 1):S24-33, 1991.

Davies P: Alz 50 as a reagent to assess animal models of Alzheimer's disease, *Neurobiol Aging* 13:613-614, 1992.

De Carli C and others: Critical analysis of the use of computer-assisted transverse axial tomography to study human brain in aging and dementia of the Alzheimer type, *Neurology* 40:872-883, 1990.

De Lacoste MC, White CL III: The role of cortical connectivity in Alzheimer's disease pathogenesis: a review and model system, *Neurobiol Aging* 14:1-16, 1993.

de Toledo-Morrell L, Morrell F: Alzheimer's disease: new developments for noninvasive detection of early cases, *Curr Opin Neurol Neurosurg* 6:113-118, 1993.

Decker MW, McGaugh JL: The role of interactions between the cholinergic system and other neuromodulatory systems in learning and memory, *Synapse* 7:151-168, 1991.

Deloncle R, Guillard O: Mechanism of Alzheimer's disease: arguments for a neurotransmitter-aluminium complex implication, *Neurochem Res* 15:1239-1245, 1990.

Derouesne C, Jouvent R: Dimensional versus nosographic approach to Alzheimer's disease: therapeutic implications, *Neuroepidemiology* 9:177-182, 1990.

Deutsch LH, Rovner BW: Agitation and other noncognitive abnormalities in Alzheimer's disease, *Psychiatr Clin North Am* 14:341-351, 1991.

Dewan MJ, Gupta S: Toward a definite diagnosis of Alzheimer's disease, *Compr Psychiatry* 33:282-290, 1992.

Dickson DW and others: Microglia and cytokines in neurological disease, with special reference to AIDS and Alzheimer's disease, *Glia* 7:75-83, 1993.

Diedrich J and others: Identifying and mapping changes in gene expression involved in the neuropathology of scrapie and Alzheimer's disease, *Curr Top Microbiol Immunol* 172:259-274, 1991.

Dillehay RC, Sandys MR: Caregivers for Alzheimer's patients: what we are learning from research, *Int J Aging Hum Dev* 30:263-285, 1990.

Domenico RA: Verbal communication impairment in dementia research frontiers in language and cognition, *Adv Exp Med Biol* 282:79-88, 1990.

Donnelly RE, Karlinsky H: The impact of Alzheimer's disease on driving ability: a review, *J Geriatr Psychiatry Neurol* 3(2):67-72, 1990.

Doraiswamy PM, Krishnan KR, Nemeroff CB: Neuropeptides and neurotransmitters in Alzheimer's disease: focus on corticotropin-releasing factor, *Baillieres Clin Endocrinol Metab* 5(1):59-77, 1991.

Doty RL: Olfactory capacities in aging and Alzheimer's disease: psychophysical and anatomic considerations, *Ann NY Acad Sci* 640:20-27, 1991.

Drachman DA, Lippa CF: The etiology of Alzheimer's disease: the pathogenesis of dementia. The role of neurotoxins, *Ann N Y Acad Sci* 648:176-186, 1992.

Drugs for Alzheimer's disease, *Drug Ther Bull* 28(11):42-44, 1990.

Dubinsky RM and others: Driving in Alzheimer's disease, *J Am Geriatr Soc* 40:1112-1116, 1992.

Duchen LW: Current status review: cerebral amyloid, *Int J Exp Pathol* 73:535-550, 1992.

Dunnett S: Cholinergic grafts, memory and ageing, *Trends Neurosci* 14:371-376, 1991.

Dunnett SB: Neural transplants as a treatment for Alzheimer's disease? [editorial] *Psychol Med* 21:825-830, 1991.

Eastwood MR, Rifat SL, Roberts D: The epidemiology of dementia in North America, *Eur Arch Psychiatry Clin Neurosci* 240:207-211, 1991.

Edwards JA: In search of the etiology of Alzheimer's disease, *Adv Exp Med Biol* 282:21-29, 1990.

Edwardson JA and others: Aluminium accumulation, beta-amyloid deposition and neurofibrillary changes in the central nervous system, *Ciba Found Symp* 169:165-179 (discussion 179-85), 1992.

Eikelenboom P and others: Distribution pattern and functional state of complement proteins and alpha 1-antichymotrypsin in cerebral beta/A4 deposits in Alzheimer's disease, *Res Immunol* 143:617-620, 1992.

Eisen A, Calne D: Amyotrophic lateral sclerosis, Parkinson's disease and Alzheimer's disease: phylogenetic disorders of the human neocortex sharing many characteristics, *Can J Neurol Sci* 19(1 suppl):117-123, 1992.

Emery VO, Oxman TE: Update on the dementia spectrum of depression, *Am J Psychiatry* 149:305-317, 1992.

Engel RR, Satzger W: Methodological problems in assessing therapeutic efficacy in patients with dementia, *Drugs Aging* 2(2):79-85, 1992.

Estus S, Golde TE, Younkin SG: Normal processing of the Alzheimer's disease amyloid beta protein precursor generates potentially amyloidogenic carboxyl terminal derivatives, *Ann N Y Acad Sci* 674:138-148, 1992.

Etienne P, Hakim A: Clinical testing of compounds modifying acute and chronic neurodegeneration in the CNS, *Prog Clin Biol Res* 361:387-407, 1990.

Evans PH, Klinowski J, Yano E: Cephaloconiosis: a free radical perspective on the proposed particulate-induced etiopathogenesis of Alzheimer's dementia and related disorders, *Med Hypotheses* 34:209-219, 1991.

Faulstich ME: Brain imaging in dementia of the Alzheimer type, *Int J Neurosci* 57:39-49, 1991.

Ferrier IN, Leake A: Peptides in the neocortex in Alzheimer's disease and ageing, *Psychoneuroendocrinology* 15(2):89-95, 1990.

Ferris SH: Therapeutic strategies in dementia disorders, *Acta Neurol Scand Suppl* 129:23-26, 1990.

Ferris SH: Alzheimer's disease. Diagnosis by specialists: psychological testing, *Acta Neurol Scand Suppl* 139:32-35, 1992.

Fiandaca MS, Gash DM: New insights and technologies in brain grafting, *Clin Neurosurg* 39:482-508, 1992.

Fibiger HC: Cholinergic mechanisms in learning, memory and dementia: a review of recent evidence, *Trends Neurosci* 14:220-223, 1991.

Fidani L, Goate A: Mutations in APP and their role in beta-amyloid deposition, *Prog Clin Biol Res* 379:195-214, 1992.

Finch CE: Mechanisms in senescence: some thoughts in April 1990, *Exp Gerontol* 27:7-16, 1992.

Fischer P, Berner P: Clinical and epidemiological aspects of dementia in the elderly, *J Neural Transm Suppl* 33:39-48, 1991.

Fisher A and others: AF102B: rational treatment strategy for Alzheimer's disease: recent advances, *Adv Neurol* 51:257-259, 1990.

Flint AJ: Delusions in dementia: a review, *J Neuropsychiatry Clin Neurosci* 3:121-130, 1991.

Flood DG, Coleman PD: Hippocampal plasticity in normal aging and decreased plasticity in Alzheimer's disease, *Prog Brain Res* 83:435-443, 1990.

Folstein MF, Warren A: Genetics of Alzheimer's disease, *Res Publ Assoc Res Nerv Ment Dis* 69:129-136, 1991.

Forette F, Boller F: Hypertension and the risk of dementia in the elderly, *Am J Med* 90(3A):14S-19S, 1991.

Forno LS: Neuropathologic features of Parkinson's, Huntington's, and Alzheimer's diseases, *Ann N Y Acad Sci* 648:6-16, 1992.

Foster AC: Physiology and pathophysiology of excitatory amino acid neurotransmitter systems in relation to Alzheimer's disease, *Adv Neurol* 51:97-102, 1990.

Fowler CJ, Cowburn RF, O'Neill C: Brain signal transduction disturbances in neurodegenerative disorders, *Cell Signal* 4:1-9, 1992.

Fowler CJ and others: Alzheimer's disease: is there a problem beyond recognition? *Trends Pharmacol Sci* 11:183-184, 1990.

Fowler CJ and others: Neurotransmitter, receptor and signal transduction disturbances in Alzheimer's disease, *Acta Neurol Scand Suppl* 139:59-62, 1992.

Francis PT, Pangalos MN, Bowen DM: Animal and drug modelling for Alzheimer synaptic pathology, *Prog Neurobiol* 39:517-545, 1992.

Francis PT, Procter AW, Bowen DM: A glycine site as therapeutic target, *Ann N Y Acad Sci* 640:184-188, 1991.

Frederickson RC: Astroglia in Alzheimer's disease, *Neurobiol Aging* 13:239-253, 1992.

Freedman M, Stuss DT, Gordon M: Assessment of competency: the role of neurobehavioral deficits, *Ann Intern Med* 115:203-208, 1991.

Freeman SE, Dawson RM: Tacrine: a pharmacological review, *Prog Neurobiol* 36:257-277, 1991.

Friston KJ, Frackowiak RS: Cerebral function in aging and Alzheimer's disease: the role of PET, *Electroencephalogr Clin Neurophysiol Suppl* 42:355-365, 1991.

Gage FH, Chen KS: Neural transplants: prospects for Alzheimer's disease, *Curr Opin Neurol Neurosurg* 5:94-99, 1992.

Galasko D, Corey-Bloom J, Thal LJ: Monitoring progression in Alzheimer's disease, *J Am Geriatr Soc* 39:932-941, 1991.

Gandy S, Greengard P: Amyloidogenesis in Alzheimer's disease: some possible therapeutic opportunities, *Trends Pharmacol Sci* 13:108-113, 1992.

Gaskin F, Fu SM: Antineurofibrillary tangle, antineural and anti-beta-amyloid-protein in Alzheimer's disease and related disorders, *Res Immunol* 143:668-670, 1992.

Gauthier L, Gauthier S: Assessment of functional changes in Alzheimer's disease, *Neuroepidemiology* 9:183-188, 1990.

Gauthier S and others: Treatment of Alzheimer's disease: hopes and reality, *Can J Neurol Sci* 18(3 suppl):439-441, 1991.

Geaney DP, Abou-Saleh MT: The use and applications of single-photon emission computerised tomography in dementia, *Br J Psychiatry Suppl* (9):66-75, 1990.

Geokas MC and others: The aging process, *Ann Intern Med* 113:455-466, 1990.

Giacobini E: The cholinergic system in Alzheimer disease, *Prog Brain Res* 84:321-332, 1990.

Giacobini E: Cholinergic receptors in human brain: effects of aging and Alzheimer disease, *J Neurosci Res* 27:548-560, 1990.

Giacobini E: Molecular genetic approaches in the therapy of Alzheimer's disease, *Adv Exp Med Biol* 265:277-281, 1990.

Giacobini E: Nicotinic cholinergic receptors in human brain: effects of aging and Alzheimer, *Adv Exp Med Biol* 296:303-315, 1991.

Gibson GE and others: The cellular basis of delirium and its relevance to age-related disorders including Alzheimer's disease, *Int Psychogeriatr* 3:373-395, 1991.

Glick JL: Dementias: the role of magnesium deficiency and an hypothesis concerning the pathogenesis of Alzheimer's disease [published erratum appears in *Med Hypotheses* 33:preceding 301, 1990] *Med Hypotheses* 31:211-225, 1990.

Goate AM and others: Genetics of Alzheimer's disease, *Adv Neurol* 51:197-198, 1990.

Goedert M, Sisodia SS, Price DL: Neurofibrillary tangles and beta-amyloid deposits in Alzheimer's disease, *Curr Opin Neurobiol* 1:441-447, 1991.

Goedert M, Spillantini MG: Molecular neuropathology of Alzheimer's disease: in situ hybridization studies, *Cell Mol Neurobiol* 10:159-174, 1990.

Goldstein S, Reivich M: Cerebral blood flow and metabolism in aging and dementia, *Clin Neuropharmacol* 14(suppl 1):S34-44, 1991.

Gorelick PB, Bozzola FG: Alzheimer's disease: clues to the cause, *Postgrad Med* 89:231-232, 237-238, 240, 1991.

Gottfries CG: Brain monoamines and their metabolites in dementia, *Acta Neurol Scand Suppl* 129:8-11, 1990.

Gottfries CG: Disturbance of the 5-hydroxytryptamine metabolism in brains from patients with Alzheimer's dementia, *J Neural Transm Suppl* 30:33-43, 1990.

Gottfries CG: Neurochemical aspects on aging and diseases with cognitive impairment, *J Neurosci Res* 27:541-547, 1990.

Gottfries CG: Pharmacological treatment strategies in Alzheimer type dementia. Department of Psychiatry and Neurochemistry, Gothenburg, *Eur Neuropsychopharmacol* 1:1-5, 1990.

Gottfries CG: Alzheimer's disease: review of treatment strategies, *Acta Neurol Scand Suppl* 139:63-68, 1992.

Gottfries CG, Karlsson I, Nyth AL: Treatment of depression in elderly patients with and without dementia disorders, *Int Clin Psychopharmacol* 6(suppl 5):55-64, 1992.

Goudsmit E, Neijmeijer-Leloux A, Swaab DF: The human hypothalamo-neurohypophyseal system in relation to development, aging and Alzheimer's disease, *Prog Brain Res* 93:237-247 (discussion 247-8), 1992.

Graves AB and others: The association between head trauma and Alzheimer's disease, *Am J Epidemiol* 131:491-501, 1990.

Greenamyre JT: Neuronal bioenergetic defects, excitotoxicity and Alzheimer's disease: "use it and lose it," *Neurobiol Aging* 12:334-336, 1991.

Grimley Evans J: From plaque to placement: a model for Alzheimer's disease [published erratum appears in *Age Ageing* 21:387, 1992] *Age Ageing* 21:77-80, 1992.

Gusella JF: The search for the genetic defects in Huntington's disease and familial Alzheimer's disease, *Res Publ Assoc Res Nerv Ment Dis* 69:75-83, 1991.

Guze BH and others: Functional brain imaging and Alzheimer-type dementia, *Alzheimer Dis Assoc Disord* 5:215-230, 1991.

Haan J, Hardy JA, Roos RA: Hereditary cerebral hemorrhage with amyloidosis—Dutch type: its importance for Alzheimer research, *Trends Neurosci* 14:231-234, 1991.

Haan J, Roos RA: Amyloid in central nervous system disease, *Clin Neurol Neurosurg* 92:305-310, 1990.

Hachinski VC: The decline and resurgence of vascular dementia, *Can Med Assoc J* 142:107-111, 1990.

Hall ST and others: Early clinical testing of cognition enhancers: prediction of efficacy, *Pharmacopsychiatry* 23(suppl 2):57-58 (discussion 59), 1990.

Ham RJ: Alzheimer's disease and the family: a challenge of the new millennium, *Adv Exp Med Biol* 282:3-20, 1990.

Hanger DP and others: Molecular pathology of Alzheimer's disease in sporadic and familial Alzheimer's disease with mutations in the amyloid precursor protein, *Biochem Soc Trans* 20:642-645, 1992.

Hanin I: Cholinergic toxins and Alzheimer's disease, *Ann N Y Acad Sci* 648:63-70, 1992.

Hardy J: Molecular genetics of Alzheimer's disease, *Acta Neurol Scand Suppl* 129:29-31, 1990.

Hardy J, Allsop D: Amyloid deposition as the central event in the aetiology of Alzheimer's disease, *Trends Pharmacol Sci* 12:383-388, 1991.

Hardy JA, Higgins GA: Alzheimer's disease: the amyloid cascade hypothesis, *Science* 256:184-185, 1992.

Harrell LE: Alzheimer's disease, *South Med J* 84(5 suppl 1):S32-40, 1991.

Harrison PJ, Roberts GW: "Life, Jim, but not as we know it"? Transmissible dementias and the prion protein [see comments], *Br J Psychiatry* 158:457-470, 1991.

Hefti F, Schneider LS: Nerve growth factor and Alzheimer's disease, *Clin Neuropharmacol* 14(suppl 1):S62-76, 1991.

Heiss WD and others: Positron emission tomography in the differential diagnosis of organic dementias, *J Neural Transm Suppl* 33:13-19, 1991.

Heiss WD and others: PET correlates of normal and impaired memory functions, *Cerebrovasc Brain Metab Rev* 4:1-27, 1992.

Hermann C and others: Diagnostic and pharmacological approaches in Alzheimer's disease, *Drugs Aging* 1:144-162, 1991.

Hershey LA: Dementia associated with stroke, *Stroke* 21(9 suppl):II9-11, 1990.

Heston LL: Alzheimer's disease: the end of the beginning? *Psychol Med* 20:7-10, 1990.

Hewitt CD, Savory J, Wills MR: Aspects of aluminum toxicity, *Clin Lab Med* 10:403-422, 1990.

Higgins GA and others: Trophic regulation of basal forebrain gene expression in aging and Alzheimer's disease, *Prog Brain Res* 86:239-255, 1990.

High DM: Research with Alzheimer's disease subjects: informed consent and proxy decision making, *J Am Geriatr Soc* 40:950-957, 1992.

Hill CD, Risby E, Morgan N: Cognitive deficits in delirium: assessment over time, *Psychopharmacol Bull* 28:401-407, 1992.

Hirsh HL: Legal and ethical considerations in dealing with Alzheimer's disease, *Leg Med*, pp. 261-326, 1990.

Hollister LE: Problems in the search for cognition enhancers, *Pharmacopsychiatry* 23(suppl 2):33-36, 1990.

Holman BL and others: Imaging dementia with SPECT, *Ann N Y Acad Sci* 620:165-174, 1991.

Holtzman DM, Mobley WC: Molecular studies in Alzheimer's disease, *Trends Biochem Sci* 16:140-144, 1991.

Husain MM, Nemeroff CB: Neuropeptides and Alzheimer's disease, *J Am Geriatr Soc* 38:918-925, 1990.

Hyman BT: Down syndrome and Alzheimer disease, *Prog Clin Biol Res* 379:123-142, 1992.

Hyman BT, Tanzi RE: Amyloid, dementia and Alzheimer's disease, *Curr Opin Neurol Neurosurg* 5:88-93, 1992.

Iqbal K, Grundke-Iqbal I: Ubiquitination and abnormal phosphorylation of paired helical filaments in Alzheimer's disease, *Mol Neurobiol* 5:399-410, 1991.

Ishiura S: Proteolytic cleavage of the Alzheimer's disease amyloid A4 precursor protein, *J Neurochem* 56:363-369, 1991.

Joachim CL, Selkoe DJ: The seminal role of beta-amyloid in the pathogenesis of Alzheimer disease, *Alzheimer Dis Assoc Disord* 6:7-34, 1992.

Jones AW, Richardson JS: Alzheimer's disease: clinical and pathological characteristics, *Int J Neurosci* 50:147-168, 1990.

Jorm AF: Cross-national comparisons of the occurrence of Alzheimer's and vascular dementias, *Eur Arch Psychiatry Clin Neurosci* 240:218-222, 1991.

Kahn N, Stoudemire A: Behavioral and pharmacologic management of patients with Alzheimer's disease, *J Med Assoc Ga* 79:287-294, 1990.

Kalaria RN: The blood-brain barrier and cerebral microcirculation in Alzheimer disease, *Cerebrovasc Brain Metab Rev* 4:226-260, 1992.

Kalaria RN: Serum amyloid P and related molecules associated with the acute-phase response in Alzheimer's disease, *Res Immunol* 143:637-641, 1992.

Kalayam B, Shamoian CA: Geriatric psychiatry: an update [see comments], *J Clin Psychiatry* 51(5):177-183, 1990.

Kaszniak AW, Keyl PM, Albert MS: Dementia and the older driver, *Hum Factors* 33:527-537, 1991.

Katzman R: Should a major imaging procedure (CT or MRI) be required in the workup of dementia? An affirmative view, *J Fam Pract* 31:401-405, 1990.

Katzman R: Education and the prevalence of dementia and Alzheimer's disease, *Neurology* 43:13-20, 1993.

Katzman R, Jackson JE: Alzheimer disease: basic and clinical advances [see comments], *J Am Geriatr Soc* 39:516-525, 1991.

Katzman R, Saitoh T: Advances in Alzheimer's disease, *FASEB J* 5:278-286, 1991.

Kawachi I, Pearce N: Aluminium in the drinking water: is it safe? [editorial], *Aust J Public Health* 15(2):84-87, 1991.

Khachaturian ZS: Overview of basic research on Alzheimer disease: implications for cognition, *Alzheimer Dis Assoc Disord* 5(suppl 1):S1-6, 1991.

Kluger A, Ferris SH: Scales for the assessment of Alzheimer's disease, *Psychiatr Clin North Am* 14:309-326, 1991.

Klunk WE, McClure RJ, Pettegrew JW: Possible roles of L-phosphoserine in the pathogenesis of Alzheimer's disease, *Mol Chem Neuropathol* 15:51-73, 1991.

Knoll J: Deprenyl-medication: a strategy to modulate the age-related decline of the striatal dopaminergic system, *J Am Geriatr Soc* 40:839-847, 1992.

Knoll J: Pharmacological basis of the therapeutic effect of (-)deprenyl in age-related neurological diseases, *Med Res Rev* 12:505-524, 1992.

Koliatsos VE and others: Biologic effects of nerve growth factor on lesioned basal forebrain neurons, *Ann N Y Acad Sci* 640:102-109, 1991.

Korczyn AD: The clinical differential diagnosis of dementia: concept and methodology, *Psychiatr Clin North Am* 14:237-249, 1991.

Kosaka K: Diffuse Lewy body disease in Japan, *J Neurol* 237:197-204, 1990.

Kosik KS: Tau protein and Alzheimer's disease, *Curr Opin Cell Biol* 2:101-104, 1990.

Kosik KS: Tau protein and neurodegeneration, *Mol Neurobiol* 4:171-179, 1990.

Kosik KS: Alzheimer plaques and tangles: advances on both fronts, *Trends Neurosci* 14:218-219, 1991.

Kosik KS: Alzheimer's disease: a cell biological perspective, *Science* 256:780-783, 1992.

Kosik KS: Cellular aspects of Alzheimer neurofibrillary pathology, *Prog Clin Biol Res* 379:183-193, 1992.

Kowall NW, McKee AC: The histopathology of neuronal degeneration and plasticity in Alzheimer disease, *Adv Neurol* 59:5-33, 1993.

Kramer SI, Reifler BV: Depression, dementia, and reversible dementia, *Clin Geriatr Med* 8:289-297, 1992.

Kraus AS, Forbes WF: Aluminum, fluoride and the prevention of Alzheimer's disease, *Can J Public Health* 83(2):97-100, 1992.

Kristensson K: Potential role of viruses in neurodegeneration, *Mol Chem Neuropathol* 16:45-58, 1992.

Krogsgaard-Larsen P: GABA and glutamate receptors as therapeutic targets in neurodegenerative disorders, *Pharmacol Toxicol* 70:95-104, 1992.

Krogsgaard-Larsen P and others: Excitatory amino acid research in Alzheimer's disease: enhancement and blockade of receptor functions, *Biochem Soc Trans* 21:102-106, 1993.

Kuhlman GJ and others: Alzheimer's disease and family caregiving: critical synthesis of the literature and research agenda, *Nurs Res* 40:331-337, 1991.

Kumar V, Calache M: Treatment of Alzheimer's disease with cholinergic drugs, *Int J Clin Pharmacol Ther Toxicol* 29:23-37, 1991.

Kung HF: Overview of radiopharmaceuticals for diagnosis of central nervous disorders, *Crit Rev Clin Lab Sci* 28:269-286, 1991.

Lai F: Clinicopathologic features of Alzheimer disease in Down syndrome, *Prog Clin Biol Res* 379:15-34, 1992.

Landfield PW, Eldridge JC: The glucocorticoid hypothesis of brain aging and neurodegeneration: recent modifications, *Acta Endocrinol (Copenh)* 125(suppl 1):54-64, 1991.

Landfield PW and others: Mechanisms of neuronal death in brain aging and Alzheimer's disease: role of endocrine-mediated calcium dyshomeostasis, *J Neurobiol* 23:1247-1260, 1992.

Larrat EP: Update on the treatment of Alzheimer's disease, *Am Pharm* NS32(9):59-67, 1992.

Larson EB, Kukull WA, Katzman RL: Cognitive impairment: dementia and Alzheimer's disease, *Annu Rev Public Health* 13:431-449, 1992.

Launer LJ, Hofman A: Studies on the incidence of dementia: the European perspective, *Neuroepidemiology* 11:127-134, 1992.

Lavretsky EP, Jarvik LF: A group of potassium-channel blockers-acetylcholine releasers: new potentials for Alzheimer disease? A review, *J Clin Psychopharmacol* 12:110-118, 1992.

Lawlor BA, Davis KL: Does modulation of glutamatergic function represent a viable therapeutic strategy in Alzheimer's disease? *Biol Psychiatry* 31:337-350, 1992.

Lee VK: Language changes and Alzheimer's disease: a literature review, *J Gerontol Nurs* 17:16-20, 1991.

Lee VM, Trojanowski JQ: The disordered neuronal cytoskeleton in Alzheimer's disease, *Curr Opin Neurobiol* 2:653-656, 1992.

Lees AJ: Selegiline hydrochloride and cognition, *Acta Neurol Scand Suppl* 136:91-94, 1991.

Lehmann HD: The puzzle of Alzheimer's disease (AD), *Med Hypotheses* 38:5-10, 1992.

Levin ED and others: Cholinergic-dopaminergic interactions in cognitive performance, *Behav Neural Biol* 54:271-299, 1990.

Levine J, Lawlor BA: Family counseling and legal issues in Alzheimer's disease, *Psychiatr Clin North Am* 14:385-396, 1991.

Lewis S: Brain imaging in psychiatry: another look, *Br J Hosp Med* 47:175-176, 178 181-183, 1992.

Li G, Silverman JM, Mohs RC: Clinical genetic studies of Alzheimer's disease, *Psychiatr Clin North Am* 14:267-286, 1991.

Lind C and others: Early diagnosis of Alzheimer dementia? *J Neural Transm Suppl* 33:53-58, 1991.

Lindvall O: Prospects of transplantation in human neurodegenerative diseases, *Trends Neurosci* 14:376-384, 1991.

Lombardini JB: Review: recent studies on taurine in the central nervous system, *Adv Exp Med Biol* 315:245-251, 1992.

Lott IT: The neurology of Alzheimer disease in Down syndrome, *Prog Clin Biol Res* 379:1-14, 1992.

Lovestone S, Anderton B: Cytoskeletal abnormalities in Alzheimer's disease, *Curr Opin Neurol Neurosurg* 5:883-888, 1992.

Maas ML, Buckwalter KC: Alzheimer's disease, *Annu Rev Nurs Res* 9:19-55, 1991.

Mahler ME, Cummings JL: Alzheimer disease and the dementia of Parkinson disease: comparative investigations, *Alzheimer Dis Assoc Disord* 4:133-149, 1990.

Maletta GJ: Treatment of behavioral symptomatology of Alzheimer's disease, with emphasis on aggression: current clinical approaches [published erratum appears in *Int Psychogeriatr* 4:271, 1992], *Int Psychogeriatr* 4(suppl 1):117-130, 1992.

Malonebeach EE, Zarit SH: Current research issues in caregiving to the elderly, *Int J Aging Hum Dev* 32:103-114, 1991.

Mann DM: Is the pattern of nerve cell loss in aging and Alzheimer's disease a real, or only an apparent, selectivity? *Neurobiol Aging* 12:340-343, 1991.

Manuelidis EE, Manuelidis L: Search for a transmissible agent in Alzheimer's disease: studies of human buffy coat, *Curr Top Microbiol Immunol* 172:275-280, 1991.

Marder K, Mayeux R: The epidemiology of dementia in patients with Parkinson's disease, *Adv Exp Med Biol* 295:439-445, 1991.

Marotta CA, Majocha RE, Tate B: Molecular and cellular biology of Alzheimer amyloid, *J Mol Neurosci* 3:111-125, 1992.

Marshak DR, Pena LA: Potential role of S100 beta in Alzheimer's disease: an hypothesis involving mitotic protein kinases, *Prog Clin Biol Res* 379:289-307, 1992.

Martignoni E and others: The brain as a target for adrenocortical steroids: cognitive implications, *Psychoneuroendocrinology* 17:343-354, 1992.

Martins RN and others: The molecular pathology of amyloid deposition in Alzheimer's disease, *Mol Neurobiol* 5:389-398, 1991.

Martyn CN: The epidemiology of Alzheimer's disease in relation to aluminium, *Ciba Found Symp* 169:69-79 (discussion 79-86), 1992.

Masters CL, Beyreuther K: Protein abnormalities in neurofibrillary tangles: their relation to the extracellular amyloid deposits of the A4 protein in Alzheimer's disease, *Adv Neurol* 51:151-161, 1990.

Mathews VP, Candy EJ, Bryan RN: Imaging of neurodegenerative diseases, *Curr Opin Radiol* 4:89-94, 1992.

Mattson MP: Calcium as sculptor and destroyer of neural circuitry, *Exp Gerontol* 27:29-49, 1992.

Mattson MP, Rydel RE: Beta-amyloid precursor protein and Alzheimer's disease: the peptide plot thickens, *Neurobiol Aging* 13:617-621, 1992.

Mayer RJ and others: Protein processing in lysosomes: the new therapeutic target in neurodegenerative disease, *Lancet* 340:156-159, 1992.

Mayeux R: Therapeutic strategies in Alzheimer's disease, *Neurology* 40:175-180, 1990.

Mazziotta JC, Frackowiak RS, Phelps ME: The use of positron emission tomography in the clinical assessment of dementia, *Semin Nucl Med* 22:233-246, 1992.

McCaddon A, Kelly CL: Alzheimer's disease: a 'cobalaminergic' hypothesis, *Med Hypotheses* 37:161-165, 1992.

McDonald WM, Nemeroff CB: Neurotransmitters and neuropeptides in Alzheimer's disease, *Psychiatr Clin North Am* 14:421-442, 1991.

McDougall GJ: A review of screening instruments for assessing cognition and mental status in older adults, *Nurse Pract* 15(11):18-28, 1990.

McEntee WJ, Crook TH: Serotonin, memory, and the aging brain, *Psychopharmacology (Berlin)* 103:143-149, 1991.

McGeer PL, McGeer EG: Complement proteins and complement inhibitors in Alzheimer's disease, *Res Immunol* 143:621-624, 1992.

McGeer PL, Rogers J: Anti-inflammatory agents as a therapeutic approach to Alzheimer's disease, *Neurology* 42:447-449, 1992.

McGeer PL and others: Reactions of the immune system in chronic degenerative neurological diseases, *Can J Neurol Sci* 18(3 suppl):376-379, 1991.

McKinney M, Coyle JT: The potential for muscarinic receptor subtype-specific pharmacotherapy for Alzheimer's disease, *Mayo Clin Proc* 66:1225-1237, 1991.

McLachlan DR, Fraser PE, Dalton AJ: Aluminium and the pathogenesis of Alzheimer's disease: a summary of evidence, *Ciba Found Symp* 169:87-98 (discussion 99-108), 1992.

McLachlan DR and others: Would decreased aluminum ingestion reduce the incidence of Alzheimer's disease? *Can Med Assoc J* 145:793-804, 1991.

McRae A, Dahlstrom A: Cerebrospinal fluid antibodies: an indicator for immune responses in Alzheimer's disease, *Res Immunol* 143:663-667, 1992.

Mendez MF, Tomsak RL, Remler B: Disorders of the visual system in Alzheimer's disease, *J Clin Neuro Ophthalmol* 10:62-69, 1990.

Mera SL: Aluminium, amyloid, and Alzheimer's disease, *Med Lab Sci* 48:283-295, 1991.

Mesulam MM, Geula C: Shifting patterns of cortical cholinesterases in Alzheimer's disease: implications for treatment, diagnosis, and pathogenesis, *Adv Neurol* 51:235-240, 1990.

Meyer JS, Kawamura J, Terayama Y: White matter lesions in the elderly, *J Neurol Sci* 110:1-7, 1992.

Michel D and others: Possible functions of a new genetic marker in central nervous system: the sulfated glycoprotein-2 (SGP-2), *Synapse* 11:105-111, 1992.

Miller FD, Geddes JW: Increased expression of the major embryonic alpha-tubulin mRNA, T alpha 1, during neuronal regeneration, sprouting, and in Alzheimer's disease, *Prog Brain Res* 86:321-330, 1990.

Miller SW, Mahoney JM, Jann MW: Therapeutic frontiers in Alzheimer's disease, *Pharmacotherapy* 12:217-231, 1992.

Mirmiran M and others: Circadian rhythms and the suprachiasmatic nucleus in perinatal development, aging and Alzheimer's disease, *Prog Brain Res* 93:151-162 (discussion 162-3), 1992.

Mirra SS, Hart MN, Terry RD: Making the diagnosis of Alzheimer's disease: a primer for practicing pathologists, *Arch Pathol Lab Med* 117:132-144, 1993.

Mohr E, Carter C, Wallin A: Neurochemical substrates of human aging and dementia, *Pharmacopsychiatry* 23(suppl 2):53-55, 1990.

Mohr E, Mann UM, Chase TN: Subgroups in Alzheimer's disease: fact or fiction? *Psychiatr J Univ Ottawa* 15:203-206, 1990.

Molchan SE and others: The dexamethasone suppression test in Alzheimer's disease and major depression: relationship to dementia severity, depression, and CSF monoamines, *Int Psychogeriatr* 2:99-122, 1990.

Moody GH, Drummond JR, Newton JP: Alzheimer's disease [see comments], *Br Dent J* 169(2):45-47, 1990.

Morley JE, Flood JF: Neuropeptide Y and memory processing, *Ann N Y Acad Sci* 611:226-231, 1990.

Morris JC: Establishing diagnostic criteria for a registry for dementing diseases, *Aging (Milano)* 2:207-215, 1990.

Morris JC, Rubin EH: Clinical diagnosis and course of Alzheimer's disease, *Psychiatr Clin North Am* 14:223-236, 1991.

Morrison JH, Hof PR, Bouras C: An anatomic substrate for visual disconnection in Alzheimer's disease, *Ann N Y Acad Sci* 640:36-43, 1991.

Mubrin Z, Kos M: Assessment of dementia flow chart approach to clinical diagnosis, *Neurol Croat* 41:141-156, 1992.

Mungas D: In-office mental status testing: a practical guide, *Geriatrics* 46(7):54-58, 63, 66, 1991.

Munoz DG: The pathological basis of multi-infarct dementia, *Alzheimer Dis Assoc Disord* 5:77-90, 1991.

Murden RA: The diagnosis of Alzheimer's disease, *Adv Exp Med Biol* 282:59-64, 1990.

Murphy DL: Neuropsychiatric disorders and the multiple human brain serotonin receptor subtypes and subsystems, *Neuropsychopharmacology* 3:457-471, 1990.

Murphy M: The molecular pathogenesis of Alzheimer's disease: clinical prospects, *Lancet* 340:1512-1515, 1992.

Murray JC, Tanner CM, Sprague SM: Aluminum neurotoxicity: a reevaluation, *Clin Neuropharmacol* 14:179-185, 1991.

Nakamura S: Senile dementia and presenile dementia, *Tohoku J Exp Med* 161(suppl):49-60, 1990.

Nalbantoglu J: Beta-amyloid protein in Alzheimer's disease, *Can J Neurol Sci* 18(3 suppl):424-427, 1991.

Nalbantoglu J, Lacoste-Royal G, Gauvreau D: Genetic factors in Alzheimer's disease, *J Am Geriatr Soc* 38:564-568, 1990.

Neary D: Non–Alzheimer's disease forms of cerebral atrophy [editorial], *J Neurol Neurosurg Psychiatry* 53:929-931, 1990.

Neve RL: Genetics of the Alzheimer amyloid protein precursor, *Adv Exp Med Biol* 265:291-299, 1990.

Neve RL and others: Genetics and biology of the Alzheimer amyloid precursor, *Prog Brain Res* 86:257-267, 1990.

Newhouse PA: Cholinergic drug studies in dementia and depression, *Adv Exp Med Biol* 282:65-76, 1990.

Newman PE: Could diet be one of the causal factors of Alzheimer's disease? *Med Hypotheses* 39:123-126, 1992.

Nordberg A: Biological markers and the cholinergic hypothesis in Alzheimer's disease, *Acta Neurol Scand Suppl* 139:54-58, 1992.

Nordberg A: Neuroreceptor changes in Alzheimer disease, *Cerebrovasc Brain Metab Rev* 4:303-328, 1992.

Odenheimer GL: Management of patients with Alzheimer's disease, *Pharmacotherapy* 11:237-241, 1991.

O'Donovan MC, Owen MJ: Advances and retreats in the molecular genetics of major mental illness, *Ann Med* 24:171-177, 1992.

Olney JW: Excitotoxin-mediated neuron death in youth and old age, *Prog Brain Res* 86:37-51, 1990.

Olton DS, Wenk L: The development of behavioral tests to assess the effects of cognitive enhancers, *Pharmacopsychiatry* 23(suppl 2):65-69, 1990.

Orrell MW, Sahakian BJ: Dementia of frontal lobe type [editorial], *Psychol Med* 21:553-556, 1991.

Osuntokun BO and others: Epidemiology of age-related dementias in the Third World and aetiological clues of Alzheimer's disease, *Trop Geogr Med* 43:345-351, 1991.

Pallett PJ: A conceptual framework for studying family caregiver burden in Alzheimer's-type dementia, *Image J Nurs Sch* 22:52-58, 1990.

Palmer AM, Gershon S: Is the neuronal basis of Alzheimer's disease cholinergic or glutamatergic? *FASEB J* 4:2745-2752, 1990.

Palmert MR and others: Analysis of the beta-amyloid protein precursor of Alzheimer's disease: mRNAs and protein products, *Adv Neurol* 51:181-184, 1990.

Parasuraman R, Nestor PG: Attention and driving skills in aging and Alzheimer's disease, *Hum Factors* 33:539-557, 1991.

Patel S, Tariot PN: Pharmacologic models of Alzheimer's disease, *Psychiatr Clin North Am* 14:287-308, 1991.

Patterson MB and others: Assessment of functional ability in Alzheimer disease: a review and a preliminary report on the Cleveland Scale for Activities of Daily Living, *Alzheimer Dis Assoc Disord* 6:145-163, 1992.

Pavlin R: Brain amyloid in Alzheimer's disease: a new experimental model, *Neurol Croat* 41:227-234, 1992.

Perl DP, Good PF: Aluminum, Alzheimer's disease, and the olfactory system, Department of Pathology, Arthur M. Fishberg Center for Neurobiology, *Ann N Y Acad Sci* 640:8-13, 1991.

Perlmutter LS, Chui HC: Microangiopathy, the vascular basement membrane and Alzheimer's disease: a review, *Brain Res Bull* 24:677-686, 1990.

Perry EK: Nerve growth factor and the basal forebrain cholinergic system: a link in the etiopathology of neurodegenerative dementias? *Alzheimer Dis Assoc Disord* 4:1-13, 1990.

Peterson C: Changes in calcium's role as a messenger during aging in neuronal and nonneuronal cells, *Ann N Y Acad Sci* 663:279-293, 1992.

Phelps CH: Neural plasticity in aging and Alzheimer's disease: some selected comments, *Prog Brain Res* 86:3-9, 1990.

Polich J: P300 in the evaluation of aging and dementia, *Electroencephalogr Clin Neurophysiol Suppl* 42:304-323, 1991.

Pomponi M, Giacobini E, Brufani M: Present state and future development of the therapy of Alzheimer disease, *Aging (Milano)* 2:125-153, 1990.

Potter H: Review and hypothesis: Alzheimer disease and Down syndrome—chromosome 21 nondisjunction may underlie both disorders, *Am J Hum Genet* 48:1192-1200, 1991.

Potter H: The involvement of astrocytes and an acute phase response in the amyloid deposition of Alzheimer's disease, *Prog Brain Res* 94:447-458, 1992.

Potter H and others: The involvement of proteases, protease inhibitors, and an acute phase response in Alzheimer's disease, *Ann N Y Acad Sci* 674:161-173, 1992.

Price DL and others: Neuronal responses to injury and aging: lessons from animal models, *Prog Brain Res* 86:297-308, 1990.

Price DL and others: Amyloid-related proteins and nerve growth factor in Alzheimer's disease and animal models, *Clin Neuropharmacol* 14 (suppl 1):S9-14, 1991.

Price DL and others: Alzheimer's disease–type brain abnormalities in animal models, *Prog Clin Biol Res* 379:271-287, 1992.

Price DL and others: Amyloidosis in aging and Alzheimer's disease, *Am J Pathol* 141:767-772, 1992.

Price DL and others: Toxicity of synthetic A beta peptides and modeling of Alzheimer's disease, *Neurobiol Aging* 13:623-625, 1992.

Pruchno RA: The effects of help patterns on the mental health of spouse caregivers, *Res Aging* 12:57-71, 1990.

Prusiner SB: Molecular biology and transgenetics of prion diseases, *Crit Rev Biochem Mol Biol* 26:397-438, 1991.

Quirion R and others: Neurochemical deficits in pathological brain aging: specificity and possible relevance for treatment strategies, *Clin Neuropharmacol* 13 (suppl 3):S73-80, 1990.

Ramsdell JW and others: Evaluation of cognitive impairment in the elderly, *J Gen Intern Med* 5:55-64, 1990.

Rapoport SI: Positron emission tomography in Alzheimer's disease in relation to disease pathogenesis: a critical review, *Cerebrovasc Brain Metab Rev* 3:297-335, 1991.

Rapoport SI and others: Abnormal brain glucose metabolism in Alzheimer's disease, as measured by position emission tomography, *Adv Exp Med Biol* 291:231-248, 1991.

Rebeck GW, Hyman BT: Neuroanatomical connections and specific regional vulnerability in Alzheimer's disease, *Neurobiol Aging* 14:45-47 (discussion 55-6), 1993.

Regland B, Gottfries CG: The role of amyloid beta-protein in Alzheimer's disease, *Lancet* 340:467-469, 1992.

Regland B, Gottfries CG: Slowed synthesis of DNA and methionine is a pathogenetic mechanism common to dementia in Down's syndrome, AIDS and Alzheimer's disease? *Med Hypotheses* 38:11-19, 1992.

Reisberg B and others: Pharmacologic treatment of Alzheimer's disease: a methodologic critique based upon current knowledge of symptomatology and relevance for drug trials, *Int Psychogeriatr* 4(suppl 1):9-42, 1992.

Reynolds CF III: Treatment of depression in special populations, *J Clin Psychiatry* 53(suppl):45-53, 1992.

Richards SJ: The neuropathology of Alzheimer's disease investigated by transplantation of mouse trisomy 16 hippocampal tissues, *Trends Neurosci* 14:334-338, 1991.

Richards SJ, Edwards P, Dunnett SB: Animal models of the neuropathology observed in Alzheimer's disease and Down syndrome, *Prog Clin Biol Res* 379:245-258, 1992.

Ritchie K, Touchon J: Heterogeneity in senile dementia of the Alzheimer type: individual differences, progressive deterioration or clinical sub-types? *J Clin Epidemiol* 45:1391-1398, 1992.

Roberts E: A systems approach to aging, Alzheimer's disease, and spinal cord regeneration, *Prog Brain Res* 86:339-355, 1990.

Rogers J and others: Complement activation and beta-amyloid-mediated neurotoxicity in Alzheimer's disease, *Res Immunol* 143:624-630, 1992.

Rohwer RG: Alzheimer's disease transmission: possible artifact due to intercurrent illness, *Neurology* 42:287-288, 1992.

Ron MA: Suspected dementia: psychiatric differential diagnosis, *J Neuropsychiatry Clin Neurosci* 2:214-220, 1990.

Roos RA, Haan J: Function of amyloid and amyloid protein precursor, *Clin Neurol Neurosurg* 94(suppl):S1-3, 1992.

Rosen J, Bohon S, Gershon S: Antipsychotics in the elderly, *Acta Psychiatr Scand Suppl* 358:170-175, 1990.

Roses AD: Molecular genetics of neurodegenerative diseases, *Curr Opin Neurol Neurosurg* 6:34-39, 1993.

Rossor M: Alzheimer's disease, *Postgrad Med J* 68:528-532, 1992.

Royston MC, Rothwell NJ, Roberts GW: Alzheimer's disease: pathology to potential treatments? *Trends Pharmacol Sci* 13:131-133, 1992.

Rozemuller JM, van der Valk P, Eikelenboom P: Activated microglia and cerebral amyloid deposits in Alzheimer's disease, *Res Immunol* 143:646-649, 1992.

Sachdev P: The neuropsychiatry of brain iron, *J Neuropsychiatry Clin Neurosci* 5:18-29, 1993.

Sadun AA, Bassi CJ: The visual system in Alzheimer's disease, *Res Publ Assoc Res Nerv Ment Dis* 67:331-347, 1990.

Saffran BN: Should intracerebroventricular nerve growth factor be used to treat Alzheimer's disease? *Perspect Biol Med* 35:471-486, 1992.

Saitoh T, Cole G, Huynh TV: Aberrant protein kinase C cascades in Alzheimer's disease, *Adv Exp Med Biol* 265:301-310, 1990.

Saitoh T and others: Degradation of proteins in the membrane-cytoskeleton complex in Alzheimer's disease. Might amyloidogenic APP processing be just the tip of the iceberg? *Ann N Y Acad Sci* 674:180-192, 1992.

Sandyk R, Anninos PA, Tsagas N: Age-related disruption of circadian rhythms: possible relationship to memory impairment and implications for therapy with magnetic fields, *Int J Neurosci* 59:259-262, 1991.

Sanger DJ, Joly D: Psychopharmacological strategies in the search for cognition enhancers, *Pharmacopsychiatry* 23(suppl 2):70-74, 1990.

Schapiro MB, Haxby JV, Grady CL: Nature of mental retardation and dementia in Down syndrome: study with PET, CT, and neuropsychology, *Neurobiol Aging* 13:723-734, 1992.

Schellenberg GD and others: Genetic heterogeneity, Down syndrome, and Alzheimer disease, *Prog Clin Biol Res* 379:215-226, 1992.

Scheltens P, Weinstein HC, Leys D: Neuro-imaging in the diagnosis of Alzheimer's disease. I. Computer tomography and magnetic resonance imaging, *Clin Neurol Neurosurg* 94:277-289, 1992.

Scher W, Scher BM: A possible role for nitric oxide in glutamate (MSG)–induced Chinese restaurant syndrome, glutamate-induced asthma, 'hot-dog headache,' pugilistic Alzheimer's disease, and other disorders, *Med Hypotheses* 38:185-188, 1992.

Schettini G: Brain somatostatin: receptor-coupled transducing mechanisms and role in cognitive functions, *Pharmacol Res* 23:203-215, 1991.

Schmage N, Bergener M: Global rating, symptoms, behavior, and cognitive performance as indicators of efficacy in clinical studies with nimodipine in elderly patients with cognitive impairment syndromes, *Int Psychogeriatr* 4(suppl 1):89-99, 1992.

Schmechel DE: New approaches to therapy for neurodegenerative diseases, *South Med J* 84(5 suppl 1):S11-23, 1991.

Schneider LS, Sobin PB: Non-neuroleptic treatment of behavioral symptoms and agitation in Alzheimer's disease and other dementia, *Psychopharmacol Bull* 28:71-79, 1992.

Schwartz G and others: Late clinical testing of cognition enhancers: demonstration of efficacy, *Pharmacopsychiatry* 23(suppl 2):60-62 (discussion 63-4), 1990.

Schwarz RD and others: Next generation tacrine, *Neurobiol Aging* 12:185-187, 1991.

Scott RB: Extraneuronal manifestations of Alzheimer's disease, *J Am Geriatr Soc* 41:268-276, 1993.

Seitelberger F, Lassmann H, Bancher C: Cytoskeleton pathology in Alzheimer's disease and related disorders, *J Neural Transm Suppl* 33:27-33, 1991.

Selkoe DJ: Deciphering Alzheimer's disease: the amyloid precursor protein yields new clues, *Science* 248:1058-1060, 1990.

Selkoe DJ: Amyloid protein and Alzheimer's disease, *Sci Am* 265(5):68-71, 74-76, 78, 1991.

Selkoe DJ: The molecular pathology of Alzheimer's disease, *Neuron* 6:487-498, 1991.

Selkoe DJ and others: Molecular relation of amyloid filaments and paired helical filaments in Alzheimer's disease, *Adv Neurol* 51:171-179, 1990.

Shimizu M: Current clinical trials of cognitive enhancers in Japan, *Alzheimer Dis Assoc Disord* 5(suppl 1):S13-24, 1991.

Shiosaka S: Attempts to make models for Alzheimer's disease, *Neurosci Res* 13:237-255, 1992.

Ship JA: Oral health of patients with Alzheimer's disease, *J Am Dent Assoc* 123:53-58, 1992.

Siegfried KR: First clinical impressions with an ACTH analog (HOE 427) in the treatment of Alzheimer's disease, *Ann N Y Acad Sci* 640:280-283, 1991.

Siman R: Proteolytic mechanism for the neurodegeneration of Alzheimer's disease, *Ann N Y Acad Sci* 674:193-202, 1992.

Singh VK: Neuroimmune axis as a basis of therapy in Alzheimer's disease, *Prog Drug Res* 34:383-393, 1990.

Sirvio J, Riekkinen PJ: Brain and cerebrospinal fluid cholinesterases in Alzheimer's disease, Parkinson's disease and aging: a critical review of clinical and experimental studies, *J Neural Transm Park Dis Dement Sect* 4:337-358, 1992.

Sisodia SS, Price DL: Amyloidogenesis in Alzheimer's disease: basic biology and animal models, *Curr Opin Neurobiol* 2:648-652, 1992.

Skelton WP III, Skelton NK: Alzheimer's disease: recognizing and treating a frustrating condition, *Postgrad Med* 90(4):33-34, 37-41, 1991.

Smyth KA, Harris PB: Using telecomputing to provide information and support to caregivers of persons with dementia, *Gerontologist* 33:123-127, 1993.

Snowden JS: Assessment of outcome in clinical trials in Alzheimer's disease, *Neuroepidemiology* 9:216-222, 1990.

Sofroniew MV, Staley K: Transgenic modelling of neurodegenerative events gathers momentum, *Trends Neurosci* 14:513-514, 1991.

Somoza E, Mossman D: Introduction to neuropsychiatric decision making: binary diagnostic tests, *J Neuropsychiatry Clin Neurosci* 2:297-300, 1990.

Spencer PS: Etiology of Alzheimer's disease: a Western Pacific view, *Adv Neurol* 51:79-82, 1990.

Spencer PS, Ludolph AC, Kisby GE: Are human neurodegenerative disorders linked to environmental chemicals with excitotoxic properties? *Ann N Y Acad Sci* 648:154-160, 1992.

Steg RE: Determining the cause of dementia, *Nebr Med J* 75(4):59-63, 1990.

Stern GM: New drug interventions in Alzheimer's disease, *Curr Opin Neurol Neurosurg* 5:100-103, 1992.

Stevenson JP: Family stress related to home care of Alzheimer's disease patients and implications for support, *J Neurosci Nurs* 22:179-188, 1990.

Stone MJ: Amyloidosis: a final common pathway for protein deposition in tissues, *Blood* 75:531-545, 1990.

Swaab DF: Brain aging and Alzheimer's disease, "wear and tear" versus "use it or lose it," *Neurobiol Aging* 12:317-324, 1991.

Swaab DF and others: The human hypothalamus in development, sexual differentiation, aging and Alzheimer's disease, *Prog Brain Res* 91:465-472, 1992.

Swash M and others: Clinical trials in Alzheimer's disease: a report from the Medical Research Council Alzheimer's Disease Clinical Trials Committee, *J Neurol Neurosurg Psychiatry* 54:178-181, 1991.

Taft LB, Barkin RL: Drug abuse? Use and misuse of psychotropic drugs in Alzheimer's care, *J Gerontol Nurs* 16(8):4-10, 1990.

Tagliavini F and others: Down syndrome as a key to the time sequence of brain changes in Alzheimer disease, *Prog Clin Biol Res* 379:143-158, 1992.

Talamo BR and others: Pathologic changes in olfactory neurons in Alzheimer's disease, *Ann N Y Acad Sci* 640:1-7, 1991.

Tanzi RE: Genetic linkage studies of human neurodegenerative disorders, *Curr Opin Neurobiol* 1:455-461, 1991.

Tanzi RE, George-Hyslop PS, Gusella JF: Molecular genetics of Alzheimer disease amyloid, *J Biol Chem* 266:20579-20582, 1991.

Tappen RM: Alzheimer's disease: communication techniques to facilitate perioperative care, *AORN J* 54:1279-1286, 1991.

Tatemichi TK: How acute brain failure becomes chronic: a view of the mechanisms of dementia related to stroke, *Neurology* 40:1652-1659, 1990.

Teri L, Logsdon R: Assessment and management of behavioral disturbances in Alzheimer's disease, *Compr Ther* 16(5):36-42, 1990.

Teri L, Wagner A: Alzheimer's disease and depression, *J Consult Clin Psychol* 60:379-391, 1992.

Teri L and others: Management of behavior disturbance in Alzheimer disease: current knowledge and future directions, *Alzheimer Dis Assoc Disord* 6:77-88, 1992.

Terry RD: Normal aging and Alzheimer's disease: growing problems, *Monogr Pathol* (32):41-54, 1990.

Terry RD: Regeneration in Alzheimer disease and aging, *Adv Neurol* 59:1-4, 1993.

Thal LJ: THA, a putative drug in the treatment of Alzheimer's disease? *Acta Neurol Scand Suppl* 129:27-28, 1990.

Thal LJ: Assessment issues in clinical trials of tetrahydroaminoacridine and studies to alter decline in Alzheimer disease, *Alzheimer Dis Assoc Disord* 5(suppl 1):S37-39, 1991.

Tolosa ES, Alvarez R: Differential diagnosis of cortical vs. subcortical dementing disorders, *Acta Neurol Scand Suppl* 139:47-53, 1992.

Tranel D: Neuropsychological assessment, *Psychiatr Clin North Am* 15:283-299, 1992.

Treves TA: Epidemiology of Alzheimer's disease, *Psychiatr Clin North Am* 14:251-265, 1991.

Trojanowski JQ and others: Vulnerability of the neuronal cytoskeleton in aging and Alzheimer disease: widespread involvement of all three major filament systems, *Annu Rev Gerontol Geriatr* 10:167-182, 1990.

Tucek S, Ricny J, Dolezal V: Advances in the biology of cholinergic neurons, *Adv Neurol* 51:109-115, 1990.

Tuszynski MH, Gage FH: Potential use of neurotrophic agents in the treatment of neurodegenerative disorders, *Acta Neurobiol Exp (Warsz)* 50:311-322, 1990.

Ulrich J: Recent progress in the characterization of the pathological hallmarks for Alzheimer's disease, *Acta Neurol Scand Suppl* 129:5-7, 1990.

van Dijk PT, Dippel DW, Habbema JD: Survival of patients with dementia, *J Am Geriatr Soc* 39:603-610, 1991.

van der Voet GB and others: Aluminium neurotoxicity, *Prog Histochem Cytochem* 23:235-242, 1991.

van Gool WA, Bolhuis PA: Cerebrospinal fluid markers of Alzheimer's disease, *J Am Geriatr Soc* 39:1025-1039, 1991.

Vandenabeele P, Fiers W: Is amyloidogenesis during Alzheimer's disease due to an IL-1-/IL-6–mediated 'acute phase response' in the brain? *Immunol Today* 12:217-219, 1991.

Vecsei L, Widerlov E: Preclinical and clinical studies with somatostatin related to the central nervous system, *Prog Neuropsychopharmacol Biol Psychiatry* 14:473-502, 1990.

Vickers AB: Role of support group for the family caregiver of dementia: recent developments in the structure of the support system, *Adv Exp Med Biol* 282:141-147, 1990.

Vinters HV: Cerebral amyloid angiopathy and Alzheimer's disease: two entities or one? *J Neurol Sci* 112:1-3, 1992.

Vitiello MV, Bliwise DL, Prinz PN: Sleep in Alzheimer's disease and the sundown syndrome, *Neurology* 42(7 suppl 6):83-93 (discussion 93-4), 1992.

Vitiello MV, Poceta JS, Prinz PN: Sleep in Alzheimer's disease and other dementing disorders, *Can J Psychol* 45:221-239, 1991.

Vogels OJ and others: Cell loss and shrinkage in the nucleus basalis Meynert complex in Alzheimer's disease, *Neurobiol Aging* 11:3-13, 1990.

Volger BW: Alternatives in the treatment of memory loss in patients with Alzheimer's disease, *Clin Pharm* 10:447-456, 1991.

Volicer L, Crino PB: Involvement of free radicals in dementia of the Alzheimer type: a hypothesis, *Neurobiol Aging* 11:567-571, 1990.

Wallin A, Blennow K: Clinical diagnosis of Alzheimer's disease by primary care physicians and specialists, *Acta Neurol Scand Suppl* 139:26-31, 1992.

Wallin A, Gottfries CG: Biochemical substrates in normal aging and Alzheimer's disease, *Pharmacopsychiatry* 23(suppl 2):37-43, 1990.

Walsh TJ, Opello KD: Neuroplasticity, the aging brain, and Alzheimer's disease, *Neurotoxicology* 13:101-110, 1992.

Warburton DM: Nicotine as a cognitive enhancer, *Prog Neuropsychopharmacol Biol Psychiatry* 16:181-191, 1992.

Warshaw GA: New perspectives in the management of Alzheimer's disease, *Am Fam Physician* 42(5 suppl):41S-47S, 1990.

Weiner MF: Advances in clinical research in Alzheimer's disease, *Compr Ther* 17(8):9-13, 1991.

Wenk GL: Animal models of Alzheimer's disease: are they valid and useful? *Acta Neurobiol Exp (Warsz)* 50:219-223, 1990.

Whitehouse PJ: Treatment of Alzheimer disease, *Alzheimer Dis Assoc Disord* 5(suppl 1):S32-6, 1991.

Whitehouse PJ: Alzheimer's disease: relationship of cognition and behavior to neurochemistry, *Int Psychogeriatr* 4(suppl 1):71-78, 1992.

Wischik CM and others: Molecular characterization and measurement of Alzheimer's disease pathology: implications for genetic and environmental aetiology, *Ciba Found Symp* 169:268-293 (discussion 293-302), 1992.

Wiseman EJ, Jarvik LF: Potassium channel blockers: could they work in Alzheimer disease? *Alzheimer Dis Assoc Disord* 5:25-30, 1991.

Wisniewski HM, Wegiel J: Alzheimer's disease neuropathology: current status of interpretation of lesion development, *Ann N Y Acad Sci* 673:270-284, 1992.

Wisniewski HM, Wegiel J: The role of perivascular and microglial cells in fibrillogenesis of beta-amyloid and PrP protein in Alzheimer's disease and scrapie, *Res Immunol* 143:642-645, 1992.

Wisniewski HM, Wen GY: Aluminium and Alzheimer's disease, *Ciba Found Symp* 169:142-154 (discussion 154-64), 1992.

Wisniewski T, Frangione B: Molecular biology of Alzheimer's amyloid—Dutch variant, *Mol Neurobiol* 6:75-86, 1992.

Yankner BA, Mesulam MM: Seminars in medicine of the Beth Israel Hospital, Boston. Beta-amyloid and the pathogenesis of Alzheimer's disease, *N Engl J Med* 325:1849-1857, 1991.

Young JK: Alzheimer's disease and metal-containing glia, *Med Hypotheses* 38:1-4, 1992.

Zandi T: Changes in memory processes of dementia patients, *Adv Exp Med Biol* 282:89-100, 1990.

Zandi T: Psychological difficulties of caring for dementia patients: the role of support groups, *Adv Exp Med Biol* 282:113-120, 1990.

Zubenko GS: Biological correlates of clinical heterogeneity in primary dementia, *Neuropsychopharmacology* 6:77-93, 1992.

Index